Cardiovascular Disease and Health in the Older Patient

Expanded from 'Pathy's Principles and Practice of Geriatric Medicine, Fifth edition'

Cardiovascular Disease and Health in the Older Patient

Expanded from 'Pathy's Principles and Practice of Geriatric Medicine, Fifth edition'

EDITED BY

David J. Stott
Institute of Cardiovascular and Medical Sciences
University of Glasgow, Glasgow Royal Infirmary
Glasgow, Scotland, UK

Gordon D.O. Lowe
Institute of Cardiovascular and Medical Sciences
University of Glasgow, Glasgow Royal Infirmary
Glasgow, Scotland, UK

FOREWORD BY STUART M. COBBE, UNIVERSITY OF GLASGOW

WILEY-BLACKWELL
A John Wiley & Sons, Ltd., Publication

Wiley-Blackwell is an imprint of John Wiley & Sons, formed by the merger of Wiley's global Scientific, Technical and Medical business with Blackwell Publishing.

Registered office: John Wiley & Sons, Ltd, The Atrium, Southern Gate, Chichester, West Sussex, PO19 8SQ, UK

Editorial offices: 9600 Garsington Road, Oxford, OX4 2DQ, UK
The Atrium, Southern Gate, Chichester, West Sussex, PO19 8SQ, UK
111 River Street, Hoboken, NJ 07030-5774, USA

For details of our global editorial offices, for customer services and for information about how to apply for permission to reuse the copyright material in this book please see our website at www.wiley.com/wiley-blackwell.

Library of Congress Cataloging-in-Publication Data

Cardiovascular disease and health in the older patient : expanded from 'Pathy's Principles and practice of geriatric medicine' / [edited by] David Stott and Gordon Lowe. – 1st ed.
p. ; cm.
Includes bibliographical references and index.
ISBN 978-0-470-97372-1 (hardback : alk. paper)
I. Stott, David, 1959- II. Lowe, G. D. O. (Gordon Douglas Ogilvie), 1949- III. Pathy's principles and practice of geriatric medicine.
[DNLM: 1. Cardiovascular Diseases–therapy. 2. Aged. WG 120]
618.97′61–dc23

2012021981

A catalogue record for this book is available from the British Library.

Wiley also publishes its books in a variety of electronic formats. Some content that appears in print may not be available in electronic books.

Cover images from iStockphoto: www.istockphoto.com

Cover Design by: Scott Graham

Typeset in 9.5/13pt Meridien by Laserwords Private Limited, Chennai, India.
Printed and bound in Malaysia by Vivar Printing Sdn Bhd

First Impression 2013

Contents

List of Contributors

Ahmed H. Abdelhafiz
Rotherham General Hospital, Rotherham, Yorkshire, UK

Suraj Alakkassery
Saint Louis University Medical Center, St Louis, MO, USA

Cristina Alonso Bouzón
Hospital Universitario de Getafe, Madrid, Spain

Wilbert S. Aronow
New York Medical College, Valhalla, NY, USA

Marco Baccini
University of Florence and Azienda Ospedaliero–Universitaria Careggi, Florence, Italy

Abhay Bajpai
St George's Hospital, University of London, London, UK

Martin M. Brown
Institute of Neurology, University College London, London, UK

A. John Camm
St George's Hospital, University of London, London, UK

Marta Castro Rodrıguez
Hospital Universitario de Getafe, Madrid, Spain

David Doig
Institute of Neurology, University College London, London, UK

Pamela M. Enderby
University of Sheffield, Sheffield, UK

Francesco Fattirolli
University of Florence and Azienda Ospedaliero–Universitaria Careggi, Florence, Italy

Jennifer K. Harrison
Glasgow Royal Infirmary, Glasgow, Scotland, UK

Lalit Kalra
King's College, London, UK

Gordon D.O. Lowe
Institute of Cardiovascular and Medical Sciences, University of Glasgow, Glasgow Royal Infirmary, Glasgow, Scotland, UK

Leocadio Rodríguez Mañas
Hospital Universitario de Getafe, Madrid, Spain

Niccolò Marchionni
University of Florence and Azienda Ospedaliero–Universitaria Careggi, Florence, Italy

Giulio Masotti
University of Florence and Azienda Ospedaliero–Universitaria Careggi, Florence, Italy

Francesco Orso
University of Florence and Azienda Ospedaliero–Universitaria Careggi, Florence, Italy

Terence J. Quinn
Institute of Cardiovascular and Medical Sciences, University of Glasgow, Glasgow Royal Infirmary, Glasgow, Scotland, UK

Michael W. Rich
Washington University School of Medicine, St Louis, MO, USA

Lucio A. Rinaldi
University of Florence and Azienda Ospedaliero–Universitaria Careggi, Florence, Italy

David J. Stott
Institute of Cardiovascular and Medical Sciences, University of Glasgow, Glasgow Royal Infirmary, Glasgow, Scotland, UK

Adam Szafranek
University Hospital of Wales, Cardiff and Vale University Health Board, University of Cardiff, Wales, UK

Anthony S. Wierzbicki
Guy's and St Thomas' Hospitals, London, UK

Adie Viljoen
Lister Hospital, Stevenage, Hertfordshire, and Bedfordshire and Hertfordshire Postgraduate Medical School, Luton, Hertfordshire, UK

Ulrich O. von Oppell
University Hospital of Wales, Cardiff and Vale University Health Board, University of Cardiff, Wales, UK

Foreword

The reduction in the age-specific mortality and morbidity from cardiovascular disease in developed countries has been one of the great medical success stories of the last 50 years. A solid foundation of epidemiology coupled with improved understanding of the pathophysiology of cardiovascular disease in general, and atherosclerosis in particular, has been achieved. Approaches to the primary and secondary prevention of cardiovascular disease, as well as medical and interventional procedures for treatment of symptomatic disease, have been developed and validated by randomized controlled trials, giving cardiovascular medicine an unrivalled evidence base of effective interventions. Unfortunately, since most cardiovascular disease is essentially progressive and degenerative, reductions in mortality in middle age have resulted in an increasing population of older individuals with overt or silent cardiovascular disease. Thus the overall prevalence of individuals with cardiac and cerebrovascular disease is rising. Although many of the treatment paradigms applicable to younger patients can be translated to the older patient, the prevalence of comorbidities, frailty and cognitive decline require a more holistic approach to the management of cardiovascular disease in elderly people.

The purpose of this book is to provide the non-specialist reader with an up-to-date review of the epidemiology, pathophysiology and management of cardiovascular disease in older people. Most of the chapters would be found in a textbook of general medicine, but the impact of physiological and pathological ageing and the importance of comorbidity and frailty on clinical management are emphasized throughout. The relative paucity of clinical trial evidence in the over-80s, or in specific groups such as those with cognitive impairment, nursing home residents or the frail, is emphasized, and should stimulate further research. The book concludes with a thoughtful discussion on the scope, limitations and appropriateness of aggressive investigation and management in older subjects.

Stuart M. Cobbe
Emeritus Professor of Medical Cardiology
University of Glasgow
May 2012

Foreword

Introduction

Prevention and treatment of cardiovascular disease in older people is an increasing part of primary and secondary care. Heart disease, stroke and peripheral vascular diseases are increasingly prevalent worldwide, due to increasing numbers of older persons; the persistence of major risk factors including tobacco smoking, hypertension and hyperlipidaemia; and the global epidemic of obesity and diabetes. Optimal management requires recognition of multiple morbidities in elderly patients, and a holistic approach to their management.

This book is based on the chapters in the Section on Cardiovascular Diseases and Health, and chapters on cerebrovascular disease in the Section on Central Nervous System Disorders, from the latest, fifth edition of *Pathy's Principles and Practice of Geriatric Medicine*, edited by Alan Sinclair and colleagues. We hope that these chapters from this standard textbook for geriatricians, together with an additional chapter on tailoring the approach to investigation and management of vascular disease in frail older subjects, will provide a useful resource to general practitioners and hospital clinicians and their teams.

We have performed some further editing to the chapters: principally some updating on recent evidence, and adding references to recent clinical practice guidelines in Europe and North America. Management of cardiovascular disease is a rapidly changing field, and readers may find the following web sites to be useful supplements to this book:

Guidelines International Network (G-I-N): www.g-i-n.net

American Heart Association (AHA): www.heart.org

American Stroke Association (ASA): www.strokeassociation.org

Canadian Heart and Stroke Foundation: www.heartandstroke.ca

American College of Chest Physicians (ACCP): www.chestnet.org

European Heart Association (EHA): www.escardio.org/guidelines

National Institute for Health and Clinical Excellence (NICE): www.nice.org.uk

Scottish Intercollegiate Guidelines Network (SIGN): www.sign.ac.uk

Australian Government, National Health and Medical Research Council: www.nhmrc.gov.au

New Zealand Guidelines Group: www.nzgg.org.nz

Guidance on systems and processes of acute medical care for frail older people is given in the Royal College of Physicians Acute Care Toolkit 3: http://rcplondon.us1.list-manage.com/track/click?u=bc4bee17da1faeabe3a951bca&id=33faac6a13&e=012fdadfb6

We welcome feedback on the usefulness of this book. We thank our colleague chapter authors; Professor Stuart Cobbe for his Foreword; Robyn Lyons and Fiona Seymour and their colleagues at Wiley-Blackwell for the original suggestion and for their efficiency in its production; and as always our families for their support.

DJS and GDOL, Glasgow
April 2012

CHAPTER 1
Epidemiology of Heart Disease

Ahmed H. Abdelhafiz
Rotherham General Hospital, Rotherham, Yorkshire, UK

Introduction

Epidemiology is defined as the study of occurrence and distribution of disease in human populations. Epidemiological research can be used to study benefits of interventions to prevent and decrease the burden of disease or to predict requirements for trained healthcare professionals, caregivers for disabled or older people, and service planning. Coronary heart disease (CHD) is an important cause of morbidity and mortality. Incidence and prevalence of CHD both rise steeply with increasing age. The older population is growing and the world's population ≥60 years old is estimated to reach 2 billion by 2050 (three times that in 2000). The development and progression of atherosclerosis is not just a function of ageing but is determined by the distribution of cardiovascular (CV) risk factors related to specific lifestyles. Heart disease may affect quality or quantity of life or both. As the population suffering from heart disease becomes older, their functional ability becomes more important. Mortality cannot be the only outcome relevant to older people: quality of life, cognitive and functional capacities are equally important endpoints. While CHD is a major cause of mortality, other heart diseases may have a significant impact on quality of life due to limitation of exercise tolerance. This chapter discusses epidemiological features of the most common heart diseases affecting older people including CHD, heart failure, valvular heart disease and rhythm disorders (Box 1.1).

Coronary heart disease

The CHD epidemic started in the 1950s affecting firstly Western countries. Prior to the 1920s CHD was not common and caused only <10% of all deaths in the United States. However, by the 1950s this had escalated to

Cardiovascular Disease and Health in the Older Patient: Expanded from 'Pathy's Principles and Practice of Geriatric Medicine, Fifth edition', First Edition. Edited by David J. Stott and Gordon D.O. Lowe.

Box 1.1 Common heart diseases in older people

- Coronary heart disease
- Heart failure
- Valvular heart disease
  Degenerative valve disease
  Infective valve disease
- Rhythm disorders
  Atrial fibrillation
  Sudden cardiac death

>30% and it is now the leading cause of death. While its mortality has fallen by 50%, its incidence has decreased to a lesser extent. Mortality from CHD has also decreased among elderly people, but information on changes in incidence in the elderly population is limited. The main reasons for the decline in morbidity and mortality are due to changes in risk factors as well as improvement of treatment. Survival after myocardial infarction has improved and significant advances have also been made in the surgical and medical treatment of CHD.

Risk factors and prevention

Major risk factors for atherosclerosis have been well established. Epidemiological studies concluded that the causes for this epidemic are genetic factors, age, smoking, hypertension, obesity, diabetes and cholesterol. Variations in disease occurrence in different nations still remain far from being fully explained.

Genetics

It is believed that CVD results from many genes, each with a relatively small effect working alone or in combination with other modifier genes and/or environmental factors. Familial hypercholesterolaemia[1] and hyperhomocysteinaemia[2] are well-described examples. Telomere length is another genetic factor associated with CV health and ageing. Telomere attrition is associated with elevated blood homocysteine and increased endothelial cell inflammatory markers and may underlie early origins of CVD. The identification and characterization of genes that enhance prediction of disease risk and improve prevention and treatment of atherosclerosis need further genetic epidemiological studies.

Age and sex

Prevalence of CHD increases with age from 2% for males and 0.5% for females at age 40–44 to peak at 18% and 12% respectively at age 85–89.

Median age at onset is 67.5 years for males and 77.5 years for females. Lifetime risk is 35% for males and 28% for females. CHD accounts for 22% of male deaths and 17% female deaths at all ages. Epidemiology of CHD is changing from a fatal disease of middle-aged men to a more chronic condition of elderly women. CHD is intimately related to normal ageing in that its incidence continues to increase indefinitely with age. In a prospective study to investigate the influence of increasing age on incidence of CVD in 22 048 male physicians aged 40–84 who were free of major disease, incidence of CVD continued to increase to age 100 over 23 years of follow-up.[3] Beginning at age 80, CVD was more likely to be diagnosed at death. The remaining lifetime risk of CVD at age 40 was 34.8%, 95% confidence interval (CI), 33.1–36.5% and at age 90 was 16.7% (95% CI, 12.9–20.6%). These findings suggest that people aged ≥80 may be living with a substantial amount of undiagnosed CVD. Additional research is needed to determine if continued screening and detection of CVD up to and beyond age 80 might help improve health in later life.

Ethnicity and race

Prevalence of CHD and related risk factors vary among different ethnic groups. The pattern of this variation is complex, and could be related to genetic or socioeconomic differences. For example, populations of African descent living in Europe and the United States have a higher incidence of stroke and lower incidence of CHD than in their white counterparts. They have higher rates of hypertension, which may explain their high rate of stroke. Similarly, in China mortality from CHD is still lower than in Western countries while mortality due to stroke is several times higher largely due to the high prevalence of hypertension. The lower rate of CHD may be explained by low rates of other risk factors including smoking.[4] In the Indian subcontinent CVD is expected to increase rapidly and it will be the host of >50% of cases of heart disease in the world within the next 15 years. Risk factors for this epidemic are similar to those elsewhere in the world; however, ~50% of CHD-related deaths occur in people <70 years compared with only 22% in the West. Also Asians living in Western countries have a 50% greater premature mortality risk from CHD than the general population.

Diet

Dietary factors are related to the risk of CHD through several biological mechanisms. For example: (i) Fish consumption provides cardio-protective benefits through favourable effects on lipid profile, threshold for arrhythmias, platelet activity, inflammation, endothelial function, atherosclerosis and hypertension. Consumption of fish 1–2 times per week or at least 5–10% of energy from polyunsaturated fatty acids reduces the risk of CHD in older people relative to lower intakes.[5] (ii) Antioxidants present in fruit and vegetables improve endothelial function, inhibit platelet activation and lower blood pressure. (iii) High salt consumption is directly related to hypertension, myocardial infarctions and strokes. Modest reductions in salt lower systolic blood pressure by at least 2 mmHg reducing the prevalence of hypertension by 17%, cardiac events by 30% and overall mortality by 20%. Older people will gain the greatest advantage from lowering their salt intake, most likely because they are more salt sensitive. (iv) Alcohol intake has a U-shaped relationship with the risk of CHD. 'Moderate drinking' defined as one drink for women and two drinks for men per day reduces the risk of CHD by 25%. Data relating to multivitamin use and the risk of CVD are inconsistent. Broader adherence to recommendations for daily intake of fruit, vegetables, low salt, alcohol in moderation and fish may take away 20–30% of the burden of CVD and result in one extra life-year if started early by the age of 40 years.[6]

Cholesterol

Cholesterol is a risk factor for CVD in the middle aged but appears to be less potent at older ages. However, dietary cholesterol is more detrimental in people with diabetes, regardless of age, because of dyslipidaemia and increased insulin resistance. In the Health, Aging and Body Composition Study of 1941 community-dwelling elderly people aged 70–79, there were no significant associations between dietary fats and CVD risk, hazard ratio (HR) 1.47, 95% CI, 0.93–2.32 for the upper versus lower tertile, p for trend 0.10 after 9 years of follow-up. However, dietary cholesterol was associated with increased CVD risk among older people with diabetes (3.66, 1.09–12.29).[7] Possible reasons for these results are attenuated association between lipids and CV risk among older people, differences in baseline CV risk between old and young, or selective survivorship of older people leading to a population sample less vulnerable to environmental factors such as dietary fat.

Exercise

Although few studies have been conducted in elderly people, most have reported physical activity to be beneficial in preventing premature mortality but with some concerns about adverse effects especially in frail elderly individuals with comorbidities. Physical activity may trigger sudden death and may have a higher risk of injury. However, in a Japanese study of 10 385 elderly (aged 65–84), most of whom were under treatment for pre-existing disease, every physical activity was associated with a reduced risk of all causes and CVD mortality after seven years of follow-up. Hazard ratios (95% CI) for CVD mortality among participants with $\geq$5 days of physical activity per week for the total sample and those with pre-existing diseases were 0.38 (0.22–0.55) and 0.35 (0.24–0.52) respectively, compared with no physical activity. In spite of possible adverse effects, this study indicated that elderly people with a pre-existing disease benefit from any level of physical activity in a dose–response relationship to mortality.[8]

Obesity

Obesity is a risk factor for CHD, poor health and excess mortality. Thresholds for normal weight or obesity defined as body mass index (BMI) were primarily based on evidence from studies in younger adults. In older people the relationship between weight and CV risk is more complex. It remains unclear whether overweight and obese cut points are overly restrictive measures for predicting mortality in older people. In a study to examine all cause and cause-specific mortality associated with underweight (BMI $<18.5\,\text{kg}\,\text{m}^{-2}$), normal weight (BMI 18.5–24.9), overweight (BMI 25.0–29.9), and obesity (BMI > or = 30.0) in an elderly cohort of 4677 men and 4563 women aged 70–75, mortality risk was lowest for overweight participants after 10 years of follow-up. Risk of death for overweight participants was 13% less than for normal weight participants (HR 0.87, 95% CI, 0.78–0.94). Minimum mortality risk was found at a BMI of 26.6 (95% CI, 25.7–27.5) in men and 26.26 (95% CI, 25.5–26.9) in women. Risk of death was similar for obese and normal weight participants (HR 0.98, 95% CI, 0.85–1.11).[9] It appears that extreme obesity is harmful but overweight older people are not at greater mortality risk, and there is little evidence that dieting in this age group confers any benefit.

Smoking

Smoking is a major modifiable risk factor for CVD and causes 11% of all CVD-related mortality. Smoking contributes to the pathogenesis of CHD through promotion of atherosclerosis, triggering of coronary thrombosis, coronary artery spasm, cardiac arrhythmias and the reduced capacity of blood to deliver oxygen. The magnitude of the burden produced by smoking increases rather than decreases with ageing. While relative risk for smoking on CHD is similar in elderly and middle-aged people, there is a twofold increase in excess absolute risk in older people. Benefits of cessation for older smokers are similar in magnitude to those of younger smokers who quit. The risk of CHD drops by 50% one year after smoking cessation and approaches that of a person who has never smoked within 3–4 years, even in individuals older than 60 years. Smoking cessation is highly cost-effective and should be viewed as a therapeutic rather than just a preventive intervention regardless of age.[10]

The prevalence of cigarette smoking in older people in the United Kingdom has declined substantially over the past 40 years, from around 1-in-3 of the over 60s smoking in the early 1970s to a stable level of 1-in-8 from around 2004 onwards. In general a lower proportion of older people are smokers compared to younger age groups.[11]

There are some important attitudinal differences to smoking in old age compared to younger people. Older smokers are less likely to accept that smoking is bad for their health, and doctors are less likely to provide smoking cessation advice to older patients despite evidence that smoking cessation is just as feasible in old age.[12]

Observational data suggests that there are substantial potential benefits for older people from stopping smoking. Compared to older continued smokers, matched ex-smokers have better mobility, greater walking speed and grip strength, reduced prevalence of chronic ill-health, better quality of life scores, reduced risk of cognitive decline and dementia, and reduced risk of death from lung cancer, stroke and cardiovascular disease.[13]

Socioeconomic factors

There is an inverse relationship between socioeconomic status (SES) and prevalence of CV risk factors. People with lower SES tend to adopt unhealthier behaviours, such as smoking and unhealthy dietary habits, and seem to have an increased prevalence of CV risk factors resulting in socioeconomic inequalities in CV health. Although there is a strong social class gradient in CHD risk in middle age, the evidence in old age is limited. In a population-based study of 3761 British men aged 60–79 years there was a graded relationship between social class and CHD incidence after 6.5 years of follow-up. The HR for CHD incidence comparing social class V (unskilled workers) with social class I (professionals) was 2.14 (95% CI, 1.06–4.33; p for trend = 0.11) after adjustment for behavioural factors. Absolute difference in CHD risk between highest and lowest social classes was 4%. Socioeconomic inequalities in CHD persist in elderly people and are at least partly explained by behavioural factors. Improving behavioural factors (especially smoking) could reduce these inequalities by one third.[14]

Hypertension

Hypertension is a major risk factor for CVD in older adults. It reduces life expectancy by 7 years. Prevalence of hypertension is 20% in developed countries. However, prevalence is significantly higher in older people affecting 70% of those >80 years. Black Americans develop hypertension earlier in life and it tends to be more severe than in the white population. There is a strong but complex association between blood pressure (BP) and age. Up to 50 years of age, systolic and diastolic BP rise in tandem. After age 50, systolic BP continues to rise, whereas diastolic BP tends to fall. Below age 50, diastolic BP is the major predictor of CHD risk, whereas above age 60, systolic BP is more important. There is also an enhanced risk for CHD associated with increased pulse pressure. The risk of a fatal CHD event doubles for every 20/10 mmHg increment above 115/75 mmHg. Absolute risk of adverse outcomes increases with age reaching 16-fold higher for persons 80–89 years than for those 40–49 years. A 10 mmHg reduction of systolic BP would predict a 50–60% lower risk of stroke death and a 40–50% lower risk of CHD death. In very old individuals (≥85 years old) the association between hypertension and mortality is weaker and treating hypertension reduces risk of death by 21%, risk of stroke by 30% and risk of cardiac failure by 64%. The target for BP is <140/90 mmHg in general and <130/80 mmHg in individuals with diabetes or chronic kidney disease. Evidence that excessive lowering of diastolic BP in older hypertensive individuals with wide pulse pressures may compromise cardiac outcomes (J curve) is inconsistent and no consensus exists regarding the minimum safe level of diastolic BP in these individuals.[15]

Diabetes mellitus

Diabetes has been recognized as an independent major CV risk factor. In spite of various known metabolic and microvascular complications of diabetes, cardiovascular disease remains the most common cause of death in diabetic persons of all age groups affecting around 65–80%. Increased risk of CVD in diabetes is not fully explained by traditional risk factors and could be related to increased insulin resistance. Risk of CHD and myocardial infarction rises by 30% and 14% respectively for every 1% increase in HbA1c. Whether hyperglycaemia itself is a risk for CHD is not very clear.

Metabolic syndrome

Metabolic syndrome is a constellation of central obesity, impaired fasting glucose, hypertension, high triglycerides and low HDL cholesterol. Pathophysiology of metabolic syndrome includes decreased physical activity and increased inflammation. In older people vitamin D deficiency,[16] leading to increased parathyroid hormone and insulin resistance, in combination with low testosterone, leading to increased waist:hip ratio, are other contributing factors. Metabolic syndrome affects >40% of persons >60 years old and is more common in men. Comparative utility of metabolic syndrome versus its individual components for predicting adverse outcomes in older populations is not well established. In an Italian study of 2910 subjects aged ≥65 years, metabolic syndrome was associated with increased all-cause mortality in all subjects (HR 1.41, 95% CI, 1.16–1.72, $p < 0.001$), in men (1.42, 1.06–1.89, $p < 0.017$), and in women (1.47, 1.13–1.91, $p < 0.004$). It was also associated with increased CV mortality in all subjects (1.60, 1.17–2.19, $p < 0.003$), in men (1.66, 1.00–2.76, $p < 0.051$), and in women (1.60, 1.06–2.33, $p < 0.025$). Among metabolic syndrome components, all-cause mortality is better predicted by high glucose in all subjects (1.27, 1.02–1.59,

$p < 0.037$) and in women (1.61, 1.16–2.24, $p < 0.005$) and by low HDL cholesterol in women (1.48, 1.08–2.02, $p < 0.014$), whereas CV mortality is better predicted by high glucose (2.17, 1.28–3.68, $p < 0.004$) and low HDL cholesterol (1.78, 1.07–2.95, $p > 0.026$) in women.[17] In a similar US study of 4258 older people ≥65 years free of CVD, those with metabolic syndrome had a 22% higher mortality, relative risk (RR) 1.22, 95% CI, 1.11–1.34 compared with persons without metabolic syndrome after multivariable adjustment. Higher risk with metabolic syndrome was confined to persons having an elevated fasting glucose level >6.1 mmol l^{-1} (RR 1.41, 95% CI, 1.27–1.57) or hypertension (RR 1.26, 95% CI, 1.15–1.39) as one of the diagnostic criteria of metabolic syndrome. Persons having metabolic syndrome without high fasting glucose or metabolic syndrome without hypertension did not have higher risk (RR 0.97, 95% CI, 0.85–1.11 and 0.92, 0.71–1.19, respectively). Persons having both hypertension and high fasting glucose had 82% higher mortality (RR 1.82, 95% CI, 1.58–10.9).

In older people individual components of metabolic syndrome predict CVD mortality with equal or higher HR when compared with metabolic syndrome. Therefore, these findings suggest that the metabolic syndrome concept is a marker of CVD risk, but may not have any more advantage in predicting cardiac risk than its individual components.[18]

Frailty and disability

Frailty is a geriatric syndrome of increased vulnerability to stress factors due to decline in function in multiple interrelated systems. Frailty is distinct from related concepts of (i) comorbidity: the burden of coexisting medical illnesses, and (ii) disability: the limited ability for self-care (Figure 1.1). Frailty reflects biological rather than chronological age leading to substantial variability in the outcomes of older people. The relationship between frailty and CVD is mutual; frailty may lead to CVD just as CVD may lead to frailty. In other words frailty is associated with CVD as a risk factor and as an outcome. Around 7% of the US population >65 years and 30% of octogenarians are frail. Domains to define frailty include mobility, strength, balance, motor processing, cognition, nutrition, endurance and physical activity. Frailty reduces a patient's ability to maintain homeostasis in the face of acute stress, predicts mortality and heralds transition to disability. In a systematic review of frailty in patients with CVD, nine studies were included encompassing 54 250 elderly patients with a mean follow-up of 6.2 years. In community-dwelling elders, CVD was associated with an odds ratio (OR) of 2.67 to 4.1 for prevalent frailty and an OR of 1.47 for incident frailty in those who were not frail at baseline. Gait velocity (a measure of frailty) was associated with an OR of 1.61 for incident CVD. In elderly patients with documented severe CHD or heart failure, the prevalence of

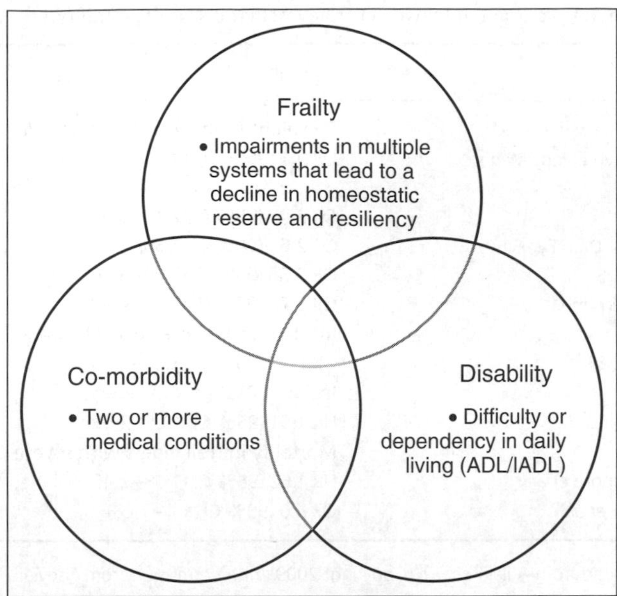

Figure 1.1 Overlap between frailty, comorbidity and disability. ADL, activities of daily living (basic self-care tasks); IADL, instrumental ADL (household management tasks). Reprinted from Afilalo *et al.*[19] Copyright 2009, with permission from Elsevier.

frailty was 50–54%, and this was associated with an OR of 1.62 to 4.0 for all-cause mortality after adjusting for potential confounders (Table 1.1). It is likely that underlying abnormalities in haematological, inflammatory and metabolic systems in frail older patients are linked to increased CV risk. Compared with non-frail counterparts, frail patients had significantly higher levels of factor VIII, D-dimer, C-reactive protein, leukocytes, fibrinogen, glucose, low vitamin D and low haemoglobin. The close correlation between frailty and biomarkers of inflammation and thrombosis resembles the correlation between CVD and these same biomarkers. This common biological pathway may explain why frailty and CVD are interrelated at clinical level. Reasons to consider frailty in older people with CVD include its early identification and anticipation of care after major cardiac events. There is overlap of frailty with comorbidity and disability. Unintended weight loss, disability in activities of daily living and presence of multiple comorbid conditions in a complex cardiac patient should alert physicians to the possibility of associated frailty. Screening of frailty may include simple tests, such as grip strength, gait speed or quadriceps strength. Early recognition of frailty will need comprehensive geriatric assessment combined with multidisciplinary interventions to slow or reverse functional decline, improve physical performance and quality of life.[19] Disability, on the other hand, is a common condition in older people and has been associated with

Table 1.1 Association between cardiovascular disease and frailty.

Study	Variable
	Prevalent frailty in elders with CVD
Zutphen Elderly Men's Study	OR 4.1 (95% CI, 1.8–9.3)
CHS	OR 2.79 (95% CI, 2.12–3.67)
Beaver Dam Eye Study	OR 2.67 (95% CI, 1.33–5.41)
WHI-OS	OR 3.36 (95% CI, 3.09–3.66)
WHAS I and II	OR 2.72 (95% CI, 1.72–4.30)
	Incident frailty in elders with CVD
WHI-OS	OR 1.47 (95% CI, 1.25–1.73)
	Incident CVD in frail elders
HABC Study	HR 1.61 (95% CI, 1.05–2.45)
	Mortality in frail elders with severe CVD
Cacciatore *et al.*	HR 1.62 (95% CI, 1.08–2.45)
Purser *et al.*	OR 4.0 (95% CI, 1.1–13.8)

Reprinted from Afilalo *et al.*[19] Copyright 2009, with permission from Elsevier.

prevalent CHD and shorter longevity. It is less clear whether disability is a risk factor for atherosclerosis development or a prognostic factor for CHD outcome. In a French multicentre prospective population-based cohort of 9294 subjects free of CVD (aged ≥65 years), the mean level of CV risk factors increased gradually with severity of disability. After a median follow-up of 5.2 years, 264 first coronary events, including 55 fatal events, occurred. After adjustment for CV risk factors, participants with moderate or severe disability had a 1.7 times (95% CI, 1.0–2.7) greater risk of overall CHD than non-disabled subjects, whereas those with mild disability were not at greater CHD risk. An association was also found with fatal CHD, for which risk increased gradually with severity of disability (HR 1.7, 95% CI, 0.8–3.6 for mild disability, 3.5, 1.3–9.3 for moderate to severe disability, p for trend = 0.01). This result reflected a specific association between disability and fatal but not with non-fatal CHD. The lack of association between disability and non-fatal CHD suggests that disability has little impact on atherosclerosis development. In other words disability even of mild severity has more to do with prognosis rather than with occurrence of CHD (Figure 1.2). However, this prognostic function of disability could be related to the possibility that disabled subjects suffering from an acute event might be treated less aggressively, too frail to cope with a vascular event and likely to die, or simply disability is associated with severe CHD with a worse prognosis. Therefore, in this population, promotion of regular physical activity seems appropriate, because physical activity has been associated with less severe acute coronary syndrome, lower in-hospital mortality, better short-term prognosis and less disability.[20]

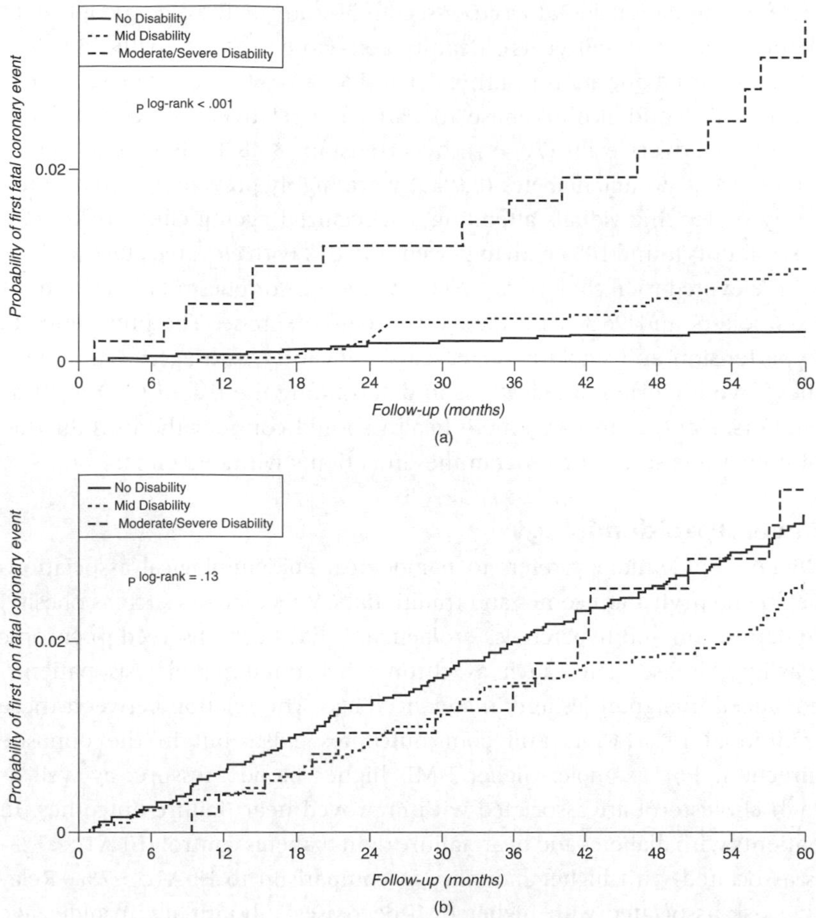

Figure 1.2 (a) Unadjusted Kaplan-Meier cumulative probability of incident fatal coronary heart disease over six years of follow-up according to baseline degree of disability. The Three-City Study. (b) Unadjusted Kaplan-Meier cumulative probability of incident non-fatal coronary heart disease over 6 years of follow-up according to baseline degree of disability. The Three-City Study. No disability (n = 54 080); mild disability: disability in mobility only (n = 52 712); moderate or severe disability: disability in mobility plus activities of daily living, instrumental activities of daily living, or both (n = 5562). Reproduced from Plichart *et al.*[20] with permission from Wiley-Blackwell.

Risk factors in the cognitively impaired

Little is known about CV risk factor profile for older people with dementia. As many CV risk factors are treatable by lifestyle changes, confirmation of the risk factor profile for older people with dementia could substantially impact upon preventive health practices for this group of patients. People with dementia often lack the ability to notice or address symptoms of disease and may not be able to understand or be appropriately concerned about vascular risk factors and may need a more active approach than the general population does. In a cross-sectional study of 470 older people with dementia (age 50–90 years), healthy behaviour was low with 98.9% of participants having an unhealthy diet and 68.3% a lack of exercise. Smoking (13.6%) and alcohol abuse (0.3%) were relatively minor problems. Abdominal overweight (70.4%), hypertension (36.8%), hypercholesterolaemia (31.8%) and diabetes (8.7%), were highly prevalent.[21] In another study of 155 individuals attending a specialized ageing clinic, risk factor assessments found 18% with hypertension, 8% with elevated glucose, 27% with elevated total cholesterol, 70% overweight or obese, 11% current or ex-smokers and 96% with inadequate daily exercise. The prevalence of hypertension and smoking increased significantly with age.[22] These profiles have important implications in determining the risk of CVD in these patients. Campaigns to promote health should consider the introduction of preventive screening programmes in patients with dementia.

Reverse epidemiology

Reverse epidemiology refers to paradoxical epidemiological associations between survival outcomes and traditional CV risk factors such as obesity, hypertension and hypercholesterolaemia. It has been observed in chronic wasting disease states such as chronic heart failure, dialysis patients, advanced malignancies and in advanced age. The relation between these traditional risk factors and poor outcomes exists but in the opposite direction. For example, higher BMI, higher blood pressure, as well as high cholesterol are associated with improved heart failure outcomes. In patients with diabetes and heart failure tight diabetes control (HbA1c <7%) is associated with higher mortality in comparison to HbA1c >7%. Relative risk associated with higher BMI decreases substantially in older age groups. Reverse epidemiology with respect to cholesterol levels has been demonstrated in elderly people; however, hypertension and poor glycaemic control in older people with diabetes remain associated with increased morbidity and mortality. In a study of 400 hospitalized individuals >60 years old, obesity did not show independent survival value. Obesity, higher blood pressure and serum cholesterol, besides being related to lower mortality both in hospital and after discharge, were associated with better nutrition and functional capacity, less intense acute phase reaction and organ dysfunction, and lower incidence of high mortality diseases such as dementia, pneumonia, sepsis or cancer. These associations may explain why obesity and other reverse epidemiology data are inversely related to mortality.

The increased mortality is related to under-nutrition and frailty manifested by low cholesterol and low BP. In hospitalized patients, weight loss and malnutrition are frequent and must be attributed to disease and to inflammatory response. Diseases such as cancer, dementia or heart failure cause malnutrition, a predisposing condition for sepsis which is often the

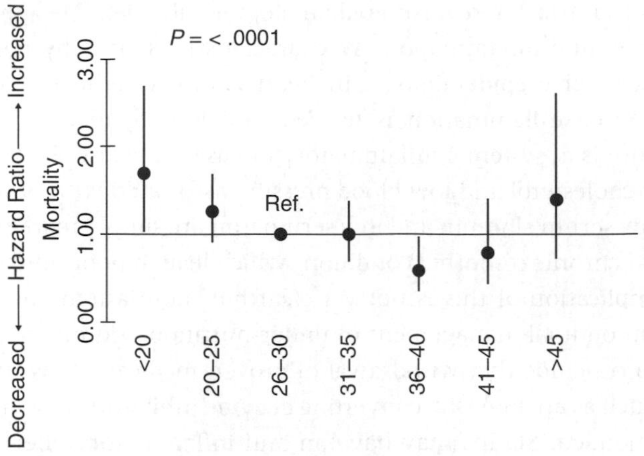

Figure 1.3 Hazard ratios for mortality by BMI after adjustment for age, history, medications, laboratory and echocardiographic findings (all $p < 0.0001$). A U-shape relationship persists between BMI and mortality. Reprinted from Kapoor *et al.*[24] Copyright 2010, with permission from Elsevier.

final cause of death. Patients with BMI <30 who died in hospital showed more weight loss than those who survived; the lower the BMI, the greater the weight loss. In contrast, patients with BMI >30 who died in hospital gained more weight than those who survived; the higher the BMI, the greater the weight gain. When BMI was <30, patients who died had lost more weight than survivors. However, above 30 the situation was the opposite: patients who died in hospital had gained more weight than those who survived. This change at 30 of the prognostic meaning of weight variation indicates a limit on the obesity paradox or a U-shaped relation.[23] Weight gain in patients with a BMI higher than 30 is unhealthy (since it is related to mortality) as is weight loss in patients with lower BMI. The U-shaped relationship between obesity and survival was also observed in community-dwelling older patients with heart failure. In a study to determine all-cause mortality for 1236 patients, mean (SD) age 71 (12) years with a prior diagnosis of heart failure and a preserved ejection fraction (≥50%) survival was better for groups with higher BMI up to a BMI >45 where the mortality increased. After adjustment for patient age, history, medications, and laboratory and echocardiographic parameters, the HR for total mortality (relative to BMI 26–30) were 1.68 (95% CI, 1.04–2.69) for BMI <20, 1.25 (95% CI, 0.92–1.68) for BMI 20–25, 0.99 (95% CI, 0.71–1.36) for BMI 31–35, 0.58 (95% CI, 0.35–0.97) for BMI 36–40, 0.79 (95% CI, 0.44–1.4) for BMI 41–45, and 1.38 (95% CI, 0.74–2.6) for BMI >45 ($p < 0.0001$) (Figure 1.3). Thus, despite the benefit of weight loss in the prevention of CHD and heart failure, there is a lack of data to support a survival benefit from weight loss in patients with established heart failure.[24]

The mechanism for reverse epidemiology is not clear. It appears that malnutrition and inflammation are characteristics shared by populations exhibiting reverse epidemiology. In heart failure weight loss associated with increased inflammation is termed cardiac cachexia. In that sense heart failure is a 'systemic inflammatory disease'. It is also likely that low BMI, low cholesterol and low blood pressure associated with other factors such as low serum albumin and low serum iron are simply markers of poor health and chronic comorbid conditions which lead to poor outcomes. The clinical implication of this is not yet clear but more attention should be focused on optimal management of under-nutrition and inflammation. It is early to conclude that withdrawal of proven medications with survival benefits such as angiotensin-converting enzyme inhibitors or beta-blockers is recommended. Statins may have an anti-inflammatory effect that can be beneficial in management of inflammation irrespective of cholesterol-lowering effects. Reverse epidemiology questions the limits of normal BMI (20–25) for ageing and chronic diseases. It seems appropriate, in diseased individuals, to restrain weight loss by improving feeding and maintaining physical activity to preserve muscle mass. Further research is still needed to clearly understand the mechanisms of reverse epidemiology to better care for these frail patients (Box 1.2).

Box 1.2 Summary–CHD

Epidemiological features

- Incidence increases indefinitely with age.
- Relationship with obesity is U-shaped and inverse with socioeconomic status.
- Hypertension-related risk is 16-fold in persons 80–89 compared to 40–49 years.
- Metabolic syndrome does not add advantage in predicting CV risk above its individual components.
- Frailty is a non-conventional risk factor with a mutual relationship to CVD.
- Disability is a poor outcome indicator for CHD.
- In frail older people a paradoxical relation exists between traditional risk factors and outcome. The mechanism of this reverse epidemiology is related to malnutrition and inflammation.
- Reverse epidemiology questions the limits of normal BMI (20–25 kg m^{-2}) for ageing and chronic diseases.

Clinical implications

- Benefits of quitting smoking persist in older people.
- A 10 mmHg reduction in systolic BP would reduce CHD mortality by 50%.
- Early recognition of frailty is important to slow or reverse functional decline, improve physical performance and quality of life through multidisciplinary interventions.

- Attention should be focused on optimal management of under-nutrition and inflammation. It seems appropriate, in diseased individuals, to restrain weight loss by improving feeding and maintaining physical activity to preserve muscle mass.
- Physical activity has a positive impact on mortality in a dose–response relationship.

Heart failure

Heart failure is characterized by systolic or diastolic ventricular dysfunction associated with evidence of circulatory failure manifested by fatigue and fluid retention. It is becoming increasingly common and is the end product of CHD, hypertension and valvular heart disease. Therefore heart failure epidemiology is related to prevalence, incidence and outcomes of these CV diseases (Figure 1.4). It mostly affects elderly people as >75% of patients are >65 years old and mean age is 75 years. In developed countries the biggest factor boosting heart failure prevalence is increasing growth of an elderly population. In the United States, the number of elderly (>65 years) is expected to grow from 35 million in the year 2000 to 70.3 million in 2030. In the United Kingdom the number of people aged >65 years has increased by 50% and those >85 has increased threefold in the last 40 years. Even if incidence remains constant, the total number of people with heart failure is expected to double increasing its prevalence. Prevalence and

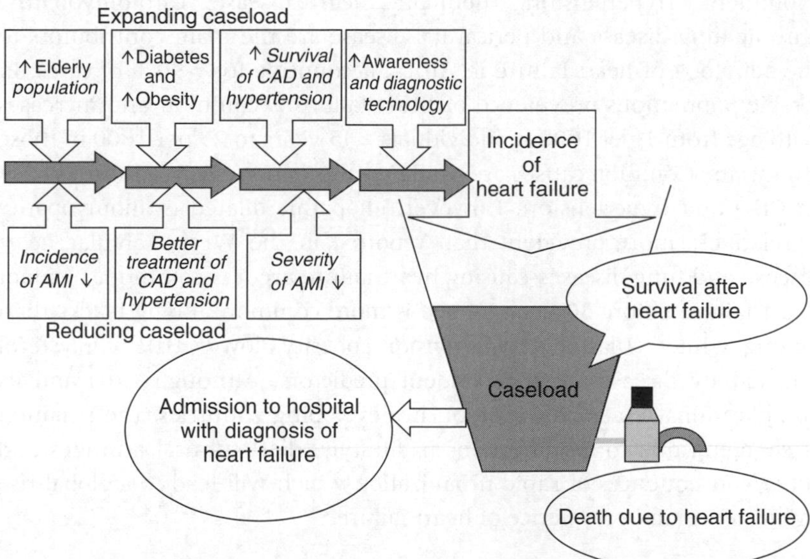

Figure 1.4 Epidemiology of heart failure. AMI, acute myocardial infarction; CAD, coronary artery disease. Reprinted from Najafi *et al.*[25] by permission of Oxford University Press.

incidence of heart failure in those aged 80–89 years is 10 times prevalence and incidence in those aged 50–59 years. In the United States 550 000 new cases of heart failure occur each year. More than 20 million people have heart failure worldwide of whom 5 million are in America and 6.5 million in Europe. Heart failure is the leading cause of hospitalization affecting >20% of acute hospital admissions of individuals >65 years. Age-adjusted annual incidence of heart failure is 0.14% in women and 0.23% in men, with better survival among women. Lifetime risk for developing heart failure at age 40 years is 21% for men and 20% for women.

Several factors contribute to the increased burden of heart failure. Improved care of acute myocardial infarctions and of those patients already diagnosed with heart failure have combined to foster a growing epidemic. Age-adjusted survival rates have improved and risk of death has declined 12% per decade. However, heart failure still carries a grave prognosis. The 2- and 5-year mortality rates are 60% and 75%, respectively. Mortality in heart failure is as high as in many common types of cancer such as bowel cancer in men and breast cancer in women. It is associated with a comparable number of expected life-years lost (6.7 years per 1000 in men and 5.1 years per 1000 in women).[25]

Ethnic variations

In developing countries ischaemic aetiology for heart failure is less common. Other causes such as rheumatic (Africa, Asia, Latin America), Chagas disease (Latin America) and hypertension (Africa) are more prominent. Hypertension, rheumatic heart disease, cardiomyopathy, chronic lung disease and pericardial disease are the main contributors to the aetiology of heart failure in Africa, accounting for >90% of cases. In Arabic populations prevalence of heart failure is common and increases with age from 1 per 1000 in individuals <45 years to 25 per 1000 in those ≥65 years. Common causes are similar to those in Western countries such as CHD and hypertension. However, idiopathic dilated cardiomyopathy is relatively more prevalent than reported in the West. Valvular heart disease and lung diseases causing heart failure are less common. Incident heart failure before 50 years of age is more common among blacks than among whites. Diastolic hypertension, obesity, lower HDL cholesterol and kidney disease are independent predictors. Although CHD and its complications remain uncommon in developing countries, the situation is changing due to modifications in lifestyle, diet, cultural attitudes and other consequences of rapid urbanization which will lead to a global rise in incidence and prevalence of heart failure.[26]

Risk factors and prevention

A large proportion of heart failure risk is attributed to modifiable risk factors. In the Health, Aging and Body Composition Study, 2934 participants were enrolled, mean (SD) age 73.6 (2.9) years, 47.9% men, 58.6% white and 41.4% black, and assessed for incidence of heart failure, population attributable risk (PAR) of independent risk factors for heart failure, and outcomes. During a median follow-up of 7.1 years, 258 participants (8.8%) developed heart failure (13.6 cases per 1000 person-years, 95% CI, 12.1–15.4). Men and black people were more likely to develop heart failure. No significant sex-based differences were observed in risk factors. CHD (PAR 23.9% for white and 29.5% for black) and uncontrolled hypertension (PAR 21.3% for white and 30.1% for black) carried the highest PAR in both races. Among black participants, six risk factors (smoking, increased heart rate, CHD, left ventricular hypertrophy, uncontrolled hypertension, and reduced glomerular filtration rate) had >5% higher PAR compared with that among white participants, leading to a higher overall proportion of heart failure attributable to modifiable risk factors in black compared to white participants (67.8% vs 48.9%). Participants who developed heart failure had higher annual mortality (18.0% vs 2.7%). No racial difference in survival after heart failure was noted; however, rehospitalization rates were higher among black participants (62.1 vs 30.3 hospitalizations per 100 person-years, $p < 0.001$).[27] In another population-based case–control study of 962 Olmsted County residents with heart failure (mean age 75.4 years; 53.7% women who were older than men 78.3 vs 72.1 years respectively, $p < 0.001$) mean (SD) number of risk factors for heart failure per case was 1.9 (1.1) and increased over time ($p < 0.001$). Hypertension was most common (66%), followed by smoking (51%). Risk of heart failure was particularly high for CHD and diabetes (OR 3.05, 95% CI, 2.36–3.95 and 2.65, 1.98–3.54) respectively (Table 1.2). However, PAR was highest for CHD and hypertension, each accounted for 20% of heart failure cases in the population, although CHD accounted for the greatest proportion of cases in men (PAR 23%) and hypertension was of greatest importance in women (PAR 28%). Preventing CHD and hypertension will have the greatest population impact in preventing heart failure. Sex-targeted prevention strategies might confer additional benefit.[28]

Table 1.2 Association between heart failure and risk factors from case/control analysis.

			Population Attributable Risk (95% CI)		
Risk Factor	OR (95% CI)	*p* Value	Overall	Women	Men
CHD	3.05 (2.36–3.95)	<0.001	0.20 (0.16–0.24)	0.16 (0.12–0.20)	0.23 (0.16–0.30)
Hypertension	1.44 (1.18–1.76)	<0.001	0.20 (0.10–0.30)	0.28 (0.14–0.42)	0.13 (0.00–0.26)
Diabetes	2.65 (1.98–3.54)	<0.001	0.12 (0.09–0.15)	0.10 (0.06–0.14)	0.13 (0.08–0.18)
Obesity	2.00 (1.57–2.55)	<0.001	0.12 (0.08–0.16)	0.12 (0.07–0.17)	0.13 (0.07–0.19)
Ever smoker	1.37 (1.13–1.68)	0.002	0.14 (0.06–0.22)	0.08 (0.00–0.15)	0.22 (0.07–0.37)

Reprinted from Dunlay *et al.*[28] Copyright 2009, with permission from Elsevier.

Diastolic heart failure

Diastolic heart failure is defined by the presence of signs and symptoms of heart failure, normal ejection fraction and evidence of abnormal left ventricular diastolic function. Echocardiographic studies in the community show that 50% of all patients with heart failure have preserved left ventricular systolic function. Prevalence of diastolic heart failure increases more sharply with age more than systolic heart failure. It is likely that age-related changes in diastolic function lower the threshold for expression of diastolic heart failure in elderly. Ageing is associated with a stiffening of large vessels and concentric hypertrophy of left ventricular myocardium with reduced early diastolic relaxation and filling rates. This combined ventricular-vascular stiffening may contribute to increased prevalence of diastolic heart failure in elderly persons. This ventricular-vascular stiffening occurs more steeply in women. It is very likely that systolic hypertension plays an important role in the genesis of diastolic heart failure by increasing both vascular and ventricular stiffness. Compared to those with reduced systolic function, patients with preserved systolic function are older, more often female, more likely to have hypertension associated with left ventricular hypertrophy and less likely to have CHD. Mortality rates are higher in these patients compared to age-matched controls without heart failure, but not as high as those in patients with reduced systolic function. In contrast, morbidity, as measured by hospitalization and re-admission, is substantial and comparable to that of patients with systolic heart failure.

Complexity and care for heart failure

Heart failure and cognition

Heart failure results in losses in memory, psychomotor speed and executive function in 25% of patients. In a study to determine types, frequency and severity of cognitive deficits among patients with heart failure compared with age and education matched healthy participants and participants with major medical conditions other than heart failure in a sample of 414 participants (249 heart failure, 63 healthy and 102 medical participants), heart-failure patients had poorer memory, psychomotor speed and executive function compared with healthy and medical participants. Significantly more heart-failure patients (24%) had deficits in three or more domains and heart failure severity was associated with more cognitive deficits. Multiple comorbidity, hypertension, depressive symptoms and medications were not associated with cognitive deficits. Older patients with more severe heart failure have more problems in executive function.[29] Future studies are needed to identify mechanisms for cognitive deficits in heart failure and to test interventions to prevent cognitive loss and decline. On the other hand, the presence of heart failure in a cognitively impaired individual further increases heart failure-related morbidity and affects functional outcomes and need for institutional care.

Heart failure and geriatric conditions

There is a high prevalence of geriatric conditions among older people with heart failure including urinary incontinence, falls and dementia. Each of these conditions suggests the presence of a high degree of disability. Geriatric conditions are strongly and independently associated with short- (30 days) and long-term (5 years) mortality among older patients hospitalized for heart failure. In a study of 62 330 hospitalized heart-failure patients, mean (SD) age 79.6 (7.8), mortality rates were 9.8% at 30 days and 74.7% at 5 years. Dementia and mobility disability were among top predictors of short (OR 1.86, 95% C I, 1.73–2.01 and 1.96, 1.81–2.12, respectively) and long-term mortality (2.01, 1.84–2.19 and 1.78, 1.70–1.87, respectively). These results enhance the relevance of cognitive and physical disabilities in heart-failure patients.[30] Despite the ageing population and the fact that heart failure primarily affects older persons in whom many complex conditions coexist, current studies and guidelines have not incorporated routine assessment or management of geriatric conditions.

Heart failure in care homes

Prevalence of heart disease in care homes is expected to be higher than in the general population due to older and frailer populations living in these settings. Little data is available because care home residents are often excluded from epidemiological studies. In a systematic review of 10 studies, prevalence of heart failure was 20% (range 15–45%). This figure is higher than in the general population (3–13%); however, it could be underestimated as both undetected and incorrect diagnosis of heart failure was common. The mean age of study populations ranged between 79–89 years. CHD and atrial fibrillation were the most common causes of heart failure. The level of associated comorbidities (dementia 9–73%, diabetes mellitus 11–38%, chronic obstructive pulmonary disease 12–36%, and hypertension 8–55%) among these patients was also high.[31] Accurate diagnosis of heart failure in these settings is difficult and hampered by concomitant comorbidity which often shows characteristic signs and symptoms similar to those of heart failure (e.g. breathlessness, ankle swelling and fatigue) making interpretation difficult. Early diagnosis and treatment may prevent progression of the disease and lead to improvement of disabling symptoms, ultimately resulting in an overall improvement in quality of life.

Care needs for heart failure

Older people with heart failure have higher rates of disability, geriatric conditions, nursing home admission, and often require a multifaceted approach of care. Promoting care delivery systems that provide a coordinated, multidisciplinary approach to older people with heart failure will be necessary to optimize care. It is important to recognize associated physical and cognitive dysfunction in heart failure patients in order to optimize care and outcome. Although geriatric conditions are chronic and incurable, physical therapy and exercise may improve mobility, and increased caregiver and nursing support can be implemented to help patients with dementia adhere to medications. Benefits of interventions to address mobility and dementia may also enhance patients' abilities to avoid or cope with other medical conditions such as falls. Older patients with severe heart failure may be severely distressed with poorly controlled symptoms. There is a growing realization that palliative and supportive care may play an important role in treatment and underpin services to improve quality of life.

Caregiver burden

Heart failure imposes a significant burden on patients, families and the long-term care system. However, social support is associated with better outcomes of heart failure. Mechanism for such better outcomes could be due to social support for enhanced self-care such as adherence to medication and healthy behaviour. Social isolation and living alone on the other hand are associated with increased heart-failure mortality, morbidity and psychosocial distress independent of possible contributing factors such as depression and severity of heart failure. The responsibilities of providing care for heart failure patients can be overwhelming, and may lead to exhaustion and depression in caregivers who may have multiple health problems of their own. Caregivers may also experience distressing symptoms such as sleep difficulties related to patient's sleep problems. Caregiver outcomes are also important, which should include both their physical and emotional health (Box 1.3).

Box 1.3 Summary–Heart failure

Epidemiological features

- Heart failure is the end product of CHD, hypertension, and valvular heart disease.
- Older people are the main sufferers (mean age 75 years).
- Prevalence and incidence in people 80–89 is 10 times those 50–59 years.
- Increasing growth of older population and improved care for CHD is leading to a growing epidemic of heart failure.
- In spite of improved survival, heart failure still carries a grave prognosis.
- Ischaemic aetiology is less common in developing countries.

- Heart failure risk is attributed to modifiable risk factors particularly CHD in men and hypertension in women.
- Diastolic heart failure is more common in older women who are likely to have hypertension, left ventricular hypertrophy and less likely to have CHD. It carries similar morbidity but less mortality than systolic heart failure.

Clinical implications

- Preventing CHD and hypertension will have an impact on reducing heart failure.
- Complex conditions tend to coexist with heart failure and are independently associated with mortality. Guidelines should incorporate routine assessment and management of these geriatric conditions.
- Prevalence in care homes is high and associated with a high level of disability. Early diagnosis and treatment in these settings may prevent progression and improve quality of life.
- Heart failure imposes a significant burden on families. It will need a multifaceted care. Caregiver outcomes are also important, and should include both their physical and emotional health.

Valvular heart disease

Prevalence and incidence of rheumatic heart disease have declined in the developed world but are still common in developing countries mainly affecting younger populations. The most common valve diseases in elderly people are either degenerative or infective.

Degenerative valve disease

The aortic valve is most commonly affected and prevalence of degenerative aortic valve disease (DAVD) rises as life expectancy increases. About 95 000 valve procedures are performed each year in the United States, and DAVD is responsible for >25 000 annual deaths. Traditional risk factors associated with atherosclerosis such as age, diabetes and cholesterol have been implicated in the development of DAVD. Early stages of DAVD are similar to the active inflammatory process of atherosclerosis including basement membrane disruption, inflammatory cell infiltration, lipid deposition and calcification. Visceral obesity also has a role in the development and progression of DAVD. In addition, visceral obesity in combination with other metabolic risk factors has been associated with degenerative changes in bioprosthetic heart valves. It seems that DAVD is related to an atherosclerotic process where interactions between lipids, inflammation and valvular tissue play an important role in the development of valvular calcification. This concept is referred to as 'valvulo-metabolic risk'. Despite these common risk factors only 50% of patients with DAVD have significant CHD, and most patients with CHD do not have DAVD suggesting that some other factors are contributing to the development of DAVD. Association of these risk factors may have implications for therapeutic interventions such as statins or angiotensin-converting enzyme inhibitors that may delay or prevent progression of DAVD. However, although 60–70% of patients with DAVD have dyslipidaemia and are already receiving statins, a substantial percentage of these patients show rapid progression. This suggests that targeting dyslipidaemia alone may not be sufficient but targeting whole metabolic risk could be more effective in slowing valve degeneration progression.

Infective valve disease

Valve infection or infective endocarditis affects patients with predisposing valvular abnormalities traditionally caused by rheumatic carditis, and *Streptococcus viridans* is the most common pathogen. This presentation is still seen in developing countries where rheumatic heart disease is prevalent. In the Western world the incidence of infective endocarditis is rising in the elderly population >65 years reaching around four times that of the general population. Factors accounting for this increase include the high prevalence of undiagnosed degenerative valve disease and increased use of invasive procedures and implanted medical devices. Infective endocarditis has a predilection for males, but the proportion of females affected progressively increases with age. Despite progress in diagnosis and treatment, mortality rates remain high reaching twice that of younger patients. Diabetes, gastrointestinal and genitourinary tract cancers are predisposing risk factors. Although the prevalence of *S. aureus* decreases with age, enterococci and *S. bovis* are emerging as major players of infective endocarditis in elderly patients.[32] The evaluation of gastrointestinal and genitourinary tract lesions frequently requires invasive procedures, which remain an important risk. These findings might affect antibiotic prophylaxis strategy by taking into account patient age in global risk assessment (Box 1.4).

Box 1.4 Summary–Valvular heart disease

Epidemiological features

- Prevalence of DAVD increases with age.
- Traditional risk factors are associated with DAVD and referred to as 'valvulo-metabolic risk'.
- Incidence of infective endocarditis in elderly population is four times and mortality is twice that of younger patients. The high prevalence of DAVD and increased use of invasive procedures and implanted medical devices are the main risks.
- Gastrointestinal and genitourinary tract cancers are predisposing factors for bacteraemia (enterococci and *S. bovis*) causing endocarditis.

Clinical implications

- Targeting metabolic risk factors may have an effect on slowing valve degeneration progression.
- Antibiotic prophylaxis strategy should take into account patient age in patients undergoing invasive gastrointestinal or genitourinary procedures.

Rhythm disorders

Abnormal heart rhythm increases with age even in those with normal hearts. Prevalence rates of atrial and ventricular ectopy reach up to 100% in older people. Left ventricular dysfunction is associated with increased prevalence of ventricular ectopy. However, there is no association between the extent or complexity of ventricular ectopy and the presence or absence of significant CHD in the absence of left ventricular dysfunction, and prognosis is good. Epidemiological features of two important rhythm disorders are discussed in this section: atrial fibrillation and sudden cardiac death believed to be due to ventricular tachycardia.

Atrial fibrillation

Atrial fibrillation (AF) is the most common sustained cardiac arrhythmia. It is characterized by uncoordinated atrial activation with consequent loss of atrial mechanical function. Hypertension is the most important single risk factor for AF, conferring a 1.5-fold increased risk in men and a 1.4-fold increased risk in women. AF affects 10% of people >80 and 20% of people ≥90 years. In developed nations, overall prevalence is 0.9% and the number of people affected is projected to be more than double over the next two decades. Incidence is 3 per 1000 person-years in men and 2 per 1000 person-years in women aged 55–64 years but increases exponentially with advancing age to 20–30 per 1000 patient-years in individuals ≥85 years. AF is 1.5 times more common in men than in women. However, onset of AF in women occurs at a later age than in men (65 vs 60 years respectively). Life-time risk of AF is 1 in 4 for both sexes from age 40 years onwards. The incidence pattern of AF may show racial and geographical variations with white subjects having twice the incidence rate of African Americans. Also incidence and prevalence appear to be lower in Asia than in the United States or Europe. The number of people with AF may reach 12.1 million by 2050 assuming no further increase in incidence, and 15.9 million assuming the continued increase in incidence rate is present. This may still be an underestimation as prevalence of sustained silent AF in people >65 years is believed to reach up to 60%.

AF is associated with a doubling of mortality ranging from 1.3–1.8-fold for men and 1.9–2.8-fold for women. Thromboembolic stroke is the most serious complication, risk of which is increased five times in patients with AF. AF is responsible for 15% of cases of strokes. Annual risk of stroke due to AF is 1.5% among patients aged 50–59 years and increases to 23.5% in those >80 years with a similar AF-related stroke mortality rate. AF also increases risk of heart failure by two- to sevenfold. As a result of increasing age and improved survival rates in patients with CHD, heart failure and hypertension, an increase in prevalence of AF is likely to be exponential and sustained in the foreseeable future. Prognosis of AF is likely to be influenced by appropriate treatment strategies such as the use of anticoagulation to reduce stroke risk as well as rate or rhythm control to prevent tachycardia-induced cardiomyopathy and heart failure.

Sudden cardiac death

Sudden cardiac death (SCD) refers to death from abrupt cessation of cardiac function due to cardiac arrest. It results from a lethal arrhythmia and usually occurs on a background of structural abnormality or CHD. The most accepted definition is sudden and unexpected death within an hour of symptom onset. Incidence of SCD is 4–5 million cases per year worldwide and 60% of cases are males.[33] There are two well-established peaks in age-related prevalence of SCD, one during infancy representing sudden infant death syndrome and the second in the geriatric age group, between ages 75–85 years. Approximately 80% of SCD are attributed to CHD. Two major mechanisms of fatal ventricular arrhythmias could result in SCD: (i) Polymorphic ventricular tachycardia resulting from acute coronary ischaemia associated with plaque rupture and occlusion of one or more main coronary arteries in patients with relatively normal left ventricular function. (ii) Monomorphic ventricular tachycardia resulting from re-entrant loops around areas of scarred myocardium in patients with established ischaemic cardiomyopathy. Either arrhythmia, if untreated, will eventually degenerate into ventricular fibrillation and SCD. A diagnosis of severe left ventricular dysfunction is the best available predictor of SCD risk and ejection fraction remains the major criterion to stratify patients for defibrillator implantation. An implantable cardiovertor defibrillator is effective therapy in the prevention of SCD. However, severe left ventricular dysfunction affects <30% of all SCD cases in the community. Almost 50% of SCD cases have normal left ventricular function and the remaining 20% have either mildly or moderately decreased left ventricular systolic function (ejection fraction >0.35 and <0.50). Impaired kidney function, as measured by cystatin C, has an independent association with SCD risk among elderly persons without clinical CVD.[34] Risk of SCD in patients with CHD is multifactorial and

Box 1.5 Summary–Rhythm disorders

Epidemiological features

- AF is the most common sustained cardiac arrhythmia.
- Hypertension is the most important risk factor for AF.
- AF affects 10% of people >80 and 20% of people ≥90 years.
- AF is 1.5 times more common in men than in women.
- It increases risk of thromboembolic stroke by 5 times, heart failure by 2–7 times, and mortality by 2 times.
- As a result of increasing age and improved survival in patients with hypertension, an increase in prevalence of AF is expected.
- Incidence of SCD is 4–5 million per year and 60% of cases are males.
- Approximately 80% of SCD are attributed to CHD.
- Ventricular tachycardia degenerating into ventricular fibrillation is the most likely cause of SCD precipitated by rupture of atherosclerotic plaque.

Clinical implications

- Prognosis of AF is likely to be improved by appropriate treatment strategies such as use of anticoagulation to reduce stroke risk as well as rate or rhythm control to prevent tachycardia-induced cardiomyopathy and heart failure.
- Stabilization of vulnerable plaques by treatment of risk factors, or by coronary interventions may reduce incidence of SCD.

one major factor is rupture of atherosclerotic plaque. By stabilization of vulnerable plaque with cholesterol-lowering and antiplatelet medications or by coronary artery bypass surgery and percutaneous angioplasty, significant decline in ejection fraction may be less common in the future. However, specific clinical risk predictors for patients with vulnerable plaque that is prone to rupture still need further studies (Box 1.5).

Conclusion

The incidence and prevalence of heart disease are increasing. As a result of the growth in an older population, combined with improvement in treatment, an increase in the number of older people living with cardiac conditions is expected. With increasing urbanization and modification of lifestyle in developing countries, the increase in heart disease is global. Unconventional risk factors are emerging in older people such as frailty and disability, which have both a predictive and prognostic effect. In the very old and frail individuals there is reversal of the effect of traditional risk factors such as obesity, hypercholesterolaemia and hypertension. The mechanism of this reverse epidemiology is likely to be due to inflammation and malnutrition. This will have clinical implications in treating malnutrition and avoiding weight loss in this group of patients with promotion of physical activity. Once heart disease is established it is likely to be associated with both physical and cognitive dysfunction and a high risk of institutionalization. Targeted care for older patients with heart disease that is multidisciplinary in nature with a focus on the whole person and outcomes relevant to them, such as quality of life, is needed.

Key points

- Epidemiology of heart disease is shifting from middle-aged men to elderly women.
- As the older population is growing combined with improvements in treatment, as well as increasing urbanization in developing countries, a global rise in prevalence of heart disease is expected.
- Once heart disease is established it is likely to be associated with physical and cognitive disability and increased risk of institutionalization.
- Care needs for older people with heart disease should take into account their complex needs and outcomes relevant to them, considering illness in the context of the whole patient rather than as a solitary entity.

References

1 Roal FJ and Santos RD. Homozygous familial hypercholesterolemia. *Atherosclerosis* 2012 Feb 16. [Epub ahead of print]

2 Clarke R. Homocysteine, B vitamins and the risk of cardiovascular disease. *Clin Chem* 2011;**57**:1201–2.

3 Driver JA, Djoussé L, Logroscino G *et al.* Incidence of cardiovascular disease and cancer in advanced age: prospective cohort study. *BMJ* 2008; DOI:10.1136/bmj.a2467.

4 Agyemang C, Addo J, Bhopal R *et al.* Cardiovascular disease, diabetes and established risk factors among populations of sub-Saharan African descent in Europe: a literature review. *Globalization and Health* 2009; DOI:10.1186/1744-8603-5-7.

5 Levitan EB, Wolk A and Mittleman MA. Fatty fish, marine omega-3 fatty acids and incidence of heart failure. *Eur J Clin Nutr* 2010 Mar 24; DOI:10.1038/ejcn.2010.50.

6 Engelfriet P, Hoekstra J, Hoogenveen R *et al.* Food and vessels: the importance of a healthy diet to prevent cardiovascular disease. *Eur J Cardiovasc Prev Rehabil* 2010;**17**:50–5.

7 Houston DK, Ding J, Lee JS *et al.* Dietary fat and cholesterol and risk of cardiovascular disease in older adults: The Health ABC Study. *Nutr Metab Cardiovasc Dis* 2009; DOI:10.1016/j.numecd.2009.11.007.

8 Ueshima K, Ishikawa-Takata K, Yorifuji T *et al.* Physical activity and mortality risk in the Japanese elderly. A cohort study. *Am J Prev Med* 2010;**38**:410–8.

9 Flicker L, McCaul KA and Hankey GJ. Body mass index and survival in men and women aged 70 to 75. *J Am Geriatr Soc* 2010;**58**:234–41.

10 Prasad D, Kabir Z, Dash A *et al.* Smoking and cardiovascular health: A review of the epidemiology, pathogenesis, prevention and control of tobacco. *Indian J Med Sci* 2009;**63**:520–33.

11 Cancer Research UK. http://info.cancerresearchuk.org/cancerstats/types/;img/smoking/lung-cancer-and-smoking-statistics (accessed June 2012).

12 Connolly MJ. Smoking cessation in old age: closing the stable door? *Age and Ageing* 2000;**29**(3):193–5.

13 Allen SC. What determines the ability to stop smoking in old age? *Age and Ageing* 2008;**37**(5):490–1.

14 Ramsay SE, Morris RW, Whincup PH *et al.* Socioeconomic inequalities in coronary heart disease risk in older age: contribution of established and novel coronary risk factors. *J Thromb Haemost* 2009;**7**:1779–86.

15 Aguado A, López F, Miravet S *et al.* Hypertension in the very old; prevalence, awareness, treatment and control: a cross-sectional population-based study in a Spanish municipality. *BMC Geriatrics* 2009; DOI:10.1186/1471-2318-9-16.

16 Barnard K and Colón-Emeric C. Extra skeletal effects of vitamin D in older adults: cardiovascular disease, mortality, mood, and cognition. *Am J Geriatr Pharmacother* 2010;**8**:4–33.

17 Zambon S, Zanonio S, Romanato G *et al.* Metabolic syndrome and all-cause and cardiovascular mortality in an Italian elderly population. *Diabetes Care* 2009;**32**:153–9.

18 Mozaffarian D, Kamineni A, Prineas RJ *et al.* Metabolic syndrome and mortality in older adults. The Cardiovascular Health Study. *Arch Intern Med* 2008;**168**:969–78.

19 Afilalo J, Karunananthan S, Eisenberg MJ *et al.* Role of frailty in patients with cardiovascular disease. *Am J Cardiol* 2009;**103**:1616–21.

20 Plichart M, Barberger-Gateau P, Tzourio C *et al.* Disability and incident coronary heart disease in older community-dwelling adults: The Three-City Study. *J Am Geriatr Soc* 2010;**58**:636–42.

21 de Winter CF, Magilsen KW, van Alfen JC *et al.* Prevalence of cardiovascular risk factors in older people with intellectual disability. *Am J Intellect Dev Disabil* 2009;**114**:427–36.

22 Wallace RA and Schluter P. Audit of cardiovascular disease risk factors among supported adults with intellectual disability attending an ageing clinic. *J Intellect Dev Disabil* 2008;http://www.informaworld.com/smpp/title~db=all~content=t713432019~tab=issueslist~branches=33 – v3333:48–58.

23 Martinn-Ponce E, Santolaria F, Aleman-Valls MR *et al.* Factors involved in the paradox of reverse epidemiology. *Clinical Nutrition* 2010; DOI:10.1016/j.clnu.2009.12.009.

24 Kapoor JR and Heidenreich PA. Obesity and survival in patients with heart failure and preserved systolic function: a U-shaped relationship. *Am Heart J* 2010;**159**:75–80.

25 Najafi F, Jamrozik K and Dobson AJ. Understanding the ‘epidemic of heart failure’: a systematic review of trends in determinants of heart failure. *Eur J Heart Fail* 2009;**11**:472–9.

26 Ntusi NB and Mayosi BM. Epidemiology of heart failure in sub-saharan Africa. *Expert Rev Cardiovasc Ther* 2009;**7**:169–80.

27 Kalogeropoulos A, Georgiopoulou V, Kritchevsky SB *et al.* Epidemiology of incident heart failure in a contemporary elderly cohort – The Health, Aging, and Body Composition Study. *Arch Intern Med* 2009;**169**:708–15.

28 Dunlay SM, Weston SA, Jacobsen SJ *et al.* Risk factors for heart failure: a population-based case–control study. *Am J Med* 2009;**122**:1023–8.

29 Pressler SJ, Subramanian U, Kareken D *et al.* Cognitive deficits in chronic heart failure. *Nurs Res* 2010;**59**:127–39.

30 Chaudhry SI, Wang Y, Gill TM *et al*. Geriatric conditions and subsequent mortality in older patients with heart failure. *J Am Coll Cardiol* 2010;**55**:309–16.

31 Daamen MAMJ, Schols JMGA, Jaarsma T *et al*. Prevalence of heart failure in nursing homes: a systematic literature review. *Scand J Caring Sci* 2010;**24**:202–8.

32 Durante-Mangoni E, Bradley S, Selton-Suty C *et al*. Current features of infective endocarditis in elderly patients. *Arch Intern Med* 2008;**168**:2095–103.

33 Chugh SS, Reinier K, Teodorescu C *et al*. Epidemiology of sudden cardiac death: clinical and research implications. *Prog Cardiovasc Dis* 2008;**51**:213–28.

34 Deo R, Sotoodehnia N, Katz R *et al*. Cystatin C and sudden cardiac death risk in the elderly. *Circ Cardiovasc Qual Outcomes* 2010;**3**:159–64.

CHAPTER 2
Cardiac Ageing and Systemic Disorders

David J. Stott and Terence J. Quinn
Institute of Cardiovascular and Medical Sciences, University of Glasgow, Glasgow Royal Infirmary, Glasgow, Scotland, UK

Introduction

Ageing is a highly heterogeneous process and deterioration in organ function, including the heart, often does not correlate well with chronological age. A complex mix of influences combine to influence cardiovascular function in older people, including intrinsic ageing, the cumulative effect of multiple underlying diseases, and many environmental or external influences (such as frequency and intensity of exercise, cigarette smoking and diet). Separating the effects of intrinsic ageing from subclinical disease is challenging, and teasing out the additional contributions of environmental and lifestyle exposures even more problematic. Accepting these difficulties, it is still important to have a basic knowledge and understanding of the effects of intrinsic ageing on the heart to enable accurate interpretation of the effect of systemic disease on cardiovascular function in older people (Figure 2.1). 'Healthy' or intrinsic cardiac ageing is associated with gradual decline in organ function and homeostatic reserve. The effects include reduced maximal aerobic exercise capacity and a decreased threshold for clinical expression of many age-related cardiac and non-cardiac diseases. However, healthy cardiac ageing by itself should not cause symptoms or limit usual activities of daily living.

Although there is no uniform ageing heart phenotype, some general principles are apparent, and we have attempted to summarize these. In this regard there are established and emergent data from multiple sources including *in vitro* work, animal models and clinical studies. This chapter aims firstly to summarize effects of ageing on cardiac structure, function and homeostatic reserve. The potential impact of these changes on the manifestation of various systemic (non-cardiac) diseases is then considered.

Cardiovascular Disease and Health in the Older Patient: Expanded from 'Pathy's Principles and Practice of Geriatric Medicine, Fifth edition', First Edition. Edited by David J. Stott and Gordon D.O. Lowe.

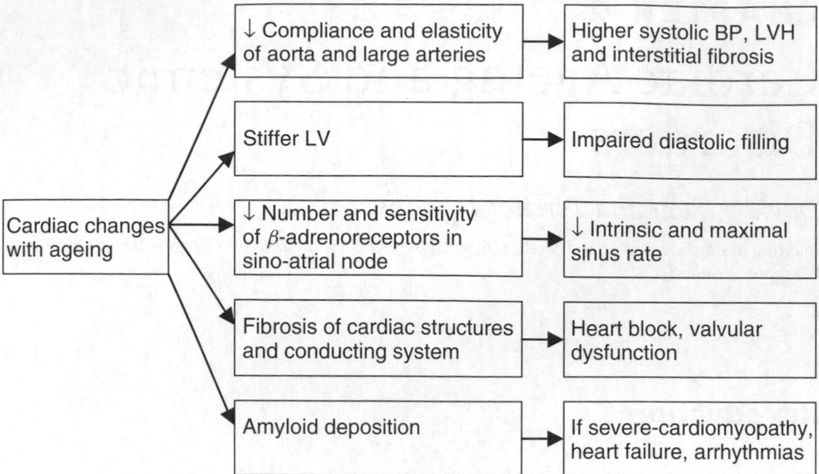

Figure 2.1 Changes in cardiovascular system with healthy ageing.

Changes in cardiac structure with ageing

For most solid organs age-related atrophy is the norm; however, magnetic resonance imaging (MRI) studies of the ageing heart show approximately 10% increase in cardiac mass from the age of 20 to 80 years in both men and women;[1] the 'healthy' older left ventricle is characterized by an increased mass-to-volume ratio.[2] Autopsy series confirm a high prevalence of left ventricular hypertrophy (LVH) in elderly subjects.[3–5] This hypertrophy is caused mainly by increased impedance to left ventricular ejection due to reduction in elasticity and compliance of the aorta and large arteries with resultant higher systolic arterial pressures; age-related degenerative aortic valve disease with sclerosis and thickening of valve leaflets and proximal bulging of the interventricular septum may also contribute; however, the contribution of these changes to LVH has not been definitively proven.

Data on cardiac changes in very elderly subjects are limited, with small numbers studied and often apparently contradictory results. Varying results are at least in part explained by differing rates of underlying disease, with coronary artery disease particularly common in males and hypertension in females.[6] As a result, in unselected very elderly subjects, reduced left ventricular systolic function and wall motion abnormalities are over-represented in males while females are particularly likely to have ventricular hypertrophy, atrial dilatation and moderate-to-severe mitral and tricuspid valve dysfunction.

Studies in older populations comprehensively screened for cardiovascular disease, particularly hypertension and coronary artery disease, have generally shown that the morphological cardiac changes described above are less marked in disease-free older hearts.[6] For example in the longitudinal Framingham cohort study, the association of LVH with increasing age was explained mainly by higher blood pressure, overweight, smoking and diabetes mellitus.[7] These findings reinforce how difficult it is to distinguish between cardiac changes secondary to intrinsic ageing and changes as a result of disease or environmental exposures. It is likely that certain structural changes classically thought to be primarily manifestations of intrinsic ageing are in fact also influenced by lifestyle or environmental factors; reports of partial reversal of age-associated changes with interventions such as exercise lends further credence to this hypothesis.[8,9]

Microscopic changes in the ageing heart are well described and include a decrease in number of myocytes with hypertrophy of remaining cells. Convincing mechanistic explanations for these changes are lacking although tissue hypoxia secondary to reduced capillary density has been postulated.[10] Contrary to previous belief, adult myocardial cells remain capable of active division and this has been demonstrated *in vitro* in response to myocardial injury.[11] There is an age-associated increase in other cardiac cell types and materials including interstitial fat, lipofuscin pigment and fibroblast numbers (and activity).[11] The magnitude and functional importance of cardiac interstitial fibrosis is debated[12] but age-related valvular fibrosis and calcification is common. The latter often causes valvular regurgitation or stenotic gradients, manifest on echocardiography or clinically as murmurs on auscultation. Previously thought to be benign, 'senile aortic sclerosis' is now recognized to be associated with significant increases in cardiovascular and total mortality.[13]

Intracellular deposits of amyloid are common in the older heart. Distinct patterns of atrial appendage amyloid and more generalized deposition are recognized.[14] In post-mortem studies amyloid deposits have been found in the majority of aged hearts with the highest prevalence (80–100%) reported in Japanese populations.[15] Although most elderly patients do not have symptoms from cardiac amyloid, some will develop extensive infiltration resulting in a clinical cardiomyopathy which can in turn be associated with heart failure and arrhythmias.[15] The electrocardiograph (ECG) may show low voltage complexes and on echocardiography, the myocardium has a characteristic bright 'speckling' appearance with other features of a restrictive physiology. In advanced cases virtually every cardiac structure can be infiltrated. Age-related reduction in the number of functional pacemaker cells in the sinoatrial node and myocyte cells in specialized conducting tissues are well described and are clinically manifest by ECG changes and predisposition to dysrhythmias such as 'sick sinus syndrome'.[16]

Biochemical changes with age have been reported including alterations in sarcoplasmic reticulum and Ca^{2+} uptake across membranes. In isolated senescent cardiac tissue slower myosin isoenzymes and decreased adenosine triphosphatase activity are also described.[17] These biochemical alterations result in prolongation of isovolumetric relaxation. These changes may be of functional importance, particularly with regard to reduced diastolic function and cardiac failure with preserved ejection fraction.

Changes in cardiac physiology with ageing

Healthy ageing is associated with little change in systolic function or cardiac output at rest. However, age-related changes in diastolic function are apparent on echocardiography or cardiac MRI.[18] There are progressive changes in the pattern of left ventricular filling, with numerous indirect measures of diastolic function showing deterioration with advancing age; the early phase of diastolic ventricular filling is delayed and maximal flow rate across the mitral valve is reduced; as a result a much greater proportion of ventricular filling occurs late in diastole during atrial contraction. These changes in diastolic function seem to be largely independent of disease. However, their precise aetiology and in particular the role of reduced left ventricular compliance and myocardial relaxation patterns remains to be definitively established.[2,19] For most older people these changes are not of major consequence. However, the development of atrial fibrillation (AF) (and loss of the late ventricular filling phase) has much more severe adverse consequences in the older heart, with greatly reduced cardiac homeostatic reserve and maximum aerobic exercise capacity.

There is an age-related reduction in cardiac responsiveness to adrenergic stimuli, resulting in a decrease in both intrinsic and maximal sinus heart rate.[20] During exercise or other stressful stimuli, the increase in heart rate is attenuated in older people; at any given submaximal work-rate the heart rate rise is reduced and the older heart relies on dilatation and increased stroke volume to increase cardiac output (working on the physiological principles of the Starling curve). This compensatory response is effective at low or moderate workloads; however, cardiac reserve is reduced, with a reduction in maximal cardiac output in the older heart. These changes appear to be due to a reduction in both the number and sensitivity of cardiac β-receptors; the age-related changes described are akin to the effects of pharmacological β-blockade.

Arterial baroreceptors responses are slowed with increasing age. As a result, aged individuals typically exhibit increased arterial pressure variability with decreased cardiac heart rate variability and responsiveness.[21] It has been postulated that these changes predispose to postural hypotension and syncope in elderly people.

It could be argued that discussion of intrinsic ageing and the disease-free heart is a somewhat academic exercise. The reality is that most older people, at least in the developed world, have clinically relevant ischaemic cardiac disease. Atherosclerosis begins in adolescence and the incidence and prevalence of ischaemic heart disease increase dramatically with age.[22] Up to 30% of the over-65s have symptoms of ischaemic heart disease with angina or previous acute myocardial infarction. However, it has been estimated that a further 30% have clinically significant but covert or unrecognized disease. A variety of factors contribute to this hidden burden of disease. There may be barriers to communication or reporting such as chronic cognitive impairment. Symptoms may be masked by comorbidities that reduce exercise capacity, or cause other more clinically obvious symptoms. In addition ageing is associated with impaired perception of ischaemic cardiac pain; on exercise there is a delay from onset of myocardial ischaemia to symptoms of angina in older people. As a result when cardiac symptoms occur they may be vague or atypical.[23] Myocardial infarction may present as a confusional state or 'collapse', while myocardial ischaemia may provoke non-specific lethargy and reduced physical capacity. Therefore, ischaemic heart disease is a common cause of reduced cardiac homeostatic reserve in older people and in the event of a physiological stressor such as systemic illness, adverse clinical consequences such as myocardial ischaemia, heart failure or cardiac arrhythmias can readily occur. The presentation, diagnosis and treatment of coronary artery disease in older people are discussed in detail in Chapter 7, Ischaemic Heart Disease.

Cardiac manifestations of non-cardiac disease

The brain

Cerebrovascular disease

Acute strokes in older people, including infarction, subarachnoid and intracranial haemorrhage are often associated with cardiac rhythm or conduction disturbances, and the 12-lead ECG may show repolarization patterns resembling acute myocardial infarction. Elevation in serum cardiac enzymes, particularly troponin, is seen in approximately 20% of patients with acute stroke and is associated with ECG changes and increased mortality. Although some patients will have underlying coronary thrombosis, these ECG and biomarker changes can occur in the absence of significant coronary arterial disease.[24] In this situation the underlying process may be a stress response with activation of the sympathoadrenal system causing patchy focal myocardial damage known as myocytolysis.[25]

Many older subjects with ischaemic cerebrovascular disease have comorbid coronary artery disease. Cardiac disease is the commonest cause of death in the first months following ischaemic stroke, with 2–6% of patients dying from cardiac causes. Risk is highest in the first days immediately post-ictus. Predictors include diabetes, LV dysfunction, renal impairment, long QTc and severe neurological impairment.[26]

Dementia and cognitive decline

Increasingly it is recognized that vascular disease is an important and potentially preventable contributor to dementia and cognitive decline in later life. Post-mortem studies have shown that Alzheimer's pathology on its own is often not sufficient to cause major cognitive decline. However, the combination of Alzheimer's pathology and ischaemic cerebrovascular disease (particularly small vessel ischaemia) carries particular risk of dementia.[27] Longitudinal population studies have shown that vascular risk factors, particularly hypertension, diabetes mellitus and cigarette smoking, are associated with increased risk of dementia.[28,29] Congestive cardiac failure (CCF) may also contribute to late-life cognitive impairment. Dementia is over-represented in CCF patients; predictors include left ventricular systolic dysfunction and arterial blood pressures below 130 mmHg.[30] A variety of mechanisms have been proposed including occult cerebral infarction, low-grade small vessel ischaemia, activated thrombosis and blood pressure variability and altered cerebrovascular reactivity. A degree of cognitive dysfunction occurs in most older patients after cardiac surgery including coronary artery bypass grafting.[31] Those with pre-existing small vessel cerebral ischaemia are at particular risk. Low blood pressure during surgery and small cerebral embolic events are thought to be the main contributors.

The respiratory system

Cardiac failure and atrial fibrillation (AF) are common complications of serious respiratory illness in older people. Chronic obstructive pulmonary disease and reduced lung function (FEV1, forced expiratory volume) are independent risk factors for arrhythmias including AF. Respiratory infections such as influenza and respiratory syncytial virus are associated with increased risk of hospitalization for heart failure and sudden death.[32] Potential mechanisms include infection-induced rises in cytokines that have negative cardiac inotropic effects, and sympathetic nervous system activation.

While there is a considerable body of research focusing on the ageing left ventricle and aorta, age-associated changes in the right heart and pulmonary circulation are less well described. Population-based studies have suggested modest increases in pulmonary systolic pressure independent of respiratory disease; greater pulmonary pressures are associated with increased risk of cardiovascular events and mortality.[33]

Gastrointestinal system

Age is an independent risk factor for circulatory collapse and death after acute gastrointestinal haemorrhage. This is likely to be due to reduced homeostatic cardiac reserve.[34] Circulatory problems to the bowel are fortunately uncommon; however, the incidence does rise markedly with increasing age. Potential mechanisms include atherosclerosis of mesenteric arteries or cardio-embolism, particularly in AF. Symptoms are usually of pain, altered bowel habit and haematochezia although clinical presentation can range from mild transient symptoms to fulminant acute abdomen with gangrenous bowel.[35] For milder cases a conservative approach is often recommended with pharmacological treatment of underlying vascular risk factors. Older age is a predictor of poor outcome.[36]

Exposure to helicobacter pylori infection becomes increasingly common with advancing age. In young subjects it has been suggested that helicobacter may be a contributory cause of ischaemic heart disease, in association with raised fibrinogen levels. However, no convincing link has been confirmed with ischaemic heart disease in elderly subjects; observational studies claiming that helicobacter eradication therapy decreases fibrinogen levels in coronary heart disease are likely to be confounded by regression to the mean.[37]

The association of aortic valvular disease (particularly aortic stenosis) with gastrointestinal angiodysplasia, the 'Heyde syndrome' has been recognized for many years. However, the nature and strength of the link has been debated as both conditions are relatively common, particularly in older age. A biological mechanism for this association involving activation of clotting factors has been postulated.[38]

Renal system

Deterioration in renal and cardiac function often occurs together in older people. Renal impairment in older people is associated with increased risk of ischaemic cardiovascular disease. The risk is inversely related to glomerular filtration rate and is significantly increased by the time biochemical alterations in serum creatinine are apparent.[39] This association is partly due to common aetiologies, including hypertension and atherosclerosis.

A cardio-renal 'vicious circle' is well recognized in older patients wherein impaired natriuretic ability of the ageing nephron results in fluid overload and CCF, while the older, diseased heart is unable to maintain adequate cardiac output and perfusion pressure to the kidneys leading to further deterioration in renal function. When elderly patients with chronic heart failure develop impaired renal function, this is an adverse prognostic factor for hospitalization and death.

Cardiovascular disease remains the leading cause of death in patients with end-stage renal disease, accounting for around half of all deaths. The risk remains elevated even after renal transplantation.[40] An association between renal impairment and modest increases in serum levels of cardiac biomarkers such as troponin has also been reported. Studies detailing the cardiac phenotype of patients with end-stage renal failure and raised troponin have shown increased incidence of cardiac risk factors and LV impairment but no excess of coronary artery disease or demonstrable ischaemic damage.[41,42] Nonetheless, elevated troponin in renal failure is associated with increased cardiovascular risk.[41]

Endocrine abnormalities and the cardiovascular system

Thyroid

Hyperthyroidism is common in older people, with cardiovascular manifestations dominating the clinical presentation; palpitations, dyspnoea, sinus tachycardia, arrhythmias and systolic hypertension are common features. Heart failure is particularly likely if pre-existing heart disease is present. The risk of AF (paroxysmal or chronic) is increased in older patients. In the absence of underlying heart disease, AF may revert to sinus rhythm when a euthyroid state is achieved. However, in older patients or when AF has been present for a long duration, the rate of reversion is lower.[43] Cardiovascular complications remain the principle cause of death, even after treatment of hyperthyroidism.

Hypothyroidism also has important cardiac manifestations in older people. Bradycardia, non-pitting peripheral oedema, pericardial effusion, CCF and low-voltage complexes on ECG are all recognized.[43] Exertional dyspnoea and easy fatigability are common complaints, resulting from a combination of systolic and diastolic dysfunction on effort.[44] Endothelial dysfunction may increase the risk of hypertension and arterial thrombotic events and there is increased risk of atherosclerosis due to hypertension and atherogenic lipid profile. Decreased metabolic demand on the myocardium and low physical activity levels in hypothyroidism make symptoms of angina less frequent even in the presence of significant coronary artery disease. Many of these cardiac manifestations of hypothyroidism reverse with thyroxine replacement therapy. However, it is recommended that extra caution is exercised in elderly patients while initiating treatment to avoid precipitating acute myocardial infarction and heart failure, as they are likely to have underlying ischaemic heart disease. The initial dose of thyroxine should normally be ~25% of the anticipated replacement dose, increased in a stepwise fashion at 6–8 week intervals.[45]

Subclinical thyroid dysfunction is common in older patients, with a prevalence of asymptomatic (biochemical) hypothyroidism of ~10% and hyperthyroidism in 1.5%. These laboratory endocrine abnormalities are associated with detrimental cardiovascular effects; prospective longitudinal studies have shown that subclinical hypothyroidism, with thyroid stimulating hormone (TSH) levels greater than $10\,\mathrm{mU\,l^{-1}}$, is associated with increased incidence of heart failure.[46] Subclinical hyperthyroidism (with low serum TSH levels) is associated with approximately two- to threefold increased risk of developing AF.[47,48] In this context this arrhythmia may be a more benign phenomenon than in primary cardiac disease.[47] However, there is some evidence that low TSH is associated with increased cardiovascular morbidity and mortality.[49] Thyroid hormones have positive inotropic and chronotropic effects and cardiac benefits for hypothyroid subjects from hormone replacement would seem likely; this is supported by imaging studies which have suggested reversal of cardiac dysfunction in patients rendered biochemically euthyroid.[50] However, no adequately powered randomized controlled trials using cardiac endpoints are available.[51] It is not certain that active treatment of subclinical hypo- or hyperthyroidism to achieve a euthyroid state prevents cardiac complications.

Other hormones

Acromegaly and associated growth hormone excess is associated with cardiac enlargement and hypertension. Chronic overproduction of growth hormone also impairs carbohydrate metabolism and leads to a state of hyperinsulinaemia and insulin resistance with consequent increased risk of diabetes mellitus. Elderly people with acromegaly are more likely to develop acromegalic cardiomyopathy with cardiac enlargement and chronic heart failure that is often refractory to treatment. Older patients with hypopituitarism and low serum levels of growth hormone also appear to be at risk of cardiac complications, including acute myocardial infarction. Growth hormone replacement therapy may ameliorate this risk.[52]

The potential link of low levels of sex hormones with cardiovascular disease has attracted considerable attention. Despite apparent beneficial effects on traditional vascular risk factors, prospective studies have shown that estrogen replacement in post-menopausal women is associated with increased incidence of vascular events.[53] In males, low serum testosterone has also been associated with cardiovascular risk factors but definitive evidence of a beneficial cardiac effect of replacement is lacking.[54]

Diabetes mellitus

A high index of suspicion is necessary for detection of myocardial ischaemia in elderly people with diabetes mellitus as they are more likely to have silent or atypical disease, particularly in females. The reported incidence of arteriosclerotic coronary heart disease in older diabetic patients is likely to be an underestimate as most studies have excluded elderly people with renal dysfunction or other comorbidities.[55] Elderly diabetics are more likely to have multivessel coronary artery disease (often unsuitable for percutaneous revascularization procedures or coronary artery bypass grafting), and have an increased risk of CCF. Diabetes is also associated with LVH independent of other common risk factors.[56] In addition, diabetic cardiomyopathy associated with small vessel disease has been described.

Metabolic syndrome

The concept of the metabolic syndrome was developed to improve understanding of links between insulin resistance and vascular disease. The components of this pre-diabetic state include raised BMI, elevated triglycerides and blood sugar, low high-density lipoprotein and hypertension. However, it appears that diagnosis of the metabolic syndrome carries limited clinical utility in older age; while it is associated with increased risk of type 2 diabetes it has weak or no associations with vascular risk in elderly populations.[57]

Systemic infections and the heart

A variety of acute and chronic systemic infections have been suggested to increase the risk of acute ischaemic vascular events. Even minor acute infections are associated with myocardial infarction and stroke. Although various specific infective agents have been implicated, the process seems most likely to be a generic systemic response to any viral or bacterial infection.[58] Factors such as dehydration, immobility and increased blood coagulability are likely to be responsible. The evidence for a strong causal link between chronic infection and vascular disease is less compelling.[59] There is a modest association between periodontal disease and risk of ischaemic vascular events (including acute myocardial infarction and stroke); the mechanism could involve systemic inflammation contributing to atherosclerosis and thrombosis. However, absence of a standard definition for periodontal disease complicates interpretation of results. In addition there are multiple potential confounding risk factors common to both conditions. Additional large-scale longitudinal epidemiological and intervention studies are necessary to validate this association and to determine causality.[60]

Cancer

Cardiac neoplasms may be primary or metastatic and although rare, as with most solid organ tumours, an age-related association is apparent. Autopsy series have found that the majority of cardiac tumours are due to secondary spread from primary neoplasms in lung, breast or from haematological malignancy.[61] Primary cardiac myxomas may present with cardiac symptoms or neurological manifestations particularly ischaemic stroke.[62]

Nutrition and cardiovascular system in elderly people

Symptomatic heart failure, especially in older people, can affect food intake, leading to malnourishment. A syndrome of cardiac cachexia is recognized and is associated with poor outcomes, independent of severity of heart failure. The weight loss seen in these patients is greater than would be expected from poor diet alone and metabolic, neurohormonal and immune abnormalities may play a role.[63] Besides presenting with significantly more comorbidity, patients with low BMI are at higher risk of post-operative complications following cardiac surgery.[64]

Conclusions

Cardiac manifestations of systemic disease are common in older people. Healthy ageing is associated with a reduction in cardiac homeostatic reserve, increasing the risk of cardiac arrhythmias and heart failure with many non-cardiac illnesses. In addition clinically significant ischaemic heart disease is present in the majority of over 65s in the developed world, further reducing cardiac reserve, and increasing the risk of myocardial ischaemia in response to almost any severe systemic non-cardiac disease. Ischaemic heart disease is linked to dysfunction in numerous other organ systems, and the classic scenario of multiple pathologies in an older person often includes cardiac disease. Optimal management of the older patient requires that the multiple interacting contributors to symptoms or functional decline are identified to allow key modifiable factors to be prevented or treated.

Key points

- Ageing is associated with a marked reduction in cardiac homeostatic reserve due to a combination of intrinsic ageing, and a high prevalence of underlying cardiac disease (particularly ischaemic heart disease).

- This reduced homeostatic reserve greatly increases the risk of cardiac dysfunction (including heart failure and arrhythmias) with non-cardiac disease in older people.
- Cardiac dysfunction in older people also places other organ systems at risk. Examples include increased risk of dementia with both atrial fibrillation and chronic heart failure.
- Frequently there is a complex interaction between different organ systems. For example deterioration in renal and cardiac functions often occurs together in older people.
- Optimal management of the older patient requires that these multiple interacting contributors to symptoms or functional decline are recognized, and key modifiable contributors prevented or treated.

References

1 He Q, Heshka S, Albu J *et al.* Smaller organ mass with greater age, except for the heart. *J Appl Physiol* 2009;**106**:1780–4.

2 Cheng S, Fernandes VRS, Bluemke DA *et al.* Age-related left ventricular remodeling and associated risk for cardiovascular outcomes. *Circ Cardiovasc Imaging* 2009;**2**:191–8.

3 Gerstenblith G, Fredriksen J, Yin FCP *et al.* Echocardiographic assessment of a normal adult aging population. *Circulation* 1977;**56**:273–8.

4 Goor D, Lillehei CW and Edwards JE. The "sigmoid septum": variation in the contour of the left ventricular outlet. *Am J Roentgenol Radium Ther Nucl Med* 1969;**107**:366–76.

5 Roberts WC. (1993) Morphological features of the elderly heart, in *Cardiovascular Disease in the Elderly Patient* (eds DD Tresh and WS Aronow), Marcel Dekker, New York.

6 Rodeheffer RJ, Gerstenblith G, Becker LC *et al.* Exercise cardiac output is maintained with advancing age in healthy human subjects: cardiac dilatation and increased stroke volume compensate for a diminished heart rate. *Circulation* 1984;**69**:203–13.

7 Lieb W, Xanthakis V, Sullivan LM *et al.* Longitudinal tracking of left ventricular mass over the adult life course: clinical correlates of short- and long-term change in the Framingham offspring study. *Circulation* 2009;**119**:3085–92.

8 Schroeder TE, Hawkins SA, Hyslop D *et al.* Longitudinal change in coronary heart disease risk factors in older runners. *Age and Ageing* 2007;**36**:57–62.

9 Inuzuka Y, Okuda J, Kawashima T *et al.* Suppression of phosphoinositide 3-kinase prevents cardiac aging in mice. *Circulation* 2009;**120**:1695–703.

10 Bernhard D and Laufer G. The ageing cardiomyocyte: a mini-review. *Gerontology* 2008;**54**:24–31.

11 Anversa P, Palackal T, Sonnenblick EH, Olivetti G and Meggs LG. Myocyte cell loss and myocyte cellular hyperplasia in the hypertrophied ageing rat heart. *Circ Res* 1990;**67**:871–85.

12 van Heerebeek L, Hamdani N, Handoko ML *et al.* Diastolic stiffness of the failing diabetic heart: importance of fibrosis, advanced glycation end products and myocyte resting tension. *Circulation* 2008;**117**:43–51.

13 Otto CM, Lind BK and Kitzman DW. Association of aortic valve sclerosis with cardiovascular mortality and morbidity in the elderly. *New Engl J Med* 1999;**341**:142–7.

14 Cornwell GG and Westermark P. Senile amyloidosis: a protean manifestation of the ageing process. *J Clin Pathol* 1980;**138**:146–52.

15 Kushwaha SS, Fallon JT and Fuster V. Restrictive cardiomyopathy. *New Engl J Med* 1997;**336**:267–76.

16 Davied MJ and Pomerance A. Quantitative study of ageing changes in human sino-atrial node and internodal tracts. *Br Heart J* 1972;**34**:150–2.

17 Judge S and Leeuwenburgh C. Cardiac mitochondrial bioenergetics, oxidative stress and ageing. *Am J Physiol* 2007;**292**:1983–92.

18 Oxenham H and Sharpe N. Cardiovascular ageing and heart failure. *Eur J Heart Fail* 2003;**5**:427–34.

19 Susic D and Frohlich ED. The ageing hypertensive heart: a brief update. *Nat Clin Pract Cardiovasc Med* 2008;**5**:104–10.

20 Kaye DM and Esler MD. Autonomic control of the ageing heart. *Neuromol Med* 2008;**10**:179–86.

21 Ferrari AU, Radaelli A and Centola M. Physiology of ageing:Ageing and the cardiovascular system. *J Appl Physiol* 2003;**95**:2591–7.

22 Elveback L and Lie JT. Continued high incidence of coronary artery disease at autopsy in Olmsted County, Minnesota 1950 to 1979. *Circulation* 1984;**70**:345–9.

23 Wenger NK. Cardiovascular disease in the elderly. *Curr Probl Cardiol* 1992;**17**:609–90.

24 Di Angelantonio E, De Castro S, Toni D *et al.* Determinants of plasma levels of brain natriuretic peptide after acute ischemic stroke or TIA. *J Neurol Sci* 2007;**260**:139–42.

25 Samuels MA. Electrocardiographic manifestations of neurological disease. *Semin Neurol* 1984;**4**:453.

26 Posser J, MacGregor L, Lees KR *et al.* Predictors of early cardiac morbidity and mortality after ischaemic stroke. *Stroke* 2007;**38**:2295–302.

27 Neuropathology Group of the Medical Research Council Cognitive Function and Ageing Study (MRC CFAS). Pathological correlates of late-onset dementia in a multicentre, community-based population in England and Wales. *Lancet* 2001;**357**:169–75.

28 Hofman A, Ott A, Breteler MMB *et al.* Atherosclerosis, apolipoprotein E, and prevalence of dementia and Alzheimer's disease in the Rotterdam study. *Lancet* 1997;**349**:151–4.

29 Ott A, Slooter AJC, Hofman A *et al.* Smoking and risk of dementia and Alzheimer's disease in a population-based cohort study: the Rotterdam study. *Lancet* 1998;**351**:1840–3.

30 Pullicino PM and Hart J. Cognitive impairment in CHF? Embolism vs hypoperfusion. *Neurology* 2001;**57**:1945–6.

31 Diegler H, Hirsch R and Schneider F. Neuromonitoring and neurocognitive outcome on off-pump versus conventional coronary bypass operation. *Ann Thorac Surg* 2000;**69**:1162–6.

32 Yap FH, Ho PL and Lam KF. Excess hospital admissions for pneumonia, chronic obstructive pulmonary disease and heart failure during influenza seasons in Hong Kong. *J Med Virol* 2004;**73**:617–23.

33 Lam CS, Borlaug BA, Kane GC *et al.* Age-associated increases in pulmonary artery systolic pressure in the general population. *Circulation* 2009;**119**:2663–70.

34 Iser DM, Thompson AJ, Sia KK *et al.* Prospective study of cardiac troponin I release in patients with upper gastrointestinal bleeding. *J Gastroenterol Hepatol* 2008;**23**:938–42.

35 Theodoropoulou A and Koutroubakis IE. Ischemic colitis: clinical practice in diagnosis and treatment. *World J Gastroenterol* 2008;**14**:7302–8.

36 Huguier M, Barrier A, Boelle PY *et al*. Ischemic colitis. *Am J Surg* 2006;**192**:679–84.
37 Yusuf SW and Mishra RM. Effect of helicobacter pylori infection on fibrinogen level in elderly patients with ischaemic heart disease. *Acta Cardiol* 2002;**57**:317–22.
38 Massyn MW and Khan SA. Heyde syndrome: a common diagnosis in older patients with severe aortic stenosis. *Age and Ageing* 2009;**38**:267–70.
39 Schillaci G, Reboldi G and Verdecchia P. High normal serum creatinine concentration is a predictor of cardiovascular risk in essential hypertension. *Arch Intern Med* 2001;**161**:886–91.
40 Foley RN, Parfrey PS and Sarnak MJ. Clinical epidemiology of cardiovascular disease in chronic renal disease. *Am J Kidney Dis* 1998;**32**:s112–19.
41 Sharma R, Gaze DC, Pellerin D *et al*. Cardiac structural and functional abnormalities in end-stage renal disease patients with elevated cardiac troponin T. *Heart* 2006;**92**:804–9.
42 deFilippi CR, Thorn EM, Aggarwal M *et al*. Frequency and cause of cardiac troponin T elevation in chronic hemodialysis patients from study of cardiovascular magnetic resonance. *Am J Cardiol* 2007;**100**:885–9.
43 Klein I and Ojamaa K. Thyroid hormone and the cardiovascular system. *New Engl J Med* 2001;**344**:501–9.
44 Biondi B and Klein I. Hypothyroidism as a risk factor for cardiovascular disease. *Endocrine* 2004;**24**:1–14.
45 Crowley WF, Ridgway EC and Bough EW. Noninvasive evaluation of cardiac function in hypothyroidism: response to gradual thyroxine replacement. *New Engl J Med* 1997;**296**:1–6.
46 Rodondi N, Bauer DC, Cappola AR *et al*. Subclinical thyroid dysfunction, cardiac function and the risk of heart failure – the cardiovascular health study. *J Am Coll Cardiol* 2008;**52**:1152–9.
47 Cappola AR, Fried LP, Arnold AM *et al*. Thyroid status, cardiovascular risk, and mortality in older adults. *JAMA* 2006;**295**:1033–41.
48 Sarwin CT, Gellar A and Wolfe PA. Low serum thyrotropin concentrations as a risk factor for atrial fibrillation in older persons. *New Engl J Med* 1994;**331**:1249–52.
49 Parle JV, Maisonneuve P, Sheppard MC *et al*. Prediction of all-cause and cardiovascular mortality in elderly people from one low serum thyrotropin result: a 10-year cohort study. *Lancet* 2001;**358**:861–5.
50 Turhan S, Tulunay C, Ozduman CM *et al*. Effects of thyroxine therapy on right ventricular systolic and diastolic function in patients with subclinical hypothyroidism: a study by pulsed wave tissue Doppler imaging. *J Clin Endocrinol Metabol* 2006;**91**:3490–3.
51 Surks MI, Ortiz E and Daniels GH. Subclinical thyroid disease: scientific review and guidelines for diagnosis and management. *JAMA* 2004;**291**:228–38.
52 Holmer H, Svensson J, Rylander L *et al*. Nonfatal stroke, cardiac disease and diabetes mellitus in hypopituitary patients on hormone replacement including growth hormone. *J Clin Endocrinol Metabol* 2007;**92**:3560–7.
53 Manson JE, Hsia J, Johnson KC *et al*. Estrogen plus progestin and the risk of coronary heart disease. *New Engl J Med* 2003;**349**:523–34.
54 Haddad RM, Kennedy CC and Caples S. Testosterone and cardiovascular risk in men: systematic review and meta-analysis of randomized placebo controlled trials. *Mayo Clin Proc* 2007;**82**:29–39.
55 Ioanitoaia LC, May C and Goldberg AP. Cardiovascular manifestations of type 2 diabetes in the elderly. *Clin Geriatr* 2001;**9**:41–51.

56 Eguchi K, Boden-Albala B, Jin Z *et al.* Association between diabetes mellitus and left ventricular hypertrophy in a multiethnic population. *Am J Cardiol* 2008;**101**:1787–91.
57 Sattar N, McConnachie A, Shaper G *et al.* Can metabolic syndrome usefully predict cardiovascular disease and diabetes? Outcome data from two prospective studies. *Lancet* 2008;**371**:1927–35.
58 Smeeth L, Thomas SL, Hall AJ *et al.* Risk of myocardial infarction and stroke after acute infection or vaccination. *New Engl J Med* 2004;**351**:2611–8.
59 Danesh J, Whincup P, Walker M *et al.* Chlamydia pneumoniae IgG titres and coronary heart disease: prospective study and meta-analysis. *BMJ* 2000;**321**:208–13.
60 Scannapieco FA, Bush RB and Paju S. Associations between periodontal disease and risk for atherosclerosis, cardiovascular disease, and stroke. A systematic review. *Ann Periodontol* 2003;**8**:38–53.
61 Butany J, Leong SW, Carmichael K and Komeda M. A 30-year analysis of cardiac neoplasms at autopsy. *Can J Cardiol* 2005;**21**:675–80.
62 Lee VH, Connolly HM and Brown RD. Central nervous system manifestations of cardiac myxoma. *Arch Neurol* 2007;**64**:1115–20.
63 Anker SD, Steinborn W and Strassburg S. Cardiac cachexia. *Ann Med* 2004;**36**:518–29.
64 Potapov EV, Loebe M, Anker S *et al.* Impact of body mass index on outcome in patients after coronary artery bypass grafting with and without valve surgery. *Eur Heart J* 2003;**24**:1933–41.

CHAPTER 3
Hypertension

Anthony S. Wierzbicki[1] *and Adie Viljoen*[2]

[1]Guy's & St Thomas' Hospitals, London, UK
[2]Lister Hospital, Stevenage, Hertfordshire, and Bedfordshire and Hertfordshire Postgraduate Medical School, Luton, Hertfordshire, UK

Definition and prevalence

Hypertension is a very prevalent disorder affecting about 1 billion people worldwide[1] and, as such, it is the most common modifiable risk factor for conditions such as atherosclerosis, stroke, heart failure, atrial fibrillation, diabetes mellitus, sudden cardiac death, acute aortic syndromes and chronic kidney failure and may cause death and disability in patients of all ages.[2]

It is thought to affect up to 70% of individuals over the age of 65 years. The exact prevalence of hypertension varies with the age, race and the overall health status of the population studied, and also the blood pressure cut-off points used to define hypertension. Hypertension in elderly patients is a complex cardiovascular disorder that affects women more than men and occurs in essentially all races, ethnic groups and countries. Although it appears to be underdiagnosed in general and particularly among women, minorities and underserved populations, clearly it is also undertreated. Elderly persons are more likely to have hypertension and isolated systolic hypertension (ISH), target organ damage (left ventricular hypertrophy, renal impairment and albuminuria, hypertensive retinopathy) and clinical cardiovascular disease (CVD), to develop new cardiovascular (CV) events, and are less likely to have hypertension controlled.

An international consensus exists about the limits of 'normal' values for brachial blood pressure at 140/90 mmHg.[3] All define a blood pressure of 160/100 mmHg as requiring therapeutic intervention and 200/120 mmHg as very high risk requiring immediate management. There is less consensus on the cut-offs for blood pressure measured by other techniques. Many groups are now beginning to recommend the use of ambulatory blood pressure monitoring (ABPM) and the recent UK NICE guidelines have

Cardiovascular Disease and Health in the Older Patient: Expanded from 'Pathy's Principles and Practice of Geriatric Medicine, Fifth edition', First Edition. Edited by David J. Stott and Gordon D.O. Lowe.

suggested that it has a primary role in the diagnosis of hypertension given its superior predictive value for CVD events compared with rather variable brachial measurements and its ability to counter stress-induced or 'white coat' hypertension.[4]

The US guidelines[5] introduced the concept of pre-hypertension, representing a systolic blood pressure (SBP) of 120–139 mmHg or diastolic blood pressure (DBP) of 80–89 mmHg, previously classified as 'normal' or 'high normal' blood pressure. Other guidelines recognize pre-hypertension as a potential risk factor but stress the role of CVD risk assessment and risk calculation as the primary guide to a requirement for any intervention – lifestyle or therapeutic. Pre-hypertension was introduced, in part, on findings of the Framingham Heart Study (FHS) suggesting that normotensive individuals at age 55 years have a 90% lifetime risk of developing hypertension.[6]

The recommendation was based on the results of 30 worldwide clinical trials conducted in 1997 and a report estimating that the risk of cardiovascular mortality doubles with each 20/10 mmHg rise in blood pressure, starting at levels as low as 115/75 mmHg.[7] In addition, evidence has accumulated which classifies individuals with comorbidities and an SBP >130–139 mmHg as suboptimal. These conditions include heart failure and left ventricular dysfunction, diabetes mellitus, chronic kidney disease and established CVD conditions such as coronary artery disease (CAD), peripheral arterial disease (PAD) and carotid artery disease.

A long-standing controversy exists about hypertension in elderly people and some argue that usual definitions of hypertension and target BP levels might not be applicable to the elderly hypertensive population. The higher prevalence of hypertension in older people partially reflects the increase in the prevalence of arterial stiffening and thus changes in reflection pressure wave timing. The new generation of hypertension diagnostic devices specifically measure pulse wave reflection, velocity and pulse amplification parameters. There is no consensus on target values or optimal measures for pulse wave diagnostics as yet although all studies show that either directly measured or inferred central blood pressures (ascending aortic arch) are better predictors of outcomes than brachial measurements. As this technology is not widely available, older measures of specific subtypes of hypertension are useful.

Pathophysiology

Blood pressure regulation is a complex process, subject to multiple interacting physiological systems, and also lifestyle and genetic factors. In its simplest conceptualization, the cardiovascular system is governed by Ohm's law, which, when adapted to a haemodynamic system, states that flow (Q)

is proportional to the pressure gradient (ΔP) and inversely proportional to the resistance (R) across a conduit.

In terms of the cardiovascular system, BP is the product of cardiac output and vascular resistance. Since cardiac output does not increase with age, hypertension in elderly people is, to a large extent, a result of increased vascular resistance. In combined systolic and diastolic hypertension (SDH), the problem arises at the site of the resistance arterioles, the smaller muscular vessels where 80–90% of arterial resistance occurs. Increased constriction at this level affects both SBP and DBP. In contrast, ISH develops as a result of large arteries that have become less compliant and therefore less able to accommodate volume changes. In young normotensive individuals, large elastic vessels contribute little resistance to blood flow. During systole, the aorta and other large arteries expand to accommodate the stroke volume, which attenuates the rise in intra-arterial pressure. During early diastole, elastic recoil of large arteries sustains forward flow, augmenting the DBP despite runoff into arterial branches. Age-related loss of elasticity increases vascular impedance, resulting in a more rapid rise in blood pressure during systole and to a higher level. The higher peak pressure, coupled with diminished elastic recoil, results in rapid runoff to the periphery, resulting in lower DBP (Figure 3.1).

A low DBP is not entirely benign. Since myocardial perfusion occurs during diastole, diastolic hypotension may result in subendocardial ischaemia. While other constituents no doubt factor into the pathogenesis

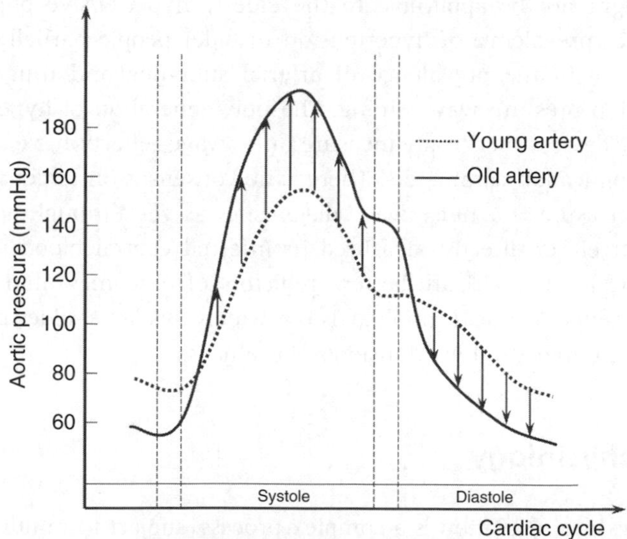

Figure 3.1 Blood pressure changes in an old versus a young artery during a cardiac cycle. The arrows indicate increased pressure during systole and decreased pressure during diastole that older arteries experience due to arteriosclerosis.

of hypertension, age-related loss of arterial elasticity successfully predicts widening of the pulse pressure (PP), ISH and the plateau in DBP that develop with ageing. Figure 3.1 depicts these changes over the course of a single cardiac cycle. Ageing blood vessels undergo a host of structural and functional changes, resulting in decreased compliance and increased resistance to flow. These changes particularly affect the intima and media of large arteries. With age, elastic fibres progressively decrease in number and elasticity and the collagen matrix increases. This fibrous transformation results in arteriosclerosis and is compounded by calcification and an increase in the number and size of vascular smooth muscle cell. The combined effect is a fall in the total cross-sectional area of peripheral vasculature. Furthermore, the dynamic nature of endothelial-derived vasoactive substances that control vascular tone is also affected by age. The delicate balance between vasoconstricting agents (such as endothelin and angiotensin II) and vasodilating agents (such as prostacyclin and nitric oxide) is offset. Nitric oxide (NO), previously termed endothelial-derived relaxing factor (EDRF), is a potent vasodilator that has been extensively studied. An age-associated decline in NO-mediated vasodilatation has been demonstrated.[8] A decreased secretion of NO and also a blunted response to NO have further been documented. Endothelial dysfunction, possibly as a direct effect of elevated peak pressure, inhibits secretion of these compounds.[9] It remains unclear to what extent the imbalance of endothelial-derived vasoactive compounds is a cause or effect of high blood pressure, but impairment of effective vasodilator agents, in the absence of appropriate compensatory mechanisms, will result in increased vascular resistance. The endothelium also secretes a number of factors that act on smooth muscles in an autocrine manner. These include interleukin-1 and insulin-like growth factor. *In vitro*, these influence the migration and proliferation of smooth muscle cells, which in turn increase vascular rigidity and decrease lumen size.

Despite increased levels of serum norepinephrine that occur in elderly people, the role of the sympathetic nervous system in the pathogenesis of hypertension appears to be more complex than mere overstimulation. The sympathetic nervous system has little clinical impact on older normotensive subjects, even with increased levels of serum norepinephrine. This is due to decreased adrenergic receptor function. Downregulation of β-adrenergic inotropic, chronotropic and vasodilatory response, and also α-adrenergic vasoconstrictor response, has been documented in elderly patients. With receptor downregulation in the face of increased norepinephrine release, α_1-adrenergic vascular tone is comparable in old and young normotensive subjects. It has been proposed by some experts that older hypertensive subjects have a relatively less degree of suppression of α_1-adrenergic relative to β_2-adrenergic activity[10] and age-related hypertension is in part due to diminishing β-mediated vasodilatation whereas α-mediated vasoconstriction continues relatively unabated. Similar findings have been observed in animal studies. Decreased carotid baroreceptor sensitivity and responsiveness occur with age. Consequently, a larger change in blood pressure is needed to trigger the appropriate compensatory response. The impaired reflex is manifested clinically as wide blood pressure fluctuations in older people compared with the young, and also increased susceptibility to clinically significant orthostatic hypotension and postprandial hypotension. The age-related baroreceptor reflex dysfunction is not necessarily limited to hypertensive persons alone, but decreased vascular distensibility at the carotid sinus, as seen in hypertensive subjects, is likely to play a central role in the process and many antihypertensive medications will further exacerbate the condition.

Ageing kidneys undergo multiple changes, which may affect blood pressure regulation. A sodium load is secreted less rapidly and less completely as renal function declines. Similarly, elderly people are more sensitive to free water depletion or repletion than the young. Angiotensin II promotes sodium reabsorption from the distal tubules directly and indirectly through aldosterone release and stimulation of the autonomic nervous system. The renin–aldosterone–angiotensin axis, however, is less responsive with age. There is a decrease in serum renin levels and activity, which may be the result of decreased functional glomeruli and a decrease in serum angiotensin II and aldosterone levels. The net effect of these changes is towards sodium retention. Free water retention ensues to maintain sodium homeostasis. It has been suggested that chronic extracellular volume expansion due to sodium and water retention leads to increased vascular resistance through the mechanism of autoregulation of organ blood flow. These observations are consistent with the high prevalence of salt sensitivity among older hypertensive individuals. Atrial natriuretic peptide (ANP) is released primarily from the atria in response to stretch due to volume overload. ANP acts both as a peripheral vasodilator and as a natriuretic/diuretic hormone. Brain natriuretic peptide (BNP) was initially identified in the brain but is also present in the ventricles. It is homologous to ANP and its serum concentration is normally approximately one-fifth that of ANP. In heart failure, levels of BNP can increase dramatically. A simple serum assay has been devised for the measurement of BNP and is now commonly used in the management of suspected heart failure.

Several variants of ANP and related hormones have been identified. Of note is a hormone with a digitalis-like effect. This putative hormone appears to be ouabain or an isomer of ouabain and binds the digitalis receptor on the sodium potassium adenosine triphosphatase pump (Na-K-ATPase) in an inhibitory manner. This hormone differs from ANP in that it increases vascular resistance. A proposed mechanism is that the Na-K-ATPase inhibitor facilitates renal sodium excretion but also diminishes intracellular sodium release, resulting in increased concentrations of sodium in smooth muscle cells. Passive sodium–calcium exchange subsequently results in increased intracellular calcium and, therefore, vascular tone.[11,12] These mechanisms may explain the high incidence of salt sensitivity in subjects with essential hypertension, but more investigation is needed to determine fully the role that this mechanism plays in the pathogenesis of hypertension.

Not all the aforementioned mechanisms have conclusively been shown to be age-related changes, independent of disease and lifestyle influences. In some populations, the incidence of hypertension changes little with age and the overall prevalence is low. To some extent, hypertension is an affliction of modern society. Until very recent history, humans employed the hunter–gatherer lifestyle for survival. Such 'primitive' peoples experienced vigorous daily physical activity and a diet rich in potassium and fibre and low in fat and sodium. Patterns of Nature led to periods of diminished food intake and obesity was virtually unheard of in these communities. Modern-day populations who enjoy relatively low incidences of hypertension tend to practice daily routines that more closely resemble the primitive lifestyle of old, particularly with regard to nutrition and physical activity. The blood pressure profiles of immigrants from such regions, however, may change over the course of a few generations to resemble that of the host community. The overabundance of foods rich in sodium, calories and fat in westernized societies, coupled with sedentary levels of activity, without doubt contributes to the epidemic of obesity and hypertension. With the abundance of effective medications available for the treatment of hypertension, these potentially modifiable risk factors receive far less attention than they deserve. Finally, there is a clear genetic role in the development of hypertension in some families. Such individuals are likely to develop hypertension early in life. The genetic contribution is complex, involves multiple interacting genes and is not fully understood at this time. Genetic factors are perhaps the strongest non-modifiable risk factor for hypertension.

Related clinical entities

Isolated systolic hypertension (ISH)

SBP rises gradually throughout adult life, whereas DBP peaks and plateaus in late middle-age, declining slightly thereafter. Therefore, the proportion of hypertensive patients with ISH increases with age, from 65% of patients with hypertension older than 60 years of age and over 90% in patients older than 70 years of age. The prevalence of ISH is higher in women than in men, whereas the proportion of hypertension attributable to ISH in older adults is similar across racial and ethnic groups. Of note, in decades past, the apparently inexorable rise in SBP with increasing age fostered the view that this was an adaptive response essential to support organ perfusion and an empirical formula '100 + age' was often used to estimate the 'appropriate' SBP. However, data from the FHS and other epidemiological investigations provide compelling evidence that SBP is a strong independent risk factor for incident CV events in all decades of life.[13] Hence the above formula should be discarded. ISH actually represents the outcome of hyaline change and increased arteriolar tone in the microvasculature with increased collagen deposition, loss of elastin and changes in endothelial function. Changes in endothelial function are driven by classical CV risk factors and some advocate its measurement as a surrogate for atherosclerotic disease burden. ISH also closely corresponds to increased wave reflection and studies of pulse wave parameters including differences between central and peripheral blood pressure may have prognostic and therapeutic consequences.[14]

Pulse pressure

After age 70 years, diastolic hypertension accounts for less than 10% of all patients with hypertension. In addition, the relationship between DBP and CV risk is bimodal in older individuals, with DBPs of greater than 90 mmHg associated with a similar increased risk to that associated with DBPs lower than about 70 mmHg.[15] As a result, at any given level of SBP, CAD risk increases as DBP decreases.[16,17] An important implication of this observation is that pulse pressure (i.e. difference between SBP and DBP), which increases with age and is a measure of the degree of age-related vascular stiffness, emerges as a potent risk factor for CAD events in older individuals. Pulse pressure has been identified as a stronger risk factor than SBP, DBP or mean pressure in older adults in some studies.[16,17] In the FHS, with increasing age, there was a gradual shift from DBP to SBP and then to PP as the strongest predictor of CAD risk. In patients younger than 50 years of age, DBP was the strongest predictor. Age 50–59 years was a transition period when all three BP indexes were comparable predictors, and from 60 to 79 years of age, DBP was negatively related to CAD risk so that PP became superior to SBP.[18] However, a falling DBP in an elderly patient correlating to an increase in PP is a bad prognostic sign.

Special populations

From the standpoint of epidemiology, pathophysiology and treatment, there are important subgroups with distinctive characteristics, including elderly women, blacks, Hispanics and Asians, that require additional focus. Hypertension prevalence is less in women than in men until 45 years of age, is similar in both genders from 45 to 64 years of age and is much higher in women than men older the 65 years of age.[19] Age-adjusted hypertension prevalence, both diagnosed and undiagnosed, from 1999 to 2002 was 78% for older women and only 64% for older men.[20]

Secondary hypertension

Although most hypertension (80–90%) is essential, that is, its pathophysiological cause is unknown, secondary causes of hypertension are being increasingly recognized as contributing to morbidity. Renal artery stenosis (RAS) is more common than is usually thought and is often associated with PAD, especially if associated with a reduction in estimated glomerular filtration rate (eGFR), signs of (micro)albuminuria. Although not contributing directly to hypertension as is the case in severe stenotic disease (>85%), it is a risk factor for angiotensin-converting enzyme inhibitor (ACE-I)/angiotensin-II receptor blocker (ARB)-induced nephrotoxicity. Any patient with these risk factors should have renal function assessed 2 weeks after starting an ACE-I/ARB or clinicians should be wary of slow progressive decreases in eGFR as a manifestation of RAS. Most endocrine causes of hypertension are rare (phaeochromocytoma, Cushing's disease or Conn's syndrome) but adrenal mineralocorticoid hyperplasia is common.[21] This manifests as aldosteronaemia allied with low renin and its prevalence varies in surveys from 5 to 10% of patients with hypertension. An increased prevalence of low-renin hypertension is found in elderly people, patients with diabetes and West African-derived populations. Most is not caused by adenomas but by generalized adrenal hypertrophy and can be diagnosed by finding a moderately raised aldosterone:renin ratio in a random sample taken in patients not receiving beta-blockade. It often responds well to treatment with an aldosterone antagonist.

Resistant hypertension

Most hypertension is treated with polypharmacy as each individual agent reduces blood pressure by about 10%. Resistant hypertension is formally defined as a BP >140/90 mmHg after treatment with three antihypertensive drugs.[5] Most commonly it is caused by poor compliance with polypharmacy, but other causes include ISH and contributory comorbidities including secondary hypertension and neurological hypertension. This can include anxiety states (see white coat hypertension in the section Clinical assessment and diagnosis, below), but also includes dysregulation of central mechanisms of BP regulation. The commonest cause of central dysregulation is sleep apnoea syndrome, which is often associated with obesity and can be diagnosed by oximetry studies and treated with continuous positive airways pressure maintenance (CPAP) allied commonly with weight loss.[22]

The effect of treating hypertension in the elderly population – an overview of clinical trials

Salient features of the pivotal clinical trials discussed below and a summary of their findings are given in Tables 3.1 and 3.2.

The benefit of treating hypertension in elderly people was evident as early as 1967. The Veterans Administration Cooperative study, which was published in three parts between 1967 and 1972, documented the benefit of treating severe[23] and mild[24] diastolic hypertension. In subjects over the age of 60 years, a 70% reduction in the incidence of stroke and 52% reduction in cardiovascular events were observed in the treatment group.[25] Similar favourable outcomes were documented in the Australian Therapeutic Trial in Hypertension, where a 33% reduction in stroke and 18% reduction in CAD were noted in the treated subgroup age 60–69 years, compared with the placebo group.[26] In the Hypertension Detection and Follow-up Program, there was a 17% reduction in all-cause mortality after a 5-year follow-up period of patients aged 60–69 years, treated for mild diastolic hypertension.[27] These and other early studies, however, primarily treated diastolic hypertension and had relatively few participants in the geriatric age group. The subgroup 60–75 years of age in the Veterans Administration Cooperative Study represented only 20% of total enrolment.

Treatment of hypertension in the elderly population remained tentative and debatable until the mid 1980s, when multiple randomized trials gave credence to the benefits and safety of aggressive BP management even in advanced age. The SHEP trial addressed ISH in subjects ≥60 years of age.[28] The treatment group received chlorthalidone, with the addition of atenolol if needed, to achieve the target BP. The impact of treatment was greatest in reducing the incident of stroke by 36% and CV events by 32%. The reduction in coronary events was 27%, but not statistically significant. Comparable results were noted in the Systolic Hypertension in Europe (Syst-Eur) trial, which also studied subjects aged 60 years or older with primarily ISH.[29] Treatment was initiated with nitrendipine, with the addition of enalapril and hydrochlorothiazide if necessary. Reductions in stroke by 42%, CV events by 31% and coronary events by 26% were noted in the treatment group compared with placebo, all of which were significant. In both studies, the reductions in CV mortality (SHEP 20%, Syst-Eur 27%) and total mortality (SHEP 13%, Syst-Eur 14%) were similar and non-significant. The Systolic Hypertension in China (Syst-China) trial[30] paralleled the Syst-Eur trial and had similar enrolment criteria, but used captopril as a second-line intervention. Treatment outcome results were in line with the previous two studies, with the exception of larger and statistically significant decreases in total and CV mortality (39% in

Table 3.1 Characteristics of treatment trials that predominantly involved older hypertensive individuals. Trial acronyms and references are found in the body of the text.

Trial	n^a	Mean age (years)	Mean baseline BP[a](mmHg)	Mean follow-up period	Treatment BP(mmHg)	Control BP(mmHg)	Mean BP difference (mmHg)	Intervention	
								First line	Second line
SHEP	4736	71.6	170/77	4.5 years	144/68	155/71	−11/−3	Chlorthalidone	Atenolol
Syst-Eur	4695	70.2	174/85	2.0 years	151/78	161/83	−10/−5	Nitrendipine	Enalapril
Syst-China	2394	66.5	171/86	3.0 years	151/81	159/84	−9/−3	Nitrendipine	Captopril
EWPHE	840	72.0	182/101	4.6 years	148/85	167/90	−19/−5	Maxzide	Methyldopa
STOP-Hyper	1627	76.0	195/102	25 months	167/87	186/96	−19/−8	Diuretic or β-blocker	Diuretic or β-blocker
MRC	4396	70.0	185/91	5.8 years	152/76	168/85	−16/−9	Diuretic or β-blocker	Diuretic or β-blocker
Coope	884	68.7	196/99	4.4 years	162/78	180/89	−18/−11	Atenolol	Diuretic
STONE	1632	66.0	168/100	30 months	146/87	156/90	−9/−5	Nifedipine	Captopril
HYVET	3845	83.6	173/90	1.8 years[b]	29.5/12.9	−14.5/6.8	−15/6.1	Diuretic	ACE inhibitor

[a] *n*, patient number; BP, blood pressure.
[b] Median follow-up.

Table 3.2 Outcome of treatment trials. Trial acronyms and references are found in the body of the text.

Trial		Stroke events (total) (%)	Cardiovascular (total) (%)	Coronary events (total) (%)	Stroke mortality (%)	Cardiovascular mortality (%)	Total mortality (%)
SHEP		−36[a]	−32[a]	−27	−29	−20	−13
Syst-Eur		−42[a]	−31[a]	−26[a]	−27	−27	−14
Syst-China		−38[a]	−37[a]	−37	−58[a]	−39[a]	−39[a]
EWPHE		−32	−38[a]	−47[a]	−32	−27[a]	−9
STOP-Hyper		−45[a]	−40[a]	−13	−76[a]	–	−43[a]
MRC		−25[a]	−17[a]	−19	−12	−9	−3
Coope		−42[a]	–	+ 3	−70[a]	−22	−3
STONE		−57[a]	−60[a]	−6	–	−26	−45[a]
HYVET	Diuretic ACE Inhibitor	−30	−34	−28	−39	−23	−21

[a]Statistically significant ($p < 0.05$).

both cases), possibly due to the slightly younger age of the participants. Similarities in trial design and enrolment criteria of these three studies lend themselves to pooling analysis. When combined, reductions in strokes (37%), coronary vascular disease (25%), CV events (32%), CV mortality (25%) and total mortality (17%) were noted in the treatment group compared with placebo, all of which were statistically significant.[31]

Other studies addressed systolic–diastolic hypertension. The Swedish Trial in Older Patients with Hypertension (STOP-Hypertension) compared beta-blockers and thiazide diuretics with placebo, in patients 70–84 years of age (average 76 years) with a mean BP of 195/102 mmHg.[32] In the treatment group, significant reductions in the incidence of stroke (45%), CV events (40%) and total mortality (43%) were documented after an average 25-month follow-up period. Myocardial infarctions were reduced by only 12%, which was not statistically significant. These findings were somewhat at odds with those of the European Working Party on High Blood Pressure in the Elderly (EWPHE) trial. The baseline SBP and DBP in the EWPHE trial ranged between 160–239 and 90–119 mmHg, respectively (average 182/101 mmHg) and treatment was with hydrochlorothiazide–triamterene for an average follow-up period of 4.6 years.[33] Unlike the STOP-Hypertension trial, the 9% decrease in total mortality and 32% decrease in stroke were not statistically significant, whereas the 47% decline in myocardial infarctions was. The significant 38% decrease in CV events was similar to that found in the STOP-Hypertension trial (40%). The Medical Research Council (MRC) Working Party trial studied both systolic and diastolic hypertension and randomized participants aged 65–74 years to a diuretic or β-blocker treatment group or to placebo.[34] After an average follow-up period of 5.8 years, the mean BPs in the two treatment groups were similar and significantly lower than in the placebo group. The combined treatment group had a statistically significant 25% reduction in stroke and 17% reduction in CV events. The 19% reduction in coronary events, 9% reduction in CV mortality and 3% reduction in total mortality were not significant. However, when treatment groups were analysed separately, stroke and cardiac events were significantly lower in the diuretic group by 31 and 44%, respectively. The β-blocker treatment group showed no such reduction in these endpoints.

It is not surprising that outcome is related not only to risk stratification but also to the choice of antihypertensive agent. From the above trials, however, it appears that treatment of hypertension in older people generally has a greater impact on stroke reduction than coronary and CV event reduction and that this effect is independent of drug choice. This pattern is seen in other trials. Both the Shanghai Trial of Nifedipine in the Elderly (STONE)[35] and the Coope and Warrender Trial[36] showed a statistically significant reduction in stroke (57 and 42%, respectively) and a non-significant reduction in coronary heart disease (CHD) (6 and 3%, respectively). Neither demonstrated a sizable change in CV mortality, but the STONE trial revealed a significant 45% decrease in total mortality compared with a non-significant 3% in the Coope and Warrender trial. Variability in treatment outcome among studies is partly due to study design, but the importance of selection criteria in treatment risk/benefit determination, independent of other study parameters, must also be stressed. Subjects with higher initial SBP and wider PP are likely to experience greater treatment benefit, as are those in a higher risk stratum. It is estimated that the reduction in all-cause mortality in the highest risk group is nine times that in the lowest risk group,[37] emphasizing the importance of establishing an individualized treatment plan based on risk stratification, rather than on generalized guidelines *per se*. The above reasoning also introduces the concept of treatment risk, a principle that until recently has largely been overlooked and will be discussed shortly.

Other endpoints have been investigated in more recent studies, notably the relationship between hypertension and cognitive decline or dementia. Data from the dementia project of the Syst-Eur trial show a significantly lower rate of development of dementia in the treatment group,[38] but the analysis was underpowered and the conclusion difficult to generalize with authority. The Study on Cognition and Prognosis in the Elderly (SCOPE) showed a non-significant 11% reduction in the incidence of cognitive decline in the group treated with candesartan compared with placebo.[39] The investigators concluded that at the very least, there is no evidence supporting a *negative* effect of treating hypertension on cognition in elderly people. The first credible evidence supporting the potential benefit of treating hypertension on dementia came from the Protection Against Recurrent Stroke Study (PROGRESS), whose primary outcome was assessing risk for recurrent stroke.[40] During a 4-year follow-up period, a 12% overall reduction in the risk of dementia was observed with treatment. This finding was not statistically significant. However, when analysed separately, the subgroup with prior stroke at baseline showed a 34% ($p = 0.3$) reduction in dementia risk, whereas the subgroup without prior stroke showed only a 1% change.

For cognitive impairment, a similar pattern was noted, with slightly more favourable results. Severe cognitive decline was defined as a drop of three or more points on the Mini Mental State Examination (MMSE). The overall risk reduction with treatment was 19% ($p = 0.01$). In the subgroup with prior stroke at baseline, the reduction in the risk of developing severe cognitive decline was 45% ($p > 0.001$), but only 9% (not significant) in the subgroup without prior stroke.

Various meta-analysis reviews have been designed for the purpose of accommodating variability among individual trials or examining smaller subgroups within larger trials. A meta-analysis of nine trials[41] confirmed treatment benefit in elderly patients. Reductions in stroke morbidity [odds ratio (RR) = 0.65; 95% confidence interval (CI), 0.55–0.76)], cardiac morbidity (RR = 0.85; 95% CI, 0.73–0.99) and total mortality (RR = 0.88; 95% CI, 0.80–0.97) were noted. Stroke and cardiac mortality individually were also significantly reduced in the treatment group. Another meta-analysis of eight ISH trials included 15 693 subjects.[42] There was a 30% reduction in combined fatal and non-fatal stroke events ($p > 0.0001$), a 26% reduction in combined CV events ($p > 0.0001$) and a 13% reduction in total mortality ($p = 0.02$). In untreated patients, after correcting for regression dilution bias and DBP, the relative hazard rates associated with a 10 mmHg higher baseline SBP were 1.26 ($p = 0.0001$) for total mortality, 1.22 ($p = 0.02$) for stroke, but only 1.07 ($p = 0.37$) for coronary events. Treatment benefit was greatest in men, patients with previous CV complications and those who had larger PPs. DBP was inversely correlated with total mortality, independently of SBP. Treatment effect was also largest in subjects over the age of 70 years, a topic of contention, which will be discussed next.

Despite compelling evidence supporting the benefit of treating hypertension in older persons,[43] the evidence for very old subjects is much less clear.[44–47] 'Very old' is arbitrarily defined as >80 years of age, since at that age the risk/benefit advantage begins to waver. Subjects over the age of 80 years are absent or under-represented in most clinical trials, even though this segment of the population is the fastest growing in the westernized world. The very old also tend to be lumped in the 65-and-over age group, whereas they clearly have diverse and distinct characteristics and data obtained in younger adults cannot instinctively be extrapolated to the very old. As early as 1986, trend analysis of EWPHE data suggested that treatment of hypertension is less effective, or even harmful, above the age of 80 years.[48] Other studies have shown mixed results. The SHEP trial found treatment benefit, particularly in stroke prevention, extending beyond the age of 80 years. In the Syst-Eur analysis, total and CV mortality were significantly lower for the treatment group under the age of 80 years, but not for those aged 80 years or older. The overall RR for CV events in the treatment group from the STOP-Hypertension trial was 0.60, but the benefit decreased with increasing age subgroups and crossed the unity point between the ages of 80 and 85 years. These trials enrolled relatively few very old subjects. A meta-analysis of randomized controlled studies that enrolled subjects older than 80 years of age included 1670 subjects followed for a mean period of 3.5 years.[49] A significant reduction in stroke (34%), CV events (22%) and heart failure (39%) occurred in the treatment group compared with the control group. No benefit in CV death and a non-significant 6% *increase* in all-cause deaths were observed in the treatment group. The trend became stronger when the analysis was limited to five double-blind trials – an 11% ($p = 0.41$) increase in CV mortality in the treatment group and a 14% ($p = 0.05$) increase in total mortality were observed.

Several population-based observational studies have demonstrated an inverse relationship between BP and mortality in the very old. One study[50] enrolled 83% of the population of Temper, Finland, aged 85 years or older ($n = 561$), and a similar study[51] enrolled 94% of the residents of Leiden, the Netherlands, aged 85 years or older ($n = 833$). In both studies, the chance of being alive after 5 years was greatest in those with the highest BP at enrolment. In the Temper study, subjects with SBP ≥200 mmHg at entry had a threefold higher survival rate than those whose SBP was 120–140 mmHg. Similar results were reported in the Helsinki Ageing Study,[52] where it was estimated that the 5-year mortality declined by 10% for every 10 mmHg increase in SBP at enrolment. These and earlier observational studies are limited to correlations and constrained by confounding variables in selection criteria. In the Leiden study, for example, low BP was associated with poor health. After adjusting for health status, the inverse relationship disappeared.

The HYVET study[53]

In the majority of studies to date, benefits in stroke reduction appear related to BP reduction, as a 10 mmHg reduction in SBP was associated with a 20–30% lower risk of stroke in individuals over 70 years of age. Furthermore, there is greater benefit with a greater reduction in BP. It is unclear whether the benefits are related solely to BP reduction or whether there are additional benefits conferred by class of BP medication. Although there was consistent benefit in stroke reduction when drugs were compared with placebo, there was little difference between drug classes.[54] The Hypertension in the Very Elderly Trial (HYVET) was the first interventional controlled trial designed to assess the risk and benefit of treating hypertension specifically in subjects older than 80 years of age.[53] Patients in the aforementioned studies consisted predominantly of the 'early elderly'. In HYVET, patients in the 'late elderly' group (>80 years of age with elevated SBP) were randomized to indapamide, with addition of perindopril if needed or placebo and followed over 2 years. This study showed major benefit in CVD events and a large reduction in new cardiac failure in those older than 80 years of age when treated with an ACE-I–indapamide combination to a target BP of 150/80 mmHg.[53] Patients in the indapamide arm had a 30% risk reduction in fatal or non-fatal stroke ($p = 0.06$). Although there have been consistent benefits in reduction of stroke with antihypertensive therapy in elderly patients, some reports have suggested that these benefits may be offset by an increase in death in treated patients.[49] The HYVET, however, found benefits consistent with a 21% risk reduction (95% CI, 4–35%; $p = 0.02$) of all-cause death in the indapamide arm.[53]

Evidence after HYVET[2]

The results of HYVET[53] modify previous recommendations for patients >80 years of age. In HYVET, 3845 patients >80 years of age with SBP >160 mmHg were randomly assigned to placebo or drug therapy. The latter included a non-thiazide sulfonamide diuretic (indapamide) supplemented by an ACE-I (perindopril) when needed for a target SBP of 150 mmHg. After 2 years, with about one-quarter of the patients using monotherapy and three-quarters combination therapy, the trial was stopped because drug treatment, although decreasing BP compared with the placebo group (144/78 vs 161/84 mmHg), reduced adverse outcomes. This consisted of reductions in the incidence of stroke (~30%), congestive heart failure (~64%) and CV morbid and fatal events (~23%). Most impressively, there was a significant reduction (~21%) in the incidence of all-cause death. Of importance, drug treatment was well tolerated. The reduction in BP in the standing position was similar to that in the sitting position. Furthermore, serum electrolyte and biochemical values were similar in drug- and placebo-treated groups. In fact, fewer serious adverse events were reported in the drug-treated than in placebo-treated patients.

The HYVET results provide clear evidence that BP-lowering by drugs is associated with definite CV benefits in patients >80 years of age. They not only refute concern that this may lead to an increase, rather than a decrease, in mortality, but also show that in this stratum of the population, there is a prolongation of life. This finding is highly relevant for public health because subjects >80 years of age represent the fastest growing fraction of the population; the prediction is that by 2050, they will account for more than one-fifth of all elderly individuals.

However, HYVET has some limitations that should be taken into account when considering antihypertensive treatment in very elderly patients. Patients with stage 1 hypertension were not included. The patients on whom HYVET results are based are not representative of the general very elderly population. First, to limit dropouts, recruitment focused on patients in relatively good physical and mental condition and with a low rate of previous CVD. This is at variance from the high rate of frail and medically compromised patients typical in this very old age range. Second, because identifying appropriate subjects was difficult, recruitment required about 6 years and was only possible through participation of Eastern European countries and China, which together accounted for 98% of the patients. Furthermore, premature interruption of the trial (because of mortality benefit) made the average follow-up relatively short (median 1.8 years). It remains unknown whether benefits of antihypertensive treatment persist or diminish after 2 or 3 years. Also, the mean age was 83 years and only a small fraction was >85 years of age, which leaves open the question of whether the benefit extends to ages much older than those investigated in previous trials. Compared with placebo, drug treatment was not accompanied by significant improvement in the incidence of dementia or cognitive dysfunction. The HYVET-COG, a HYVET substudy, found a non-significant 14% decrease in dementia with active treatment versus placebo.[55] Although no specific class of antihypertensive drugs has been definitively linked with cognitive decline in elderly patients, inadequate BP reduction is associated with cognitive decline. Although benefits in HYVET-COG were limited to CV outcomes, hypertension treatment was not associated with negative effects on cognition. Although there is clear evidence of the benefits of hypertension treatment in the reduction of both ischaemic and haemorrhagic stroke, the benefits in reducing cognitive impairment and dementia have only been demonstrated in the early elderly. In the patients, mean age 64 years, in PROGRESS, a perindopril-based BP-lowering regimen among patients with previous ischaemic stroke or TIA significantly reduced stroke-related dementia (34%) and severe cognitive decline (19%).[56] Finally, the optimal BP goal for reducing CV events and mortality was not investigated.

Clinical assessment and diagnosis[2]

Diagnosis of hypertension should be based on at least three different BP measurements, taken on two or more separate office visits. At least two measurements should be obtained once the patient has been seated comfortably for at least 5 minutes with the back supported, feet on the floor, arm supported in the horizontal position and the BP cuff at heart level. With the switch from mercury to aneroid sphygmomanometers, adjustment is required to cut-offs and many societies now validate individual instruments to ensure accurate reporting.[57] All societies recommend measurement on at least three occasions as biological variation in BP is extensive and stress or exercise effects can be substantial.

Pseudohypertension is a falsely increased SBP that results from markedly sclerotic arteries that do not collapse during cuff inflation (e.g. 'non-compressible'). Although this occurs more commonly in elderly people, the actual prevalence is unclear. Identification of pseudohypertension is necessary to avoid overtreating high BP and should be suspected in elders with refractory hypertension, no organ damage and/or symptoms of overmedication and in patients with chronic renal disease with secondary hyperparathyroidism with marked arterial classification as defined by much raised ankle-brachial BP or extreme pulse wave velocities.

White coat hypertension is more common in the elderly population and frequent among centenarians. The white coat effect is directly related to the seniority of the measurer, with greater effects shown for consultants (SBP +6 mmHg) than primary care practitioners (+4 mmHg) or nurses (reference group).

Ambulatory BP monitoring is recommended to confirm a diagnosis of white coat hypertension in patients with persistent office hypertension but no organ damage. Ambulatory BP monitoring (ABPM) is indicated when hypertension diagnosis or response to therapy is unclear from office visits, when syncope or hypotensive disorders are suspected and for evaluation of vertigo and dizziness and as the primary diagnostic assessment in the United Kingdom.[4] The optimum ABPM technique uses both day and night values,[58] but a 12 h day BP may be sufficient for diagnostic purposes. The equivalence points for ambulatory compared with brachial measurements are more controversial, ranging from 5/5 mmHg correction[4] to 10/5 mmHg (ISH[5]) or 12/6 mmHg depending on the studies. Some patients cannot tolerate the BP cuff used in ABPM nor do they have significant white coat effects in any clinical setting, and in these subjects home BP measurement can be useful even using wrist BP monitors, which are less accurate than brachial measures.

The case for using out-of-office BP readings in elderly individuals, particularly home BP measurements, is strong owing to potential hazards of excessive BP reduction in older people and better prognostic accuracy versus office BP. It is recommended that 12–14 measurements of BP are gathered at different times over 5–7 days to determine average home blood pressure.[59]

All patients should undergo a CVD risk assessment, including ascertainment of a family history of hypertension, diabetes or CVD, smoking status and history, measurement of weight and ideally waist circumference and measurement of lipids (total cholesterol; HDL-cholesterol), glucose (or HbA1c) and creatinine for determination of an estimated GFR using the Modified Diet in Renal Disease (MDRD) equation. If eGFR is significantly reduced ($<45\,\text{ml}\,\text{min}^{-1}$ per $1.73\,\text{m}^2$) in a hypertensive patient then a formal measurement should be made of urine albumin concentration to allow subclassification of the degree of renal impairment present. CVD risk should be calculated in all cases and total appropriate risk factor treatment instituted if the CVD risk exceeds 20%[4] or if the CHD risk exceeds 20% for the next decade.[3] In some groups, it may be appropriate to calculate lifetime CHD/CVD risk.

Management

Differences exist between guidelines about the optimal therapeutic strategies for hypertension.[2–4] All antihypertensive drugs deliver ~5–10% reduction of initial BP. The only comparative trial of different major drug classes, the ALLHAT study, showed equivalence of a thiazide diuretic (chlorthalidone), an ACE-I and a calcium channel blocker (CCB). Alpha-blockade was not recommended given its worse prognostic outcome.[60] Meta-analyses of BP trials have suggested that all classes are equivalent provided that BP reduction is achieved.[7] Guidelines have diverged in their recommendations, with an emphasis on diuretics and beta-blockers by some (JNC-7[5]), and an age-differentiated strategy recommending the use of CCBs and diuretics in elderly people. This has recently been revised following the results of the CAFE sub-study of ASCOT[61] and the results of the ACCOMPLISH study.[62] CAFE showed that, as previously suspected, beta-blockers were less effective at reducing central BP and thus stroke than other agents, and these drugs have been demoted to second-line status.[4] In ACCOMPLISH, an ACE-I–CCB combination was compared with an ACE-I–thiazide combination therapy, with superior results for the ACE-I–CCB on CVD events. Hence ACE-I and CCBs are the preferred initial antihypertensive drugs. Controversy exists about thiazide diuretics as they may not be therapeutically equivalent. Recent guidelines have suggested that chlorthalidone (not bendroflumethiazide or hydrochlorothiazide) should be the preferred thiazide and that an independent evidence base exists for indapamide (a non-thiazide diuretic).[4] There is no benefit to combining ACE-Is with ARBs and this combination causes excess hypotension.[63]

Evidence for individual SBP targets remains poor and is derived from meta-analyses and indirectly from the DBPs achieved in the HOT study.[64] Evidence suggests that populations at higher CVD risk should be targeted to lower BP levels, but clinicians need to remain mindful that BP targets are based primarily on observational data in middle-aged patients and optimal targets for elderly patients, especially those with systolic hypertension and normal or low DBP (e.g. ISH), remain to be defined from randomized trial data.

The mantra of 'lower is better' suggested by the epidemiology of BP has been investigated in some high-risk groups. Both the ADVANCE and ACCORD BP trials found that among patients with type 2 diabetes mellitus at high risk for CV events, targeting SBP below 120 mmHg, as compared with below 140 mmHg, did not reduce the rate of fatal and non-fatal major CVD events and resulted in an increase in adverse experiences attributed to BP medications.[65,66]

Because hypertension increases with ageing and is also associated with longevity, there is often uncertainty about its management in very elderly patients. Until very recently, this was a particular dilemma for the very elderly because most hypertension management trials had upper age thresholds for enrolment (<70 years) and/or did not present age-specific results. However, the HYVET showed major benefit in CVD events and a large reduction in new cardiac failure in those older than 80 years of age when treated with an ACE-I–indapamide combination to a target BP of 150/80 mmHg.[53] No difference was found in outcomes between those with generalized hypertension and ISH, despite a greater therapeutic efficacy of the combination in ISH.[67]

Conclusion

Hypertension in the elderly population is a major and increasing problem that should be assessed in parallel with other comorbidities and should be managed in the context of total CVD risk with no special allowance being made for chronological age.

Key points

- The prevalence of hypertension and wide PP increases with age.
- Treatment of high BP can significantly reduce the risk of CV mortality and morbidity in older persons, and the evidence for this is now also available for treating the very old.
- On the basis of current interventional trials, significant cardiovascular benefit may result from relatively small reductions in BP and the optimal SBP in older people may be 140–160 mmHg.
- The results from HYVET provide clear evidence that BP-lowering by drugs is associated with definite CV benefits in patients >80 years of age.
- The benefits of treatment of hypertension need to be weighed against the hypotensive conditions commonly seen in the elderly population, such as postprandial hypotension and postural hypotension, which can lead to syncope and falls.

Acknowledgement

The authors would like to acknowledge the excellent chapter on hypertension written by Ramzi R. Hajjar for the fourth edition of *Principles and Practice of Geriatric Medicine*, on which this chapter is based.

References

1 Kearney PM, Whelton M, Reynolds K *et al*. Global burden of hypertension: analysis of worldwide data. *Lancet* 2005;**365**:217–23.

2 Aronow WS, Fleg JL, Pepine CJ *et al*.; ACCF Task Force. ACCF/AHA 2011 Expert Consensus Document on Hypertension in the Elderly: a report of the American College of Cardiology Foundation Task Force on Clinical Expert Consensus Documents. *Circulation* 2011;**123**:2434–506.

3 Graham I, Atar D, Borch-Johnsen K *et al*.; European Society of Cardiology (ESC); European Association for Cardiovascular Prevention and Rehabilitation (EACPR); Council on Cardiovascular Nursing; European Association for Study of Diabetes (EASD); International Diabetes Federation Europe (IDF-Europe); European Stroke Initiative (EUSI); Society of Behavioural Medicine (ISBM); European Society of Hypertension (ESH); WONCA Europe (European Society of General Practice/Family Medicine); European Heart Network (EHN); European Atherosclerosis Society (EAS). European guidelines on cardiovascular disease prevention in clinical practice: full text. Fourth Joint Task Force of the European Society of Cardiology and other societies on cardiovascular disease prevention in clinical practice (constituted by representatives of nine societies and by invited experts). *Eur J Cardiovasc Prev Rehabil* 2007;**14**(Suppl. 2):S1–113.

4 National Institute for Health and Clinical Excellence (NICE) (2011) NICE clinical guidelines. Hypertension (update). *Hypertension: Clinical management of primary hypertension in adults*, NICE, London, http:// publications.nice.org.uk/ hypertension-cg127 (last accessed June 2012).

5 Bakris GL, Black HR, Cushman WC *et al*.; National Heart, Lung and Blood Institute Joint National Committee on Prevention, Detection, Evaluation and Treatment of High Blood Pressure; National High Blood Pressure Education Program Coordinating Committee. The Seventh Report of the Joint National Committee on Prevention, Detection, Evaluation and Treatment of High Blood Pressure: the JNC 7 report. *JAMA* 2003;**289**:2560–72.

6 Vasan RS, Beiser A, Seshadri S *et al*. Residual lifetime risk for developing hypertension in middle-aged women and men: the Framingham Heart Study. *JAMA* 2002;**287**:1003–10.

7 Blood Pressure Lowering Treatment Trialists' Collaboration. Effects of different regimens to lower blood pressure on major cardiovascular events in older and younger adults: meta-analysis of randomised trials. *BMJ* 2008;**336**:1121–3.

8 Cooper LT, Cook JP and Dzau VJ. The vasculopathy of aging. *J Gerontol Biol Sci* 1994;**49**:B191–6.

9 Panza JA, Casino PR, Kilcoyne CM and Quyyumi AA. Role of nitric oxide in the abnormal endothelium-dependent vascular relaxation of patients with essential hypertension. *Circulation* 1993;**87**:1468–74.

10 Supiano MA, Hogikyan RV, Sidani MA *et al.* Sympathetic nervous system activity and α-adrenergic responsiveness in older hypertensive humans. *Am J Physiol* 1999;**276**:E519–38.

11 Blaustein MP. Endogenous ouabain: role in the pathogenesis of hypertension. *Kidney Int* 1996;**49**:1748–53.

12 Jackson WF. Ion channels and vascular tone. *Hypertension* 2000;**35**:173–8.

13 Stokes J III,, Kannel WB, Wolf PA *et al.* Blood pressure as a risk factor for cardiovascular disease: the Framingham Study – 30 years of follow-up. *Hypertension* 1989;**13**(5 Suppl.):I13–8.

14 Vlachopoulos C, Aznaouridis K, O'Rourke MF *et al.* Prediction of cardiovascular events and all-cause mortality with central haemodynamics: a systematic review and meta-analysis. *Eur Heart J* 2010;**31**:1865–71.

15 Staessen JA, Gasowski J, Wang JG *et al.* Risks of untreated and treated isolated systolic hypertension in the elderly: meta-analysis of outcome trials. *Lancet* 2000;**355**:865–72.

16 Franklin SS, Lopez VA, Wong ND *et al.* Single versus combined blood pressure components and risk for cardiovascular disease: the Framingham Heart Study. *Circulation* 2009;**119**:243–50.

17 Franklin SS, Khan SA, Wong ND *et al.* Is pulse pressure useful in predicting risk for coronary heart disease? The Framingham Heart Study. *Circulation* 1999;**100**:354–60.

18 Franklin SS, Larson MG, Khan SA *et al.* Does the relation of blood pressure to coronary heart disease risk change with aging? The Framingham Heart Study. *Circulation* 2001;**103**:1245–9.

19 National Center for Health Statistics (2007) *Health, United States, 2007. With Chartbook on Trends in the Health of Americans*, National Center for Health Statistics, Hyattsville, MD.

20 Robinson K. (2007) *Trends in Health Status and Health Care Use Among Older Women*. Aging Trends, No. 7, National Center for Health Statistics, Hyattsville, MD, http://www.cdc.gov/nchs/data/ahcd/agingtrends/07olderwomen.pdf (last accessed August 2011).

21 Young WF Jr,. Endocrine hypertension: then and now. *Endocr Pract* 2010;**16**:888–902.

22 Acelajado MC and Calhoun DA. Resistant hypertension, secondary hypertension and hypertensive crises: diagnostic evaluation and treatment. *Cardiol Clin* 2010;**28**:639–54.

23 Veterans Administration Cooperative Study Group on Antihypertensive Agents. Effects of treatment on morbidity in hypertension. Results in patients with diastolic blood pressure averaging 115 through 125 mmHg. *JAMA* 1967;**202**:1028–34.

24 Veterans Administration Cooperative Study Group on Antihypertensive Agents. Effects of treatment on morbidity in hypertension. II: results in patients with diastolic blood pressure averaging 90 through 114 mmHg. *JAMA* 1970;**213**:827–38.

25 Veterans Administration Cooperative Study Group on Antihypertensive Agents. Effects of treatment on morbidity in hypertension. III: influence of age, diastolic blood pressure and prior cardiovascular disease: further analysis of side effects. *Circulation* 1972;**45**:991–1004.

26 Management Committee of the Australian Therapeutic Trial in Hypertension. Treatment of mild hypertension in the elderly. *Med J Aust* 1981;**2**:398–402.

27 Hypertension Detection and Follow-up Program Cooperative Group. Five-year findings on the Hypertension Detection and Follow-up Program. II. Mortality by race, sex and age. *JAMA* 1979;**242**:2572–7.

28 Systolic Hypertension in the Elderly Program Cooperative Research Group. Prevention of stroke by antihypertensive drug treatment in older persons with isolated systolic hypertension. Final results of the Systolic Hypertension in the Elderly Program (SHEP). *JAMA* 1991;**265**:3255–64.

29 Staessen JA, Fagard R, Thijs L *et al.*; The Systolic Hypertension in Europe (Syst-Eur) Trial Investigators. Randomised double-blind comparison of placebo and active treatment for older patients with isolated systolic hypertension. *Lancet* 1997;**350**:757–64.

30 Liu L, Wang JG, Gong L *et al.* Comparison of active treatment and placebo in older Chinese patients with isolated systolic hypertension. *J Hypertens* 1998;**16**:1823–9.

31 Staessen JA, Thijs L, Fagard R *et al.*; The Systolic Hypertension in Europe Trial Investigators. Predicting cardiovascular risk using conventional vs ambulatory blood pressure in older patients with systolic hypertension. *JAMA* 1999;**282**:539–46.

32 Dahlof B, Lindholm LH, Hannson L *et al.* Morbidity and mortality in the Swedish trial in patients with hypertension (STOP-Hypertension). *Lancet* 1991;**338**:1281–5.

33 Amery A, Birkenhäger W, Brixko P *et al.* Mortality and morbidity results from the European Working Party on High Blood Pressure in the Elderly trial. *Lancet* 1985;**i**:1349–54.

34 MRC Working Party. Medical Research Council trial of treatment of hypertension in older adults: principal results. *BMJ* 1992;**304**:405–12.

35 Gong L, Zhang W, Zhu Y *et al.* Shanghai trial of nifedipine in the elderly (STONE). *J Hypertens* 1996;**14**:1237–45.

36 Coope J and Warrender TS. Randomized trial of treatment of hypertension in the elderly patient in primary care. *BMJ* 1986;**293**:1145–8.

37 Ogden LG, He J, Lydick E and Whelton PK. Long-term absolute benefit of lowering blood pressure in hypertensive patients according to the INC VI risk stratification. *Hypertension* 2000;**35**:539–43.

38 Forette F, Seux ML, Staessen JA *et al.*; The Syst-Eur Investigators. Prevention of dementia in randomised double-blind placebo-controlled Systolic Hypertension in Europe (Syst-Eur) trial. *Lancet* 1998;**352**:1347–51.

39 Lithell H, Hannson L, Skoog I *et al.*; SCOPE Study Group. The Study on Cognition and Prognosis in the Elderly (SCOPE): principal results of a randomized double-blind intervention trial. *J Hypertens* 2003;**21**:875–86.

40 PROGRESS Collaborative Group. Randomised trial of a perindopril-based blood-pressure-lowering regimen among 6105 individuals with previous stroke or transient ischaemic attack. *Lancet* 2001;**358**:1033–41.

41 Insua JT, Sacks HS, Lau T-S *et al.* Drug treatment of hypertension in the elderly: a meta-analysis. *Ann Intern Med* 1994;**121**:355–62.

42 Staessen JA, Gasowski J, Wang JG *et al.* Risks of untreated and treated isolated systolic hypertension in the elderly: meta-analysis of outcome trials. *Lancet* 2000;**355**:865–72.

43 Leonetti G and Zanchetti A. Results of antihypertensive treatment trials in the elderly. *Am J Geriatr Cardiol* 2002;**11**:41–7.

44 Goodwin JS. Embracing complexity: a consideration of hypertension in the very old. *J Gerontol A Biol Sci Med Sci* 2003;**58**:653–8.

45 Heikinheimo RJ, Haavisto MV, Kaarela RH *et al.* Blood pressure in the very old. *J Hypertens* 1990;**8**:361–7.

46 Langer RD, Ganiats TG and Barrett-Conner E. Factors associated with paradoxical survival at higher blood pressures in the very old. *Am J Epidemiol* 1991;**134**:29–38.

47 Satish S, Freeman DH, Ray L and Goodwin JS. The relationship between blood pressure and mortality in the oldest old. *J Am Geriatr Soc* 2001;**49**:367–74.

48 Amery A, Birkenhäger W, O'Brien E *et al*. Influence of antihypertensive drug treatment on morbidity and mortality in patients over the age of 60 years. EWPHE results: sub-group analysis based on entry stratification. *J Hypertens* 1986;**4**(Suppl.):S642–7.
49 Gueyffier F, Bulpitt C, Boissel JP *et al*. Antihypertensive drugs in very old people: a subgroup meta-analysis of randomised controlled trials: INDANA Group. *Lancet* 1999;**353**:793–6.
50 Mattila K, Haavisto M, Rajala S and Heikinheimo R. Blood pressure and five-year survival in the very old. *BMJ* 1998;**296**:887–9.
51 Boshuizen HC, Isaks GJ, van Buuren S *et al*. Blood pressure and mortality in elderly people aged 85 and over: community-based study. *BMJ* 1998;**316**:1780–4.
52 Hakala S-M, Tilvis RS and Strandbert TE. Blood pressure and mortality in an older population: a 5-year follow-up of the Helsinki Ageing Study. *Eur Heart J* 1997;**18**:1019–23.
53 Beckett NS, Peters R, Fletcher AE *et al*.; HYVET Study Group. Treatment of hypertension in patients 80 years of age or older. *New Engl J Med* 2008;**358**:1887–98.
54 Lawes CM, Bennett DA, Feigin VL *et al*. Blood pressure and stroke: an overview of published reviews. *Stroke* 2004;**35**:776–85.
55 Peters R, Beckett N, Forette F *et al*. Incident dementia and blood pressure lowering in the HYpertension in the Very Elderly Trial COGnitive function assessment (HYVET-COG): a double-blind, placebo controlled trial. *Lancet Neurol* 2008;**7**:683–9.
56 Chalmers J and MacMahon S. Perindopril pROtection aGainst Recurrent Stroke Study (PROGRESS): interpretation and implementation. *J Hypertens Suppl* 2003;**21**:S9–14.
57 Stergiou GS, Karpettas N, Atkins N and O'Brien E. European Society of Hypertension International Protocol for the validation of blood pressure monitors: a critical review of its application and rationale for revision. *Blood Press Monit* 2010;**15**:39–48.
58 O'Brien E, Asmar R, Beilin L *et al*.; European Society of Hypertension Working Group on Blood Pressure Monitoring. Practice guidelines of the European Society of Hypertension for clinic, ambulatory and self blood pressure measurement. *J Hypertens* 2005;**23**:697–701.
59 Parati G, Stergiou GS, Asmar R *et al*.; ESH Working Group on Blood Pressure Monitoring. European Society of Hypertension practice guidelines for home blood pressure monitoring. *J Hum Hypertens* 2010;**24**:779–85.
60 ALLHAT Officers and Coordinators for the ALLHAT Collaborative Research Group. The Antihypertensive and Lipid-Lowering Treatment to Prevent Heart Attack Trial. Major outcomes in high-risk hypertensive patients randomized to angiotensin-converting enzyme inhibitor or calcium channel blocker vs diuretic: The Antihypertensive and Lipid-Lowering Treatment to Prevent Heart Attack Trial (ALLHAT). *JAMA* 2002;**288**:2981–97.
61 Williams B, Lacy PS, Thom SM *et al*.; CAFE Investigators; Anglo-Scandinavian Cardiac Outcomes Trial Investigators; CAFE Steering Committee and Writing Committee. Differential impact of blood pressure-lowering drugs on central aortic pressure and clinical outcomes: principal results of the Conduit Artery Function Evaluation (CAFE) study. *Circulation* 2006;**113**:1213–25.
62 Jamerson K, Bakris GL, Dahlöf B *et al*.; ACCOMPLISH Investigators. Exceptional early blood pressure control rates: the ACCOMPLISH trial. *Blood Press* 2007;**16**:80–6.
63 ONTARGET Investigators, Yusuf S, Teo KK, Pogue J *et al*. Telmisartan, ramipril, or both in patients at high risk for vascular events. *N Engl J Med* 2008;**358**:1547–59.

64 Hansson L, Zanchetti A, Carruthers SG *et al.* for the HOT study group. Effects of intensive blood-pressure lowering and low-dose aspirin in patients with hypertension: principal results of the Hypertension Optimal Treatment (HOT) randomised trial. *Lancet* 1998;**351**:1755–62.

65 Patel A, ADVANCE Collaborative Group, MacMahon S *et al.* Effects of a fixed combination of perindopril and indapamide on macrovascular and microvascular outcomes in patients with type 2 diabetes mellitus (the ADVANCE trial): a randomised controlled trial. *Lancet* 2007;**370**:829–40.

66 ACCORD Study Group, Cushman WC, Evans GW, Byington RP *et al.* Effects of intensive blood-pressure control in type 2 diabetes mellitus. *New Engl J Med* 2010;**362**:1575–85.

67 Bulpitt CJ, Beckett NS, Peters R *et al.* Blood pressure control in the Hypertension in the Very Elderly Trial (HYVET). *J Hum Hypertens* 2012; **26**: 157–63.

CHAPTER 4
Lipid Management

Adie Viljoen[1] *and Anthony S. Wierzbicki*[2]

[1]Lister Hospital, Stevenage, and Bedfordshire and Hertfordshire Postgraduate Medical School, Luton, Hertfordshire, UK
[2]Guy's & St Thomas' Hospitals, London, UK

Introduction

Atherosclerosis is a disease of ageing. Cardiovascular event rates increase in a curvilinear fashion after age 65 years in men and 75 years in women.[1,2] The decline in age-standardized cardiovascular disease (CVD)-associated death rates has shifted mortality to increasingly advanced age, with the number of cardiovascular events in those aged >80 years having increased by 60% since 1970.[3] Numerous epidemiological studies have shown that age is the principal unmodifiable risk factor for events.[4–6] Both diabetes and hypertension are strongly age-related risk factors.[7] In parallel with these risk factors levels of total cholesterol rise with age especially after middle age or the menopause. The increasing incidence of metabolic syndrome and obesity with age means that high density lipoprotein cholesterol (HDL-C) levels tend to fall and triglyceride levels rise.[8] Thus hyperlipidaemia is an increasing risk factor for coronary events, aortic valve disease, stroke, peripheral vascular disease including abdominal aortic aneurysm and possibly dementia (multi-infarct type). As many elderly patients have suffered one cardiovascular event they are at high risk of another, often in a different vascular bed. Thus patients with strokes more often have coronary events than second strokes.

As life expectancy increases, preventive efforts will become increasingly important for preventing morbidity, improving quality of life, and reducing healthcare expenditures for older persons. Clinicians need to consider additional factors in elderly people which most often are not applicable in younger individuals when faced with treatment decisions. These include comorbid conditions, polypharmacy, drug–drug interactions and differential safety and tolerability profiles; all of which could lead to

Cardiovascular Disease and Health in the Older Patient: Expanded from 'Pathy's Principles and Practice of Geriatric Medicine, Fifth edition', First Edition. Edited by David J. Stott and Gordon D.O. Lowe.

alterations in the benefit-harm balance. This highlights the importance of considering both the treatment options and the evidence for their use in the elderly population.

Cholesterol in elderly people

Ageing is associated with a progressive increase in cholesterol levels in men and in many women profound changes in lipids follow the menopause with substantial increases in low density lipoprotein cholesterol (LDL-C) secondary to possibly changes in proprotein convertase subtilisin kexin-9 (PCSK-9) levels which are under the control of sex steroids and a reduction in HDL-C most probably caused by changes in sex steroids.[9] However, most hyperlipidaemia in the elderly population is still caused by dietary and lifestyle choices. The slowly declining metabolic rate of the older people, associated with reduced levels of activity due to concurrent ageing or osteological problems means that many show features of the metabolic syndrome. Dietary conservatism also tends to mean that currently elderly people are less likely to consume a diet rich in fruit and vegetables and are more likely to eat a diet rich in saturated fat.

Secondary causes of hyperlipidaemia are more common in elderly people. The most common cause of mixed hyperlipidaemia is insulin resistance and/or type 2 diabetes. Rates of chronic renal disease also increase in elderly people, which allied to greater arterial stiffness, result in increases in pulse pressure, isolated systolic hypertension and secondary cardiovascular risk. Other causes that tend to be associated with ageing include alcohol-induced hyperlipidaemia which is more commonly due to a reduction in liver-related detoxification in older adults and its frequent association with depression, especially in single men. Alcohol-induced hyperlipidaemia may show a profile varying between mixed hyperlipidaemia to pure hypercholesterolaemia depending on the frequency of alcohol intake. Non-alcoholic steatitic hepatitis, which is often associated with a mixed hyperlipidaemia, is more common in centrally obese elderly people.

The most common cause of pure secondary hypercholesterolaemia is hypothyroidism. The significance of this is that prescription of a lipid-lowering drug to a grossly hypothyroid patient massively increases their risk of drug-associated rhabdomyolysis.

However, despite these factors the positive association between total and LDL-C and cardiovascular risk attenuates with advancing age.[10] In epidemiological studies a 1 $\text{mmol}\,\text{l}^{-1}$ lower total cholesterol (TC) is associated with approximately 50% reduction in coronary heart disease (CHD) mortality in patients aged 40–49 years, 33% in those aged 50–69 and 15% in those aged 70–89 years.[11] Yet, though the relative risk reduction associated with lower cholesterol decreases with age, the absolute effects of lower cholesterol on annual ischaemic heart disease mortality rates are greater in the elderly population given the higher prevalence of atheroma. Also cholesterol levels decline in acute and chronic disease states, inflammation, malnutrition and cancer, all of which are more common in older people and thus this attenuated association may be partly due to confounding.[12]

Clinical signs

Clinical signs present differently in elderly population. Arcus senilis is associated with familial hypercholesterolaemia in the young but not in older people. Xanthelasma are associated with mixed dyslipidaemia and reduced skin thickness and elasticity and thus are more common in older individuals. Tendon xanthomata may be confused with gout tophi or Heberden's nodes which are common in elderly people but may be clinically distinguished by their movement with the underlying tendon.

Lipoproteins and their measurement

Blood lipids are transported in macromolecular complexes called lipoproteins. Figure 4.1 shows a schematic representation of these complex molecules. Their function is to transport triglycerides (energy) and fat soluble vitamins to sites of storage or metabolism, the principal function of the apolipoprotein B group (chylomicrons, very low density lipoprotein, low density lipoprotein (LDL)). They also function to detoxify lipopolysaccharide toxins and remove potentially toxic fatty acid metabolites – principally through reverse transport by apolipoprotein A-1 containing high density lipoproteins (HDLs). Blood lipids are most often measured as TC, LDL, HDL as well as plasma total triglyceride (TG) components. Only the cholesterol fraction (-C) of the major lipoprotein fractions is measured routinely and the concentrations of the cholesterol subfractions do not necessarily reflect the activity of these dynamic pathways – as is most true of HDL. LDL-C is generally not measured by laboratories but calculated instead, using the Friedewald equation [LDL-C (mmol l^{-1}) = TC − (HDL-C + TG/2.20)].[13] This approximation becomes less reliable at higher triglyceride concentrations (TG > 4.5 mmol l^{-1}) and cannot be used in non-fasting samples.[14]

Alternatively the concentrations of the principal proteins – apolipoproteins (apo) B and A1 can be measured and can be better measures of total CVD risk[12] analogous to the use of non-HDL cholesterol and HDL-C.[14]

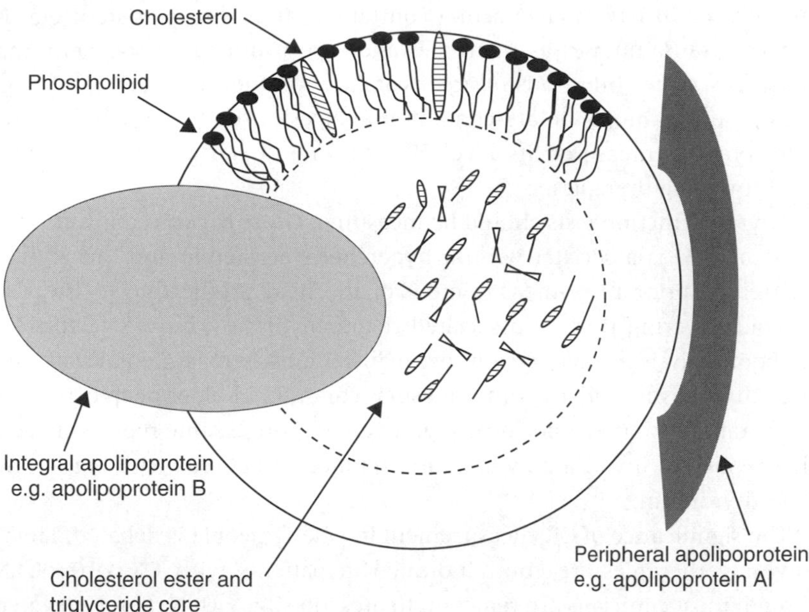

Figure 4.1 Schematic representation of a lipoprotein molecule.

Diagnosis

Lipid screening in elderly people should comprise a full profile of TC, TG and HDL-C with a calculated LDL-C. At lower levels of TC, current recommendations from the UK National Institute for Health and Clinical Excellence[15] and the Joint British Societies guidelines[16] recommend risk assessment using the Framingham (1991) equation. Treatment is recommended for any cardiovascular risk factor at 20%/future decade risk of CVD (15%/future decade risk of CHD). This approach differs from European[17] and US guidelines[18] where risk is assessed at the chronological age and treatment instituted at 20% CHD risk. It should be noted that risk assessment is an imprecise art with any estimate having a wide confidence interval.[19] The UK guidelines also adjust the risk assessment to age 70 to reduce prescribing in otherwise fit elderly people given the strong association of risk with age whereby almost any 75-year-old would require lipid lowering. This statement is controversial and many would recommend direct assessment of plaque burdens using non-invasive techniques, for example carotid intima media thickness or coronary calcium scores.[20,21]

The risk assessment biochemical profile should include measurement of transaminases (AST/ALT), thyroid function tests and a baseline creatine kinase (CK). Lipid-lowering therapy with a statin or fibrate is contraindicated if AST/ALT exceeds 3 x upper reference limit of normal (ULN) (usually >150 IU l^{-1}). The actual contraindication is to persistent elevations in transaminases as many elevations turn out to be transient and caused by either infections or are secondary to other drug therapies (e.g. heavy paracetamol or opiate-containing analgesic use). If gamma-glutamyl transferase is measured its level is irrelevant to starting or continuing lipid-lowering therapies.

Thyroid function tests should be measured. Gross hypothyroidism (TSH > 20 mU l^{-1}) is associated with a hypercholesterolaemia and this should be treated prior to re-measurement of the lipid profile due to the risk of lipid-lowering therapy-associated rhabdomyolysis. The risk factors for rhabdomyolysis are age, creatinine, reduced muscle mass, female sex and hypothyroidism. Mild hypothyroidism is common in older people and not a contraindication to lipid-lowering therapies though some reports suggest that reports of myalgia may be more common in patients with borderline hypothyroidism.

The significance of CK measurement in elderly people is debated. Lipid-lowering therapies are contraindicated in patients with CK > 10 × ULN though most clinicians are reluctant to prescribe if 5 × ULN. Some elevated CK measurements, for example in Africans or Afro-Caribbeans, represent normal variants. In other patients a mildly elevated CK allied with a mild adverse reaction to lipid-lowering therapies should prompt investigation for rheumatological causes of disease as the lipid-lowering therapy may have uncovered this predisposition.

LDL-C as a target of therapy with statins

Epidemiological studies incriminate high levels of LDL-C as being atherogenic with the serum TC as a good correlate for LDL-C levels.[18] However, the definitive proof has come from clinical trial work of lipid-lowering interventions which has been hailed as one of the major advances in clinical medicine. Whether cholesterol is lowered by diet, drugs or other means, CVD risk decreases.[22] Comparing earlier trials of statins, and other treatment modalities such as bile acid sequestrant resins and ileal bypass surgery with more recent statin trials, the benefit of absolute LDL-C reduction is present across a wide range of baseline concentrations.

Statins

Statins form the cornerstone of pharmaceutical CVD prevention. These agents have shown to reduce the risk of both CHD and stroke in clinical trials enrolling persons aged up to 80 years (Table 4.1). A meta-analysis of 90 056 patients which included 14 randomized trials showed that those aged >65 years (n = 6446) had 19% reduction in the risk of major

Table 4.1 Notable statin trials.

Year	1994	1995	1996	2002	2002	2004	2008
Study	4S	WOSCOPS	CARE	HPS	PROSPER	CARDS	JUPITER
Setting	secondary prevention	primary prevention	secondary prevention	combined	combined	type 2 diabetes	primary prevention
Statin	Simvastatin	Pravastatin	Pravastatin	Simvastatin	Pravastatin	Atorvastatin	Rosuvastatin
Number patients	4444	6595	4159	20 536	5804	2838	17 802
Diabetes	202 (4.5%)	76 (1%)	586 (14%)	5963 (29%)	623 (11%)	2838 (100%)	(0) 0%
Follow-up (mean)	5.4 years	4.9 years	5 years	5 years	3.2 years	3.9 years	1.9 years
LDL-C lowering	36%	26%	28%	31%	34%	40%	50%
Age range (yrs)	35–70	45–64	21–75	40–80	70–82	40–75	60–71
>65 years	23%	0%	31%	52%	100%	40%	32%[a]
Primary endpoint	Total mortality 12% → 8%	CHD death/ non-fatal MI 8% → 5.5%	CHD death/ non-fatal MI 13% → 10%	Total mortality 15% → 13%	CHD death/ non-fatal MI and stroke 16% → 14%	CHD event or stroke 9% → 6%	CHD event or stroke 1.8% → 0.9%

4S, Scandinavian Simvastatin Survival Study; WOSCOPS, West of Scotland Coronary Prevention Study; CARE[25]. Cholesterol and Recurrent Events; HPS, Heart protection study; PROSPER, Prospective Study of Pravastatin in the Elderly at Risk; CARDS, Collaborative Atorvastatin Diabetes Study; JUPITER, Justification for the Use of statins In prevention: an intervention Trial Evaluating Rosuvastatin

[a]Percentage of subjects older than 70 years.

cardiovascular events, a benefit similar to the 22% reduction in risk experienced by those aged <65 years (n = 7902).[23] Earlier secondary prevention statin trials, such as the Scandinavian Simvastatin Survival Study (4S),[24] Cholesterol and Recurrent Events (CARE),[25] and Long-term Intervention with Pravastatin in Ischemic Disease (LIPID),[26] support a benefit of lipid lowering after MI. Although these trials excluded patients >75 years of age (4S upper age limit, 69 years), subgroup analysis demonstrated a benefit of statins among younger elderly patients.[27,28] More data on statin therapy in the elderly population became available following the Heart Protection Study which randomized more than 20 000 participants with known CVD or diabetes to either simvastatin 40 mg or placebo in the age range 40–80 (85 by trial end).[29] Simvastatin reduced the risk of cardiovascular events by 18% in those aged 70–80 years (n = 5806) compared with 24% in those aged <65 years. The apparent attenuated impact of simvastatin in the older age group was not statistically significant. As elderly people have a higher absolute risk of events the number of events prevented in those aged >70 years and in those aged <70 years were similar. More evidence on the benefits of statin intervention in older adults accumulated following the Prospective Study of Pravastatin in the Elderly at Risk (PROSPER), which was specifically aimed at evaluating the efficacy of statin use in elderly people.[30] In this study 5804 subjects between the ages 70–82 years with pre-existing CHD or at high risk for CHD were randomized to 40 mg of pravastatin or placebo. Over an average of more than 3 years follow-up, the pravastatin group had significantly fewer combined cardiovascular outcomes (CHD death or non-fatal or fatal myocardial infarction, fatal or non-fatal stroke). The question as to whether older individuals without evidence of CVD will benefit from statin treatment (i.e. in the primary prevention setting)[31] was answered by the recent Justification for the Use of Statins in Prevention: an Intervention Trial Evaluating Rosuvastatin (JUPITER) trial.[32] This study compared rosuvastatin 20 mg to placebo in 17 802 apparently healthy participants with relatively low LDL-C levels of <3.4 mmol l^{-1} and high sensitivity C-reactive greater than 2 mg l^{-1}. The composite primary cardiovascular endpoint showed a relative risk reduction of 44% (hazard ratio: 0.56; 95% CI, 0.46–0.69). 5644 (32%) of participants were older than 70 years making this by far the most representative primary prevention data of the benefits of statin treatment in the elderly population.

Heart failure is common in elderly people secondary to ischaemia, hypertension and cardiomyopathy. A number of statin trials have been conducted in populations with grade 2–3 heart failure after post hoc analyses of general CHD prevention trials suggested benefits in grade 1–2 disease.[33] The Controlled Rosuvastatin Multinational Study in Heart Failure CORONA[34] and GISSI-Heart Failure (GISSI-HF)[35] studies showed no benefits of adding statin therapy in advanced heart failure but also that these drugs were not toxic in these populations.

Specific prescribing points in elderly patients

Data from the large trials shows little difference in side-effect rates between statin and placebo arms.[36,37] However, many patients recruited to the trials have previous experience of statins and the designs of many trials incorporate an active run-in period in which those who suffer side effects are identified early. Thus side-effect rates may be underestimated especially in elderly populations. No specific dose reduction is advised or necessary for elderly patients with statins though many general practitioners worldwide initiate therapy at low doses but unfortunately do not titrate the dose to efficacious levels resulting in a persistent under-treatment of lipids in the elderly population. Drug interactions vary between compounds in the statin class. The most significant interaction is of cytochrome P450 3A4 metabolized statins (lovastatin, simvastatin, atorvastatin) with other drugs metabolized by this pathway – conazole antifungals, erythromycin, and in specialist practice, cyclosporine and HIV protease inhibitors (Table 4.2). Simvastatin interacts with amiodarone at doses >20 mg and other statins should be used if amiodarone therapy is necessary (e.g. for atrial fibrillation). A weaker interaction 3A4 can occur with diltiazem through this pathway but is not usually clinically significant. Drug interactions of this type are less significant for the other statins.

All statins frequently cause gastrointestinal disturbance by a transient dysregulation of bile acid metabolism through the farnesoid-X receptor pathway. This problem may be exacerbated in patients with diverticulosis or irritable bowel disease. Gastrointestinal side effects may be accompanied by a transient increase in bilirubin and transaminases. This problem is usually self-limiting within 2–3 weeks and on repeat measurement liver profiles have usually normalized.

Myalgia occurs in 5% of patients with statin therapy and is not associated with any change in CK.[37] Again often it is self-limiting but if symptoms persist then the statin therapy should be changed to the weaker agents that show predictably better side-effect profiles (pravastatin, fluvastatin). Myositis (raised CK, muscle pain) and rhabdomyolysis (CK > 20 x ULN; muscle pain; myoglobinuria) are rare side effects of statin therapy. The risk factors for rhabdomyolysis are age, creatinine, muscle mass, female sex, hypothyroidism and concomitant therapy with drugs interacting through the relevant cytochrome pathway (usually 3A4); likely to displace statins from plasma proteins; or sharing a myopathic tendency (e.g. other lipid-lowering drugs).

Table 4.2 Practical therapeutics of lipid-lowering drugs.

DRUG	Start dose	Usual dose	Pharmaco-kinetics	Metabolism	Important interactions	Important adverse events	Other tips
Atorvastatin	10 mg	20 mg (10–80)	Y $t_{1/2} = 14$ hrs E $t_{1/2} > 16$ hrs AUC +30%	CYP3A4	Conazoles Erythromycin Ciclosporin	GI disturbance Myalgia-myositis-rhabdomyolysis	
Fluvastatin	80 mg	80 mg (20–80)	Y $t_{1/2} = 0.6$ hrs E $t_{1/2} = 0.6$ hrs AUC – nil	CYP2C9	Nil	GI disturbance Myalgia-myositis-rhabdomyolysis	
Lovastatin	40 mg	80 mg (20–80)	Y $t_{1/2} = 3$ hrs E $t_{1/2} > 3$ hrs AUC +45%	CYP3A4	Conazoles Erythromycin Ciclosporin	GI disturbance Myalgia-myositis-rhabdomyolysis	
Pravastatin	40 mg	40 mg (10–40)	Y $t_{1/2} = 2$ hrs E $t_{1/2} > 2$ hrs AUC +19–27%	$3 - \alpha$-isomer	Nil	GI disturbance Myalgia-myositis-rhabdomyolysis	
Rosuvastatin	10 mg	10 mg (10–20)[40]	Y $t_{1/2} = 19$ hrs E $t_{1/2} = 19$ hrs AUC – nil	CYP2C19 (10%)	Nil	GI disturbance Myalgia-myositis-rhabdomyolysis	
Simvastatin	40 mg	40 mg (10–80 mg)	Y $t_{1/2}$ 1.9 hrs E $t_{1/2} - 3$ hrs AUC +45%	CYP3A4	Conazoles Erythromycin Amiodarone Ciclosporin	GI disturbance Myalgia-myositis-rhabdomyolysis	

Bezafibrate	400 mg	400 mg	Y $t_{1/2} = 4$ hrs E $t_{1/2} = 8$ hrs AUC +160%	Glucuronide	Warfarin Statins	GI disturbance, rash Myalgia-myositis-rhabdomyolysis	
Ciprofibrate	100 mg	100 mg	Y $t_{1/2} = 81$ hrs E $t_{1/2}$ = NA AUC = NA	Glucuronide	Warfarin Statins	GI disturbance, rash Myalgia-myositis-rhabdomyolysis	
Fenofibrate	Various 122/160/ 200 mg	Various 122/145/160/200 mg (122–267)	Y $t_{1/2} = 20$ hrs E $t_{1/2} > 20$ hrs AUC +10%	Glucuronide UGT A2	Warfarin Statins	GI disturbance, rash Myalgia-myositis-rhabdomyolysis	
Gemfibrozil	300 mg bd	600 mg bd	Y $t_{1/2} = 3.0$ hrs E $t_{1/2} = 3.0$ hrs AUC +10%	Glucuronide UGT A1 & UGT A3 **NB. CYP 2C8 inhibitor**	Warfarin Statins	GI disturbance, rash Myalgia-myositis-rhabdomyolysis	Avoid with statin combination therapy
Nicotinic acid (Niacin)	375–500 mg	1000–2000 mg (500–2000)	Y $t_{1/2} = 0.5$ hrs E $t_{1/2}$ = NA AUC = NA	10% nicotinuric acid	–	Flush, rash, hyperglycaemia Hypophos-phataemia Gout	Reduce flush with aspirin/ indomethacin.

(*continued overleaf*)

Table 4.2 *(continued)*

DRUG	Start dose	Usual dose	Pharmaco-kinetics	Metabolism	Important interactions	Important adverse events	Other tips
Ezetimibe	10 mg	10 mg	Y $t_{1/2} = 22$ hrs E $t_{1/2} > 22$ hrs AUC +200%	Glucuronide	Ciclosporin	GI disturbance, rash	Add to low dose statin in myalgia
MaxEPA	1 g	10 g	Y $t_{1/2}$ = NA E $t_{1/2}$ = NA	Beta-oxidation	–	Bloating, weight gain	–
Omacor	1 g	1–2 g	Y $t_{1/2}$ = N/A E $t_{1/2}$ = N/A	Beta-oxidation	–	Bloating	–

Y, Young; E, Elderly

Recently, a meta-analysis of randomized trials showed that statin therapy increases the risk of diabetes.[38] While one risk is unlikely to counter the benefit, it is prudent to check blood glucose annually.

Ezetimibe

The cholesterol absorption inhibitor, ezetimibe, works by reducing the upper intestinal cholesterol absorption to produce in monotherapy around 20% reduction in LDL-C. This drug has proven to be very successful in the market due to its low side-effect profile with its main benefit being add-on therapy to statins to achieve targets.[39] Currently no CVD outcomes data is available on ezetimibe and the importance of this has recently been highlighted.[40] The Simvastatin-Ezetimibe in Aortic Stenosis trial[41] investigated the efficacy of a simvastatin–ezetimibe combination in 1873 patients with aortic stenosis – a common disease in elderly people. No benefit was shown on the combined valve disease-CVD events primary outcome or on valve progression-related endpoints, though a 20% reduction was seen in cardiovascular events. The data in advanced aortic stenosis from SEAS parallels that from other surrogate outcome trials. The Study of Heart And Renal Protection (SHARP) trial investigated the efficacy of simvastatin 20 mg and ezetimibe in 9270 patients with chronic renal failure including those on dialysis and showed a 17% reduction in cardiovascular events.[42]

An ongoing trial namely, IMPROVE-IT (the Improved Reduction of Outcomes: Vytorin Efficacy International Trial), in which simvastatin plus ezetimibe is compared with simvastatin plus placebo, is underway in a middle-aged population with acute coronary syndromes. This study will hopefully provide answers with respect to the benefits of ezetimibe monotherapy on CVD outcomes.

Bile acid sequestrants

Bile acid sequestrants reduce cholesterol absorption and reduce LDL-C by 15–20%. They can be used in monotherapy or combination therapy with any lipid-lowering drug except ezetimibe. They may raise TG levels and have modest positive effects on levels of HDL-C. They are not often used in elderly people as gastrointestinal side effects are common and interact with irritable bowel syndrome and diverticulitis to cause bloating, diarrhoea and constipation. Endpoint evidence exists for bile acid sequestrants from the Lipid Research Clinics trial where they reduced coronary events by 15%.[43]

Bile acid sequestrants have multiple drug interactions as they interfere with the absorption of all lipid-soluble drugs. A 4-hour clear interval is recommended between taking these drugs and taking any other medication. Bile acid sequestrants cause gastrointestinal disturbance in 40% of patients. This may be accompanied by a liver-X-receptor (LXR)-induced hypertriglyceridaemia. Myalgia, myositis (raised CK, muscle pain) and rhabdomyolysis (CK > 20 x ULN; muscle pain; myoglobinuria) are rare side effects of bile acid sequestrant therapy and usually occur when it is prescribed with a concomitant statin.

Intervention on triglycerides

Several meta-analyses have found that TGs are an independent risk factor for CHD.[44,45] Raised serum TG levels (>1.7 mmol l^{-1}) are associated with abnormal lipoprotein metabolism giving rise to increased atherogenicity. The lipid triad of high TG, low HDL-C and increased atherogenic particle numbers (high apo B, low apo A-1 concentrations) is associated with the metabolic syndrome found in many patients with obesity, insulin resistance or diabetes mellitus. Highly elevated TG levels (>9–10 mmol l^{-1}) are a risk factor for pancreatitis.[46]

No specific trials have addressed hypertriglyceridaemia and most exclude patients with this condition. Thus there is no clear consensus on the benefits of directly targeting hypertriglyceridaemia in order to reduce CVD risk. Three drug classes are commonly prescribed for hypertriglyceridaemia namely: fibrates, niacin and omega-3 fatty acids. Statin therapy is still recommended first line for TGs <4.6 mmol l^{-1} as statins reduce TGs in direct proportion to their efficacy on LDL-C and the baseline TG level.[47] At higher TG levels fibrates and niacin are more efficacious and are recommended first-line therapies.[18,48] Guidelines suggest TGs are viewed as risk indicators for intensifying LDL-C-reducing therapy commonly stating an indication with a residual TG >2.3 mmol l^{-1} after initial statin therapy.

Fibrates

Fibrates are used to lower TG and raise HDL-C though their principal action is to increase lipoprotein particle sizes (which is well marked by TG). They reduce TG by 30–50%, raise HDL-C by 2–15% and reduce LDL-C by 0–10% depending on the drug and dose. Four drugs are available (Table 4.1). The evidence base for fibrates is contradictory.[49] The World Health Organization clofibrate trial[50,51] showed decreased cardiovascular events but an increase in total mortality due mostly to an excess of pancreatitis/cholecystitis. Later fibrate trials with gemfibrozil in primary prevention (Helsinki Heart Study)[52] and in secondary prevention patients with low HDL-C (<0.95 mmol l^{-1}) (Veterans Administration-HDL Intervention Trial)[53] showed reductions in cardiovascular events. Data with bezafibrate in the Bezafibrate Infarct Prevention (BIP) study[54] showed a non-significant slight reduction in events concentrated in a high triglyceride group (>2.3 mmol l^{-1}) though this was not reproduced in the patients with peripheral vascular disease in the Northwick Park Study. Fenofibrate reduced CHD events non-significantly and CVD significantly by 11% in patients with type 2 diabetes in the Fenofibrate Intervention in Event Lowering in Diabetes (FIELD) study.[55] The Action to Control Cardiovascular Risk in Diabetes (ACCORD) study also in 5518 patients with type 2 diabetes of fenofibrate added to baseline statin therapy showed a non-significant 8% reduction in CHD events with combination therapy which was, however, safe.[56] A subgroup hinted at a benefit in patients with TG $>2.3\,\text{mmol}\,\text{l}^{-1}$ and HDL-C $<0.88\,\text{mmol}\,\text{l}^{-1}$. Meta-analyses of fibrate trials tend to suggest they are beneficial delivering a 11% reduction in CVD events mostly in smaller non-fatal events in all age groups but at the price of increases in cholecystititis, deep venous thrombosis and pulmonary embolism.[57,58]

Specific prescribing points

No specific dose reduction is advised or necessary for elderly people with fibrates. Fibrate therapy needs to be used with caution in patients with creatinine $>150\,\mu\text{mol}\,\text{l}^{-1}$ (eGFR$<30\,\text{ml}\,\text{min}^{-1}$) as these drugs are renally cleared. Atrial fibrillation is common in elderly patients and guidelines recommend the use of warfarin for stroke prevention. Fibrates show a significant interaction with warfarin such that warfarin doses need to be decreased by 33%. Fibrates can interact with other lipid-lowering therapies to increase the risk of rhabdomyolysis. This is a particular problem with gemfibrozil which has a unique mechanism of glucuronidation and this causes increases in free statin acid concentrations (lovastatin, simvastatin) as well as causing problems with other drugs (e.g. pioglitazone). Gemfibrozil is not recommended to be used in combination therapy (especially statins) for any lipid disorder.[59,60]

Omega-3 fatty acids

Omega-3 fatty acids reduce TG by 20–25% at high doses.[61] The active components are docosahexaenoic acid (DHA) and eicosapentenoic acid (EPA). Epidemiological studies show a progressive reduction in events with fish intake, the greatest effects being seen with minimal intake as opposed to none.[62,63] At moderate doses omega-3 fatty acids have proportionally lesser effects but seem to reduce cardiovascular events especially sudden cardiac death. They can be used in monotherapy or combination therapy with any lipid-lowering drug. The endpoint evidence with omega-3 fatty acids is controversial. In the GISSI-Prevention study (DHA/EPA)[64] and DART-1 (fish oil capsules) studies they reduced CHD events by 13–25% but in the DART-2 study an increase in CVD events was seen. More recently in the Japanese Eicosapentaenoic Lipid Intervention Study (JELIS)[65] 1 g EPA reduced CVD events by 22% in a predominantly female, mostly primary prevention Japanese population with raised LDL-C and a high fish intake. The benefits, however, were concentrated in men and those with prior CHD. The second arm of the GISSI heart failure trial (GISSI-HF)[66] in grade 2–3 heart failure showed that 1 g EPA reduced cardiovascular events and death or heart failure admission by 9% with a number need to treat of 44.

Specific prescribing points

Omega-3 fatty acids have few significant drug interactions but can cause gastrointestinal disturbance and bloating. They may be associated with weight gain if given in preparations that require taking multiple capsules – usually less pure forms of DHA-EPA.

HDL-cholesterol

The inverse relationship between HDL-C levels and atherosclerotic CVD provides the epidemiological basis for the widely accepted hypothesis that HDL is atheroprotective. Based on this epidemiological data, HDL-C measurement forms part of routine CVD risk prediction tools. However, the biology of HDL is more complex than LDL and a single measurement is not necessarily a guide to HDL fluxes. Thus some HDL-raising therapies such as hormone replacement therapy or with a specific cholesterol ester transfer protein inhibitor (CETPi) (torcetrapib) have not reduced CVD events but showed increases while others associated with reduced HDL levels (e.g. apo A1 Milano infusion) show decreases in atheroma burden. The meta-analyses of HDL do show some benefits but rely heavily on the niacin trials as other agents have modest effects.[67] Guidelines are disparate when it comes to treatment targets for HDL-C. An international consensus exists that HDL-C should be $>1\ \mathrm{mmol\,l^{-1}}$.[68] International guidelines state that low HDL-C is in indicator of increased CVD risk but argue that there is no specific treatment for HDL-C as it is only altered modestly, and not independently of changes in other lipid parameters, in the clinical trials.

Niacin

Nicotinic acid (niacin) is used to raise HDL-C and reduce TG. It raises HDL-C by 10–25%, reduces TG by 20–40%, and reduces LDL-C by 10–20% depending on the dose. It can also reduce lipoprotein (a) levels by 10–25%.[69] There is endpoint evidence when the immediate release formulation used a $3\,\mathrm{g\ day^{-1}}$ in the Coronary Drug Project where it reduced CHD events by 22%.[70] In subsequent studies niacin added to statins reduced rates of atherosclerosis progression in coronary (HDL Atherosclerosis Treatment Study; HATS)[71] and carotid arteries (Arterial Biology for the Investigation of the Treatment Effects of Reducing Cholesterol; ARBITER-2)[72] even compared to ezetimibe (ARBITER-6).[73] Endpoint studies of niacin added to optimized LDL-C-lowering therapies are underway in patients with dyslipidaemia and CHD (AIM-HIGH)[74] or mixed secondary prevention and diabetes population (Heart Protection Study-2; treatment of HDL to reduce the incidence of cardiovascular events; HPS2-THRIVE[75]). In the underpowered AIM-HIGH study no benefit was seen with adding niacin to statin on CVD events in patients optimized to LDL-C $<2\,\mathrm{mmol\,l^{-1}}$ both prior to and post-randomization.[74] Given the problems with flushing with the immediate release form a modified release formulation (up to $2\,\mathrm{g\,day^{-1}}$) or one co-formulated with the prostaglandin D2 type 1 receptor antagonist flush suppressant (laropiprant) are commonly used these days. These have similar lipid-lowering efficacy but lesser rates of flushing compared to immediate release niacin.

Specific prescribing points

No specific dose reduction is advised or necessary for elderly people with niacin. Niacin needs to be used with caution in patients with creatinine $>150\,\mu\mathrm{mol\,l^{-1}}$ (eGFR$<30\,\mathrm{ml\,min^{-1}}$) as this drug is renally cleared. Niacin interacts with warfarin such that warfarin doses need to be decreased by 20%. It can interact with other lipid-lowering therapies to increase the risk of rhabdomyolysis but the effect is less than with statin or fibrate monotherapy. The principal side effect of nicotinic acid is facial flushing. This can extend beyond erythema to a burning sensation. Though spectacular this is not a serious side effect. It occurs in 80% of patients commencing niacin therapy and the frequency and intensity of flushes habituate with time. Flushing can be decreased by slow dose titration, concurrent aspirin therapy (150 mg) or by indomethacin (200 mg) except if laropiprant is used, and by slowing absorption using a snack.

Niacin has variable effects on glycaemic control in diabetes.[76] In most patients it has no or a transient effect though in some patients increases of up to $1\,\mathrm{mmol\,l^{-1}}$ in glucose (0.5% in HbA1c) are seen. Transient increases in bilirubin and transaminases are rarer with nicotinic acid than with other lipid-lowering agents. Myalgia occurs in 0.1% of patients on niacin and is not associated with any change in CK. Again often it is self-limiting but if symptoms persist then the therapy should be changed to another drug class. Myositis (raised CK, muscle pain) and rhabdomyolysis (CK > x 20 ULN; muscle pain; myoglobinuria) are very rare side effects of niacin therapy. The risk factors for rhabdomyolysis are similar to those described for statins.

Patients older than 80 years

Very little trial evidence exists for individuals older than 80 years. Ever since the early landmark statin trials such as 4S, CARE and LIPID excluded patients older than 75 years (<70 years for 4S) there has been a paucity of data on older elderly people. The PROSPER trial, which was specifically designed to evaluate statin therapy in elderly patients, included patients aged 70–82 years and the mean age was 75 years.[30] The majority of patients were, however, younger than 80 years. This randomized placebo-controlled trial extended the treatment strategy already employed to younger individuals at the time to older individuals and confirmed the suggested benefits from subgroup analysis of the earlier studies. The question of whether elderly patients will benefit from primary statin intervention was answered by the recent JUPITER study where 5644 patients were aged >70 years.[32] These two recent studies confirm the benefit of statins in older individuals and suggest the benefit to those older than 80 years. A recent meta-analysis of 10 randomized controlled trials which assessed the benefits of statins in people without established cardiovascular disease but with cardiovascular risk factors found that the benefits were similar irrespective of age group (younger versus individuals >65 years).[23] Little compelling trial evidence for lipid lowering in individuals >80 years is therefore available. However, the data available on elderly people suggests that the benefit demonstrated should extend to those >80 years.

Conclusion

Any clinical treatment decision requires consideration of the benefit to risk ratio. As is the case with cardiovascular risk estimation, this remains an inexact science. Statins have revolutionized preventative cardiovascular medicine and their benefits are undisputed following primary and secondary intervention trials which have now included a significant proportion of older individuals. The initiation of lipid-lowering therapy needs to be considered in the context of other CVD risk factors as CVD is multifactorial in origin with clustering of risk factors that have a multiplicative effect on CVD risk. Therefore, total cardiovascular risk management which includes factors such as lifestyle modification and blood pressure management are required in order to maximize cardiovascular risk reduction. Modifying lipids is only one of the essential components of this approach. When deciding on a therapeutic treatment option, clinicians have to weigh up the envisaged benefits against the potential detriment. Clinical acumen is therefore paramount when making a treatment decision in elderly patients as these factors need to be considered.

Key points

- Cardiovascular disease (CVD) increases in a curvilinear fashion after 65 years in men and 75 years in women and the majority of all cardiovascular events occur in individuals older than 65 years.

- There are notable differences in the clinical assessment of cardiovascular risk as well as the safety and tolerability profiles of drug treatment in elderly people compared to younger individuals.
- Randomized controlled clinical trials have demonstrated benefits of statin treatment in elderly people both for primary and secondary prevention. There are, however, limited data to inform decisions for individuals older than 80 years. Few data are available on other lipid-modifying medication in elderly people.
- With continuing increases in average life expectancy, prevention of cardiovascular disease is likely to become increasingly important for improving quality of life and reducing healthcare expenditure for older people.

References

1 World Health Organization (WHO). (2008) Top 10 causes of death. *World Health Statistics, 2008,* WHO, Geneva. Available at: www.who.int/whosis/whostat/EN_WHS08_Full.pdf (last accessed June 2012).

2 Rothwell PM, Coull AJ, Silver LE *et al.* Population-based study of event-rate, incidence, case fatality, and mortality for all acute vascular events in all arterial territories (Oxford Vascular Study). *Lancet* 2005;**366**:1773–83.

3 Jemal A, Ward E, Hao Y and Thun M. Trends in the leading causes of death in the United States, 1970–2002. *JAMA* 2005;**294**:1255–9.

4 Menotti A, Blackburn H, Kromhout D *et al.* Cardiovascular risk factors as determinants of 25-year all-cause mortality in the seven countries study. *Eur J Epidemiol* 2001;**17**:337–46.

5 Menotti A and Giampaoli S. A single risk factor measurement predicts 35-year mortality from cardiovascular disease. *G Ital Cardiol* 1998;**28**:1354–62.

6 The multiple risk factor intervention trial (MRFIT). A national study of primary prevention of coronary heart disease. *JAMA* 1976;**235**:825–7.

7 Vascular Programme. (2008) Putting prevention first – vascular checks: risk assessment and management. Report No.: 287093. UK Department of Health, London, 1 April 2008.

8 Eckel RH, Alberti KG, Grundy SM and Zimmet PZ. The metabolic syndrome. *Lancet* 2010;**375**:181–3.

9 Baass A, Dubuc G, Tremblay M *et al.* Plasma PCSK9 is associated with age, sex, and multiple metabolic markers in a population-based sample of children and adolescents. *Clin Chem* 2009;**55**:1637–45.

10 Anum EA and Adera T. Hypercholesterolemia and coronary heart disease in the elderly: a meta-analysis. *Ann Epidemiol* 2004;**14**:705–21.

11 Lewington S, Whitlock G, Clarke R *et al.* Blood cholesterol and vascular mortality by age, sex, and blood pressure: a meta-analysis of individual data from 61 prospective studies with 55 000 vascular deaths. *Lancet* 2007;**370**:1829–39.

12 Corti MC, Guralnik JM, Salive ME *et al.* Clarifying the direct relation between total cholesterol levels and death from coronary heart disease in older persons. *Ann Intern Med* 1997;**126**:753–60.

13 Friedewald WT, Levy RI and Fredrickson DS. Estimation of the concentration of low-density lipoprotein cholesterol in plasma, without use of the preparative ultracentrifuge. *Clin Chem* 1972;**18**:499–502.

14 Walldius G, Jungner I, Holme I *et al.* High apolipoprotein B, low apolipoprotein A-1, and improvement in the prediction of fatal myocardial infarction (AMORIS study): a prospective study. *Lancet* 2001;**358**:2026–33.

15 National Institute for Health and Clinical Excellence (NICE). (2008) Lipid modification. Report No.: CG67, NICE, London.

16 British Cardiac Society, British Hypertension Society, Diabetes UK, HEART UK, Primary Care Cardiovascular Society, The Stroke Association. JBS 2: the Joint British Societies' guidelines for prevention of cardiovascular disease in clinical practice. *Heart* 2005;**91**(Suppl. V):v1–v52.

17 De Backer G, Ambrosioni E, Borch-Johnsen K *et al.* European guidelines on cardiovascular disease prevention in clinical practice. Third Joint Task Force of European and Other Societies on Cardiovascular Disease Prevention in Clinical Practice. *Eur Heart J* 2003;**24**:1601–10.

18 Expert Panel on Detection Evaluation and Treatment of High Blood Cholesterol in Adults (Adult Treatment Panel III). Executive Summary of the Third Report of the National Cholesterol Education Program (NCEP). *JAMA* 2001;**285**:2486–97.

19 British Cardiac Society, British Hypertension Society, Diabetes UK, HEART UK, Primary Care Cardiovascular Society, The Stroke Association. JBS2: Joint British Societies' guidelines on prevention of cardiovascular disease in clinical practice. *Heart* 2005; DOI:10.1136/hrt.2005.079988.

20 de Groot E, van Leuven SI, Duivenvoorden R *et al.* Measurement of carotid intima-media thickness to assess progression and regression of atherosclerosis. *Nat Clin Pract Cardiovasc Med* 2008;**5**:280–8.

21 Folsom AR, Kronmal RA, Detrano RC *et al.* Coronary artery calcification compared with carotid intima-media thickness in the prediction of cardiovascular disease incidence: the Multi-Ethnic Study of Atherosclerosis (MESA). *Arch Intern Med* 2008;**168**:1333–9.

22 Bucher HC, Griffith LE and Guyatt GH. Systematic review on the risk and benefit of different cholesterol-lowering interventions. *Arterioscler Thromb Vasc Biol* 1999;**19**:187–95.

23 Baigent C, Keech A, Kearney PM *et al.* Efficacy and safety of cholesterol-lowering treatment: prospective meta-analysis of data from 90 056 participants in 14 randomised trials of statins. *Lancet* 2005;**366**:1267–78.

24 The Scandinavian Simvastatin Survival Study (4S) investigators. Baseline serum cholesterol and treatment effect in the Scandinavian Simvastatin Survival Study (4S). *Lancet* 1995;**345**:1274–5.

25 Sacks FM, Pfeffer MA, Moye LA *et al.* The effect of pravastatin on coronary events after myocardial infarction in patients with average cholesterol levels. Cholesterol and Recurrent Events Trial investigators. *New Engl J Med* 1996;**335**:1001–9.

26 Long-Term Intervention with Pravastatin in Ischemic Disease (LIPID) Study Investigators. Prevention of cardiovascular events and death with pravastatin in patients with coronary heart disease and a broad range of initial cholesterol levels. The Long-Term Intervention with Pravastatin in Ischaemic Disease (LIPID) Study Group. *New Engl J Med* 1998;**339**:1349–57.

27 Miettinen TA, Pyorala K, Olsson AG *et al.* Cholesterol-lowering therapy in women and elderly patients with myocardial infarction or angina pectoris: findings from the Scandinavian Simvastatin Survival Study (4S). *Circulation* 1997;**96**:4211–8.

28 Sacks FM, Tonkin AM, Shepherd J *et al.* Effect of pravastatin on coronary disease events in subgroups defined by coronary risk factors: the Prospective Pravastatin Pooling Project. *Circulation* 2000;**102**:1893–900.

29 MRC/BHF Heart Protection Study Investigators. MRC/BHF Heart Protection Study of cholesterol lowering with simvastatin in 20 536 high-risk individuals: a randomised placebo-controlled trial. *Lancet* 2002;**360**:7–22.

30 Shepherd J, Blauw GJ, Murphy MB *et al.* Pravastatin in elderly individuals at risk of vascular disease (PROSPER): a randomised controlled trial. *Lancet* 2002;**360**:1623–30.

31 Robinson JG, Bakris G, Torner J, Stone NJ and Wallace R. Is it time for a cardiovascular primary prevention trial in the elderly? *Stroke* 2007;**38**:441–50.

32 Ridker PM, Danielson E, Fonseca FA *et al.* Rosuvastatin to prevent vascular events in men and women with elevated C-reactive protein. *New Engl J Med* 2008;**359**:2195–207.

33 Kjekshus J, Dunselman P, Blideskog M *et al.* A statin in the treatment of heart failure? Controlled rosuvastatin multinational study in heart failure (CORONA): study design and baseline characteristics. *Eur J Heart Fail* 2005;**7**:1059–69.

34 Kjekshus J, Apetrei E, Barrios V *et al.* Rosuvastatin in older patients with systolic heart failure. *New Engl J Med* 2007;**357**:2248–61.

35 Gissi-HF Investigators, Tavazzi L, Maggioni AP *et al.* Effect of rosuvastatin in patients with chronic heart failure (the GISSI-HF trial): a randomised, double-blind, placebo-controlled trial. *Lancet* 2008;**372**:1231–9.

36 Law M and Rudnicka AR. Statin safety: a systematic review. *Am J Cardiol* 2006;**97**(8A):S52–S60.

37 Joy TR and Hegele RA. Narrative review: statin-related myopathy. *Ann Intern Med* 2009;**150**:858–68.

38 Preiss D and Sattar N. Statins and the risk of new-onset diabetes: a review of recent evidence. *Curr Opin Lipidol* 2011;**22**:460–6.

39 Mikhailidis DP, Wierzbicki AS, Daskalopoulou SS *et al.* The use of ezetimibe in achieving low density lipoprotein lowering goals in clinical practice: position statement of a United Kingdom consensus panel. *Curr Med Res Opin* 2005;**21**:959–69.

40 Wierzbicki AS. Muddy waters: more stormy SEAS for ezetimibe. *Int J Clin Pract* 2008;**62**:1470–3.

41 Rossebo AB, Pedersen TR, Boman K *et al.* Intensive lipid lowering with simvastatin and ezetimibe in aortic stenosis. *New Engl J Med* 2008;**359**:1343–56.

42 Baigent C, Landray MJ, Reith C *et al.* The effects of lowering LDL cholesterol with simvastatin plus ezetimibe in patients with chronic kidney disease (Study of Heart and Renal Protection): a randomised placebo-controlled trial. *Lancet* 2011;**377**:2181–92.

43 The Lipid Research Clinics (LRC) Coronary Primary Prevention Trial Investigators. The Lipid Research Clinics Coronary Primary Prevention Trial results. I. Reduction in incidence of coronary heart disease. *JAMA* 1984;**251**:351–64.

44 Hokanson JE and Austin MA. Plasma triglyceride level is a risk factor for cardiovascular disease independent of high-density lipoprotein cholesterol level: a meta-analysis of population-based prospective studies. *J Cardiovasc Risk* 1996;**3**:213–9.

45 Sarwar N, Sandhu MS, Ricketts SL *et al.* Triglyceride-mediated pathways and coronary disease: collaborative analysis of 101 studies. *Lancet* 2010;**375**:1634–9.

46 Mao EQ, Tang YQ and Zhang SD. Formalized therapeutic guideline for hyperlipidemic severe acute pancreatitis. *World J Gastroenterol* 2003;**9**:2622–6.

47 Stein EA, Lane M and Laskarzewski P. Comparison of statins in hypertriglyceridemia. *Am J Cardiol* 1998;**81**(4A):66B–9B.

48 National Institute for Health and Clinical Excellence (NICE). (2008) Type 2 diabetes: the management of type 2 diabetes (update). Report No.: CG66, NICE, London.

49 Wierzbicki AS. FIELDS of dreams, fields of tears: a perspective on the fibrate trials. *Int J Clin Pract* 2006;**60**:442–9.

50 Committee of Principal Investigators. A co-operative trial in the primary prevention of ischaemic heart disease using clofibrate. Report from the Committee of Principal Investigators. *Br Heart J* 1978;**40**:1069–118.

51 Committee of Principal Investigators. WHO cooperative trial on primary prevention of ischaemic heart disease with clofibrate to lower serum cholesterol: final mortality follow-up. Report of the Committee of Principal Investigators. *Lancet* 1984;**2**:600–4.

52 Frick MH, Elo O, Haapa K *et al*. Helsinki Heart Study: primary-prevention trial with gemfibrozil in middle-aged men with dyslipidemia. Safety of treatment, changes in risk factors, and incidence of coronary heart disease. *New Engl J Med* 1987;**317**:1237–45.

53 Rubins HB, Robins SJ, Collins D *et al*. Gemfibrozil for the secondary prevention of coronary heart disease in men with low levels of high-density lipoprotein cholesterol. Veterans Affairs High-Density Lipoprotein Cholesterol Intervention Trial Study Group. *New Engl J Med* 1999;**341**:410–8.

54 Bezafibrate Infarction Prevention Study Group. Secondary prevention by raising HDL cholesterol and reducing triglycerides in patients with coronary artery disease: the Bezafibrate Infarction Prevention (BIP) study. *Circulation* 2000;**102**:21–7.

55 Keech A, Simes RJ, Barter P *et al*. Effects of long-term fenofibrate therapy on cardiovascular events in 9795 people with type 2 diabetes mellitus (the FIELD study): randomised controlled trial. *Lancet* 2005;**366**:1849–61.

56 The ACCORD study group. Effects of combination lipid therapy in type 2 diabetes mellitus. *New Engl J Med* 2010;**362**:1563–74.

57 Saha SA, Kizhakepunnur LG, Bahekar A and Arora RR. The role of fibrates in the prevention of cardiovascular disease – a pooled meta-analysis of long-term randomized placebo-controlled clinical trials. *Am Heart J* 2007;**154**:943–53.

58 Jun M, Foote C, Lv J *et al*. Effects of fibrates on cardiovascular outcomes: a systematic review and meta-analysis. *Lancet* 2010;**375**(9729):1875–84.

59 Shek A and Ferrill MJ. Statin-fibrate combination therapy. *Ann Pharmacother* 2001;**35**:908–17.

60 Wierzbicki AS, Mikhailidis DP, Wray R *et al*. Statin-fibrate combination: therapy for hyperlipidemia: a review. *Curr Med Res Opin* 2003;**19**:155–68.

61 Hartweg J, Farmer AJ, Perera R, Holman RR and Neil HA. Meta-analysis of the effects of n-3 polyunsaturated fatty acids on lipoproteins and other emerging lipid cardiovascular risk markers in patients with type 2 diabetes. *Diabetologia* 2007;**50**:1593–602.

62 Hooper L, Thompson RL, Harrison RA *et al*. (2004) Omega 3 fatty acids for prevention and treatment of cardiovascular disease. *Cochrane Database Syst Rev* **4** (Art no.:CD003177).

63 Wierzbicki AS. A fishy business: omega-3 fatty acids and cardiovascular disease. *Int J Clin Pract* 2008;**62**:1142–6.

64 Gruppo Italiano per lo Studio della Sopravvivenza nell'Infarto miocardico. Dietary supplementation with n-3 polyunsaturated fatty acids and vitamin E after myocardial infarction: results of the GISSI-Prevenzione trial. *Lancet* 1999;**354**:447–55.

65 Yokoyama M, Origasa H, Matsuzaki M *et al*. Effects of eicosapentaenoic acid on major coronary events in hypercholesterolaemic patients (JELIS): a randomised open-label, blinded endpoint analysis. *Lancet* 2007;**369**:1090–8.

66 Tavazzi L, Maggioni AP, Marchioli R *et al.* Effect of n-3 polyunsaturated fatty acids in patients with chronic heart failure (the GISSI-HF trial): a randomised, double-blind, placebo-controlled trial. *Lancet* 2008;**372**:1223–30.

67 Birjmohun RS, Hutten BA, Kastelein JJ and Stroes ES. Efficacy and safety of high-density lipoprotein cholesterol-increasing compounds: a meta-analysis of randomized controlled trials. *J Am Coll Cardiol* 2005;**45**:185–97.

68 Sacks FM. The role of high-density lipoprotein (HDL) cholesterol in the prevention and treatment of coronary heart disease: expert group recommendations. *Am J Cardiol* 2002;**90**:139–43.

69 Chapman MJ, Assmann G, Fruchart JC, Shepherd J and Sirtori C. Raising high-density lipoprotein cholesterol with reduction of cardiovascular risk: the role of nicotinic acid – a position paper developed by the European Consensus Panel on HDL-C. *Curr Med Res Opin* 2004;**20**:1253–68.

70 The Coronary Drug Project Research Group. Clofibrate and niacin in coronary heart disease. *JAMA* 1975;**231**:360–81.

71 Brown BG, Zhao XQ, Chait A *et al.* Simvastatin and niacin, antioxidant vitamins, or the combination for the prevention of coronary disease. *New Engl J Med* 2001;**345**:1583–92.

72 Taylor AJ, Sullenberger LE, Lee HJ *et al.* Arterial Biology for the Investigation of the Treatment Effects of Reducing Cholesterol (ARBITER) 2: a double-blind, placebo-controlled study of extended-release niacin on atherosclerosis progression in secondary prevention patients treated with statins. *Circulation* 2004;**110**:3512–7.

73 Taylor AJ, Villines TC, Stanek EJ *et al.* Extended-release niacin or ezetimibe and carotid intima-media thickness. *New Engl J Med* 2009;**361**:2113–22.

74 AIM-HIGH Investigators: Boden WE, Probstfield JL, Anderson T *et al.* Niacin in patients with low HDL cholesterol levels receiving intensive statin therapy. *New Engl J Med* 2011;**365**:2255–67.

75 HPS2-THRIVE Investigators. (2009) A randomized trial of the long-term clinical effects of raising HDL cholesterol with extended release niacin/laropiprant. Heart Protection Study 2-Treatment of HDL to Reduce the Incidence of Vascular Events (HPS2-THRIVE). ClinicalTrials.gov [last updated 19 July 2010]. Available at: http://clinicaltrials.gov/ct2/show/NCT00461630 (last accessed June 2012).

76 Vogt A, Kassner U, Hostalek U and Steinhagen-Thiessen E. Evaluation of the safety and tolerability of prolonged-release nicotinic acid in a usual care setting: the NAUTILUS study. *Curr Med Res Opin* 2006;**22**:417–25.

CHAPTER 5
Arrhythmias

Abhay Bajpai and A. John Camm
St George's, University of London, London, UK

Introduction

The population is ageing and, as the heart ages, pathophysiological changes occur that predispose to numerous rhythm disturbances. Prognostic improvements made in the management of heart disease have further increased the burden by prolonging exposure to conditions that promote the development of arrhythmias. Arrhythmias are associated with a substantial risk of morbidity and mortality and the management of arrhythmias in elderly people presents important challenges. Clinical presentation can vary from one extreme (asymptomatic incidental finding) to the other (acute haemodynamic collapse) and includes a myriad of non-specific symptoms common to many disorders. The general principles of arrhythmia management in the elderly population are the same as with other ages, but plans must be individualized as there is a vast scope amongst older people for comorbidity, polypharmacy, impaired cognition, poor exercise tolerance and other factors that modify the risk–benefit ratio. This chapter reviews arrhythmias in elderly people and their associated morbidity and mortality, with increased emphasis on the commonest rhythm disorder, atrial fibrillation (AF).

The elderly heart

Ageing of the heart is associated with the deposition of amyloid in the atrial myocardium, a gradual loss of the specialized pacemaker myocytes of the sinoatrial (SA) node and the deposition of collagen and fibrous tissue in the specialized ventricular conduction tissue. These ageing processes are associated with a pathological outcome in some patients. For instance, loss of SA node pacemaker cells contributes to the development of sick sinus syndrome. This process is augmented by pathological changes secondary to

Cardiovascular Disease and Health in the Older Patient: Expanded from 'Pathy's Principles and Practice of Geriatric Medicine, Fifth edition', First Edition. Edited by David J. Stott and Gordon D.O. Lowe.

cardiovascular disease such as hypertension and coronary atherosclerosis, both of which increase in incidence with age. In reviewing 12-lead and 24 h electrocardiogram (ECG) survey findings in elderly patients, it can be difficult to distinguish between whether purely ageing or pathological processes are responsible.

12-Lead and ambulatory ECG surveys

Findings of a prolonged PR interval, left-axis deviation and bundle branch block (BBB) are more common in elderly people. First-degree heart block, as a lone finding in an asymptomatic patient, is not associated with an adverse prognosis. Left-axis deviation is associated with cardiovascular disease but in the absence of clinical disease does not carry a worse prognosis. Increases in left ventricular hypertrophy and left BBB with age correspond to the increased incidence of cardiovascular disease and clearly are associated with an increased mortality. Right BBB is more common than left in older adults, but has no prognostic impact *per se*.

In the absence of medication, a sustained bradycardia is not a normal finding in an elderly individual. However, elderly subjects do show a significant reduction in 24 h heart rate variability.[1] A survey of 500 asymptomatic individuals aged 50–80 years[2] found no association between heart rate and age, and a study of 1372 individuals aged 65 years and older[3] found no association between bradycardia and age. Various studies have shown a small decline in mean heart rate with age,[4] but even in healthy subjects aged 80–99 years, mean heart rate is still >70 bpm.[1] A persistent and significant bradycardia should alert the clinician to the possibility of sinus node disease. There is a low incidence of sinus arrhythmia in elderly people, but ectopic activity is considerably increased. Specific brady- and tachyarrhythmias are discussed individually below.

Symptomatic bradycardias

Cardiac impulse originates in the SA node, propagates through the atria and is normally conducted to the ventricles via the atrioventricular (AV) node and bundle of His. Bradycardia can result from abnormalities at any level: dysfunction of SA node automaticity, conduction disturbances within the AV node or bundle of His. These are discussed individually below. Bundle branch or fascicular blocks may prolong ventricular depolarization (QRS complex width) or cause electrical axis deviation, but will not result in a bradycardia unless conduction through all fascicles is interrupted, equivalent to complete AV block. The autonomic nervous system regulates sinus node automaticity and AV nodal conduction. The balance of parasympathetic and sympathetic tone is subject to influence from a host of extrinsic factors: physiological (e.g. sleep), pathological (e.g. hypothyroidism) and iatrogenic (e.g. medication). The causes of a bradycardia are summarized in Table 5.1.

Presentation

Episodes of bradycardia are common in all age groups. However, a sustained bradycardia is not a normal finding in older people and, as discussed above, implies pathology. The presence or absence of symptoms is principally determined by the heart's ability to compensate for a bradycardia. Cardiac output is the product of heart rate and left ventricular stroke volume. If the latter cannot increase sufficiently to match demand and peripheral and/or cerebral perfusion falls, this will result in symptoms. These vary from understated symptoms such as lack of concentration, fatigue, poor memory, dizziness and myalgia to more pressing concerns of syncope and heart failure.

Assessment

Documentation of a bradycardia (rhythm strip, 12-lead ECG or ambulatory monitoring) is not sufficient. The symptoms described above are

Table 5.1 Causes of bradycardia.

System	Cause
Cardiovascular	Ischaemia/infarction
	Infiltrative disorders (e.g. sarcoid, amyloid, haemochromatosis)
	Inflammatory disorders (e.g. systemic lupus erythaematosus, rheumatoid)
Respiratory	Obstructive sleep apnoea
Medication	β-Blockers (including topical eye preparations)
	Anti-arrhythmics (e.g. digoxin, amiodarone)
	Antihypertensives (e.g. calcium channel antagonists)
Iatrogenic	Valve replacement
	Catheter/surgical ablation
	Correction of congenital heart disease
Endocrine	Hypokalaemia
	Hyperkalaemia
	Hypothyroidism
Neurological	Raised intracranial pressure
	Increased vagal tone (e.g. micturition, defecation, coughing)
	Carotid sinus hypersensitivity
Infectious disease	Infective endocarditis
	Lyme disease
	Chagas disease
Miscellaneous	Hypothermia
	Metastatic disease

SLE, systemic lupus erythaematosus.

all non-specific and differential diagnoses are extensive, especially in the elderly population. It is essential to establish a correlation between the patient's symptoms and the occurrence of bradycardia, otherwise treatment of the arrhythmia may be successful (e.g. pacemaker implantation), but without any symptomatic benefit. History, examination and investigations should be targeted at confirming the presence of arrhythmia, its association with symptoms, to differentiate physiology from pathology and to recognize reversible risk factors (such as medication, hypothyroidism, sleep apnoea).

Sinus node dysfunction (sick sinus syndrome)

The term sick sinus syndrome confers the impression of a constellation of multiple electrocardiographic manifestations such as sinus bradycardia, inappropriate sinus node response to exercise (chronotropic incompetence), sinoatrial block and periods of sinus arrest, particularly occurring after paroxysms of atrial tachyarrhythmias ('tachy-brady syndrome'). Dysfunction may progress to the stage that no sinus beats occur (Figure 5.1). Both paroxysmal and chronic AF are commonly associated with sinus node disease. Sinus node dysfunction is primarily a disease of elderly people resulting from degenerative or ischaemic causes which may also affect other conductive tissue including the AV node. The majority of patients experience recurrent syncope from sinus pauses with inadequate escape rhythm or marked sinus bradycardia. Mortality appears to be unaffected by sinus node dysfunction[5] and survival is influenced by associated pathology such as ischaemic heart disease.

The main indications for pacing in sinus node dysfunction are as follows:[6]

- Sinus node dysfunction with documented symptomatic bradycardia, symptomatic chronotropic incompetence or where bradycardia is the result of medication necessary to treat other medical conditions, such as in the treatment of tachyarrhythmias (class I recommendation).
- Sinus node dysfunction and heart rate <40 bpm, where an association between symptoms consistent with bradycardia and the presence of bradycardia has not been clearly established; syncope of unknown origin

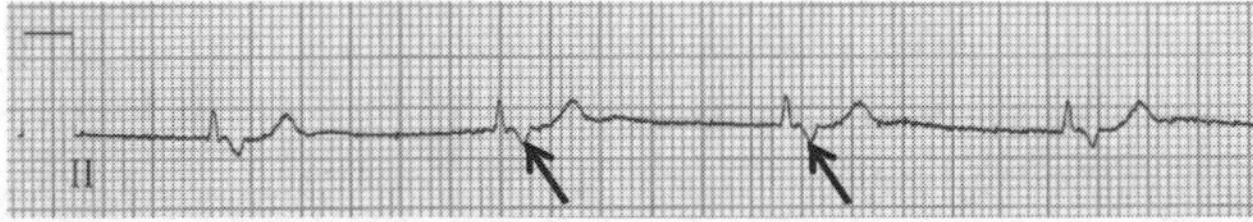

Figure 5.1 Junctional bradycardia: failure of sinus beats has resulted in a junctional escape rhythm. The junctional impulses are seen conducting antegradely causing ventricular depolarization, but also retrogradely into the atria causing inverted P waves, seen immediately after the QRS complex (arrows).

in presence of significant sinus node abnormalities on electrophysiological testing (class IIa recommendations).

Atrioventricular blocks

First-degree heart block

The PR interval (time from onset of P wave to onset of QRS complex) corresponds to the time from initiation of atrial depolarization, conduction through the atria and into the bundle branch system via the AV node and bundle of His. A prolonged PR interval (>0.2 s) with preservation of 1:1 AV conduction is termed *first-degree heart block*. The incidence of first-degree AV block increases with ageing. Moderate prolongation of the PR interval in this fashion is a benign condition,[7] but PR intervals >0.3 s can be symptomatic.[8] Marked first-degree AV block could cause loss of synchrony between the atria and the ventricles leading to incomplete atrial and ventricular filling and increased capillary wedge pressure.

Indications for pacing in first-degree AV block are as follows:[6]

- First-degree heart block associated with symptoms of a delay in AV synchronous contraction or haemodynamic compromise (class IIa recommendation).
- First-degree heart block in association with neuromuscular diseases due to unpredictable progression of AV disease; drug-related AV block where the block is expected to persist even after withdrawal of the drug (class IIb recommendation).

Second-degree heart block

This is an intermittent failure of atrial depolarization to result in ventricular depolarization and tends to occur in various patterns. Mobitz type I second-degree heart block (Wenckebach) is present when there is progressive lengthening of the PR interval with each beat until an atrial depolarization is not conducted, resulting in a dropped beat. The PR interval resets and the cycle resumes. Mobitz type II second-degree heart block occurs when atrial depolarizations are intermittently blocked without preceding progressive PR interval prolongation. AV conduction occurring in a 2:1 fashion (or higher) represents another pattern of second-degree heart block. If block of two or more consecutive P waves occurs, this is termed *advanced second-degree heart block* (Figure 5.2).

Indications for pacing in second-degree AV block are as follows:[6]

- Any form of second-degree heart block associated with symptomatic bradycardia or ventricular arrhythmias presumed to be secondary to the AV block (class I recommendation).
- Advanced second-degree AV block in symptom-free patients with documented significant periods of pauses or asystole lasting ≥3.0 s or

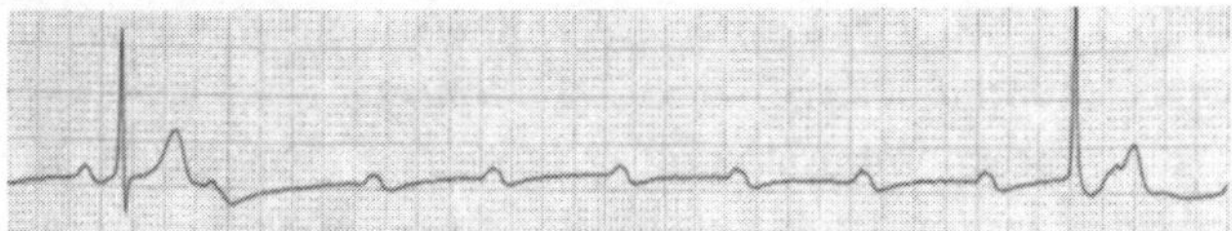

Figure 5.2 Rhythm strip showing advanced second-degree heart block. The second ventricular complex is a junctional escape beat.

any escape rhythm of rate <40 bpm in an awake patient (class I recommendation).

- Advanced second-degree AV block associated with arrhythmias and other medical conditions that require drug therapy that results in symptomatic bradycardia (class I recommendation).
- Unresolving advanced second-degree block following cardiac surgery or catheter ablation of AV junction (class I recommendation).
- AV block during exercise in the absence of myocardial ischaemia.
- Type II second-degree heart block with a wide QRS complex (class I recommendation).
- Asymptomatic type II second-degree heart block with narrow QRS complex (class IIa recommendation).
- Associated with symptoms of a delay in AV synchronous contraction or haemodynamic compromise (class IIa recommendation).
- In association with neuromuscular diseases due to unpredictable progression of AV disease; drug-related AV block where the block is expected to persist even after withdrawal of the drug (class IIb recommendation).

Third-degree heart block (complete heart block)

Third-degree heart block is a complete block of conduction between the atria and ventricles resulting in regular atrial activity and the presence of an independent escape rhythm. The escape rhythm is generally ventricular in origin with a wide QRS complex and rate of ~30–40 bpm. Nodal or junctional escape rhythms imply that the anatomical level of block is higher within the AV node or the bundle of His (Figure 5.3). The lower the origin of the escape rhythm, the less specialized and hence less reliable is the conduction tissue.

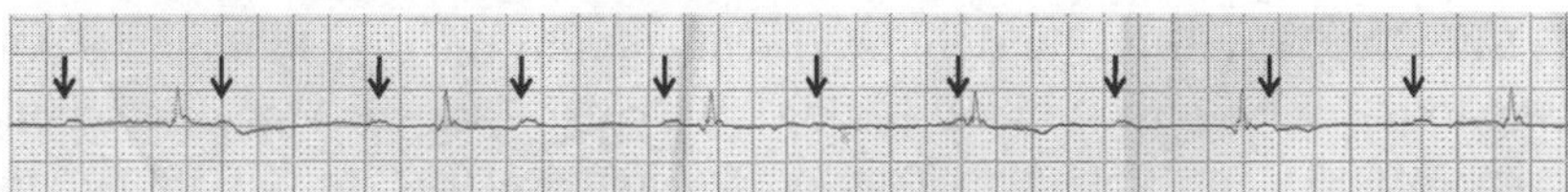

Figure 5.3 Complete heart block. Rhythm strip showing P waves (arrows) that are independent and unrelated to QRS complexes. The QRS complexes are relatively narrow, suggestive of junctional escape rhythm.

Indications for pacing in complete AV block are as follows:[6]

- Third-degree heart block with one of the following features: symptomatic bradycardia; documented asystole ≥3.0 s or any escape rhythm of rate <40 bpm in symptom-free awake patients; unresolving block following cardiac surgery or catheter ablation of AV junction; asymptomatic third-degree heart block, especially in the context of LV dysfunction or cardiomegaly; AV block during exercise in the absence of myocardial ischaemia (class I recommendations).
- Asymptomatic heart block in the absence of cardiomegaly (class IIa recommendation).
- Drug-related AV block where the block is expected to persist even after withdrawal of the drug (class IIb recommendation).

Choice of pacemaker

Once the decision to implant a pacemaker has been made, consideration should be given to the appropriate pacemaker mode. The choice lies between single-chamber ventricular-only pacing (VVI/R), dual chamber atrial plus ventricular pacing (DDD/R) or single-chamber atrial-only pacing (AAI/R). DDD or AAI pacing allow the preservation of normal physiology by maintaining AV synchrony. Single-chamber AAI pacing is indicated in patients with pure sinus node disease with no evidence of either existing or future development of disease elsewhere in the conduction system. However, elderly patients, who may initially present with apparently pure sinus node dysfunction, have a greater likelihood of more widespread conduction system involvement and therefore generally will not benefit from atrial-only pacing. Physiological pacing may improve haemodynamics, but dual-chamber systems can be technically more challenging as two leads are required with greater potential for late complications. A series of large prospective, randomized trials have compared ventricular pacing (VVI/R) with physiological systems (DDD/R or AAI/R) for sinus node dysfunction or AV block (see Table 5.2 for a summary of these trials). A key limitation of these trials is that a significant number of patients either crossed over between treatment arms or dropped out of their assigned pacing mode. Meta-analysis of these five trials shows that there is no difference in overall mortality between ventricular and physiological pacing systems and no difference in new-onset heart failure or improvement or progression of any existing heart failure.[9]

However, a statistically significant reduction in the development of AF was found with physiological pacing, particularly in the Mode Selection Trial (MOST) and Canadian Trial of Physiological Pacing (CTOPP) trial. There was borderline reduction in thromboembolic stroke with physiological pacing. Some cross-over studies with intra-patient comparison

Table 5.2 Characteristics of trials comparing ventricular and physiological pacing.

Trial[a]	*n*	Age (years)	Indication[a]	Follow-up (years)	Results
CTOPP	2568	73	SND or AVB	3.1	No significant difference in stroke, cardiovascular death or hospitalization for heart failure Annual rate of AF significantly lower in physiological group, but higher perioperative complication rate
CTOPP (long-term)	2568	73	SND or AVB	6	No significant difference in cardiovascular death, stroke or total mortality Persistent significantly lower rate of AF in physiological group
MOST	2010	74 (median)	SND	2.8	No significant difference in death, non-fatal stroke or hospitalization for heart failure Incidence of AF significantly lower in physiological group
PASE	407	76	SND or AVB	2.5	No significant difference in stroke, stroke or all-cause mortality, stroke, death or hospitalization for heart failure No significant difference in the development of AF
UKPACE	2021	80	AVB	4.6	No significant difference in all-cause mortality No significant difference in secondary end-points of AF or heart failure

[a]CTOPP, Canadian Trial Of Physiologic Pacing:[13] CTOPP (long-term), Canadian Trial Of Physiologic Pacing long-term follow-up:[14] MOST, Mode Selection Trial:[15] PASE, pacemaker selection in the elderly:[16] UKPACE, United Kingdom Pacing and Cardiovascular Events; SND, sinus node dysfunction: AVB, atrioventricular block.

between the two pacing modes have shown improved functional capacity and increased patient preference for dual-chamber pacing.[10]

Therefore, elderly patients with sinus node dysfunction who require pacing should be considered for a dual-chamber system. No clear evidence exists for benefit of dual-chamber pacing over simple ventricular pacing for AV block in elderly patients, but given the overall findings from trials, physiological pacing should be considered for those likely to be pacemaker dependent. Active elderly patients over 70 years of age appear to benefit from DDD pacing in terms of improvement in quality of life.[11] However, the final decision in the elderly population depends on an individual basis after taking into account patient preferences, comorbidities and the available resources.

Complications of pacemaker implantation

Complications can occur during implantation and include pneumothorax (1–2% with subclavian vein approach; <0.1% with cephalic or axillary vein approach), bleeding, myocardial perforation and tamponade (<0.2%), lead dislodgement and failure to sense or capture. Post-procedure complications are bruising, wound haematoma, infection (<1%), device erosion, lead fracture and box or lead dislodgement. In a recent series, early complications (within 2 weeks of implantation) occurred in 6.7% of patients and late complications in 7.2% of patients.[12] The majority of these patients required an invasive correction of the complication. Despite the reduction in size of the modern pacemaker, special considerations have to be made for elderly patients. Devices are generally implanted subcutaneously between the skin and the pectoral muscle in the infra-clavicular region, but skeletal deformities resulting from osteoarthritis or osteoporosis of the shoulder, spine or pectoral region may occasionally prevent this. In addition, wound healing and device erosion through the skin are more likely to occur with cachexia and thinning skin. In such patients, the pacemaker may be better positioned under the pectoral muscle. Clearly, as with any procedure, a risk–benefit assessment has to be made on an individual basis.

Atrial tachyarrhythmias

Atrial ectopic beats

These are a common finding in elderly people and, if frequent, can result in a pulse that could be confused with AF. No specific treatment is required, but if symptomatic, patients generally respond to beta-blocker therapy.

Atrial tachycardia

Short bursts of atrial tachycardia are common in elderly people (Figure 5.4). In many cases, no symptoms are associated and no treatment may be

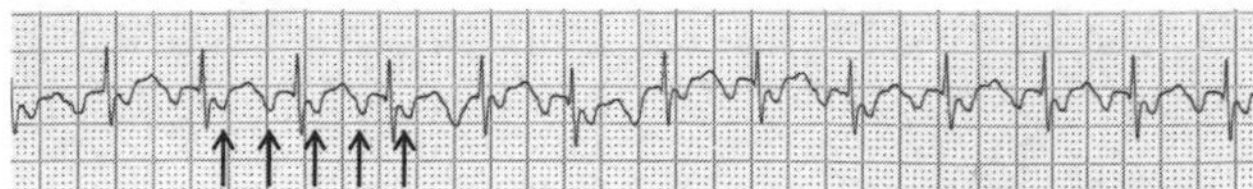

Figure 5.4 Atrial tachycardia. Abnormal, inverted P waves are seen (arrows) with 2:1 conduction to the ventricles. The tracing may appear like atrial flutter, but note that the P wave rate or cycle length is less than the typical flutter cycle length of 300 bpm.

needed. Sometimes the atrial tachycardia triggers AF or causes rapid ventricular rates when treatment of the tachycardia may become necessary. Most elderly patients will achieve symptomatic benefit from beta-blocker therapy, and some may require anti-arrhythmic medication (e.g. amiodarone, sotalol) or urgent direct current cardioversion (DCC) if haemodynamically unstable. Percutaneous catheter ablation utilizing radiofrequency or cryo energy is increasingly used, but success rates are generally higher in younger patients and therefore not currently a preferred option in older people.

Multifocal atrial tachycardia (MAT)

Another common atrial arrhythmia in elderly people, multifocal atrial tachycardia (MAT), is characterized by the appearance of diverse P wave morphologies as complexes originate from different foci within the atria. This can result in irregular R–R intervals and hence clinically mimic AF. There is an association with chronic airways disease and drug toxicity (digoxin, theophyllines and tricyclic antidepressants). Treatment should be aimed at the underlying cause.

Atrial flutter

Atrial flutter and AF are two ends of the same spectrum. Whereas the atria are activated in a chaotic manner in AF, atrial flutter consists of organized atrial activation seen on the ECG as a regular saw-tooth pattern of flutter waves with typically a flutter-wave rate of ~300 bpm (Figure 5.5). A physiological 2:1 AV block frequently occurs and atrial flutter should always be suspected in a patient with a ventricular rate of 150 bpm. In the elderly population, variable 4:1, 8:1 or other AV ratios may also be seen. Vagal manoeuvres or intravenous adenosine can temporarily increase the AV block, making flutter waves more visible. With typical (counterclockwise) atrial flutter, flutter waves are seen inverted in the inferior limb leads, giving rise to the characteristic saw-tooth appearance on the ECG. Atrial flutter commonly occurs in patients with AF and vice versa. Anti-arrhythmic medication prescribed for AF can convert the AF into atrial flutter. Management of the two conditions is essentially similar and although the stroke risk associated with atrial flutter may not be as high as for AF, there is still a substantial risk[17] and a high likelihood of coexisting AF requiring the use of anticoagulation. In a given elderly

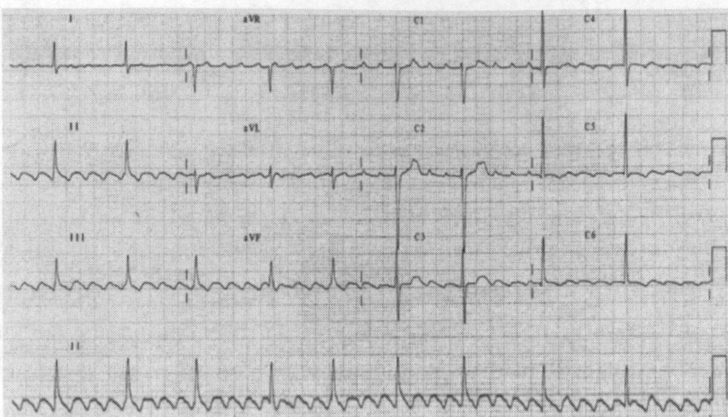

Figure 5.5 12-Lead ECG of typical atrial flutter with variable AV block. Note the inverted P waves (flutter waves) in the inferior leads II, III and aVF. The flutter wave cycle length is 300 bpm.

patient, unlike other atrial arrhythmias, catheter ablation of typical atrial flutter may be performed with relative ease and high curative rates.

Atrial fibrillation

AF is characterized by disorganized atrial activity confirmed on the ECG by the substitution of regular P-wave activity by rapid fibrillatory waves varying in shape, amplitude and timing. If AV node conduction is intact, the chaotic atrial activation will result in a rapid and irregular ventricular response. In elderly patients, AV conduction may be impaired. A slower ventricular rate is common and sometimes verges on a symptomatic bradycardia (Figure 5.6). The presence of regular rhythm on the ECG with a fibrillatory baseline implies development of complete AV block in a patient with AF, the regularity arising from the escape rhythm (Figure 5.7).

Classification

AF can be classified into five types based on the presentation, duration and choice of treatment strategy. When the first episode is detected, it is important to understand that its duration may be uncertain and there may have been previous episodes, which were not symptomatic, remembered

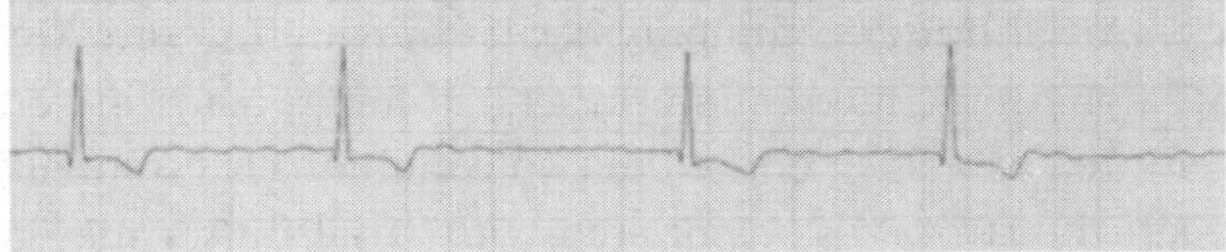

Figure 5.6 Rhythm strip of patient in AF with a slow ventricular response.

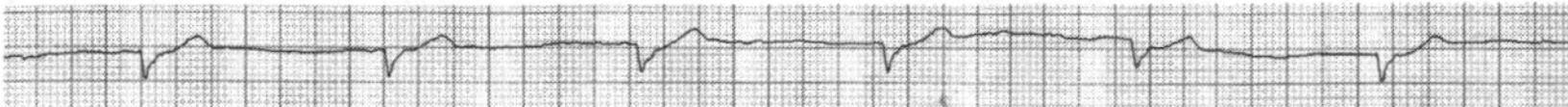

Figure 5.7 Lead II rhythm strip of a patient with chronic AF who presented with syncope. The rhythm is regular with fibrillatory baseline and absence of P waves, suggestive of complete heart block in the setting of AF.

or documented. After first detection, AF is then subclassified into the following categories according to its time course and intervention: *paroxysmal (PAF), persistent, long-standing persistent* and *permanent* atrial fibrillation. PAF is characterized by recurrent episodes of AF alternating with sinus rhythm. The characteristic feature of PAF is that the episodes terminate spontaneously, usually within 48 h. If the episodes of fibrillation continue for more than 7 days or patients require intervention to restore sinus rhythm, this is termed persistent AF. When AF has lasted for ≥1 year and when it is decided to adopt a rhythm-control strategy, AF is termed long-standing persistent AF. Permanent AF is more a statement of intent rather than a duration or pathological-based description and is reserved for patients in whom AF is resistant to conversion or accepted for rate control by the patient and there are no further attempts to achieve sinus rhythm. Permanent AF is redesignated long-standing persistent AF if there is a change of plan towards adopting a rhythm-control strategy.[18]

Epidemiology

AF affects 1–2% of the general population and is the commonest sustained arrhythmia in elderly people. The true prevalence of AF may be closer to 2% as many patients remain asymptomatic and may never present to a hospital. The prevalence of AF increases with age from <0.5% at 40–50 years to 5–15% at 80 years.[19]

Men are more often affected than women. An analysis of 1.4 million patients registered with 211 general practices in England and Wales showed that prevalence rates increased with age from <1 in 1000 in those under 35 years of age to >100 in 1000 in those aged 85 years and older.[20] The prevalence of AF is estimated to double in the next 50 years.[21]

We are in part victims of our own success owing to prognostic improvements made in coronary heart disease and heart failure, conditions known to predispose to the development of AF. This, together with an ageing population, has led to the description of a near-epidemic of AF.[22] AF increases the risk of stroke fivefold. In 2000, the projected direct cost of AF to the UK National Health Service (NHS) was calculated at £459 million, 0.98% of total NHS expenditure,[23] a conservative estimate as costs related to stroke rehabilitation and anticoagulant-related haemorrhage were not considered.

Aetiology

Valvular AF

It is essential to make a distinction between valvular and non-valvular AF because of the consequence for stroke risk. Valvular heart disease is present in about 30% of patients with AF.[24]

Mitral stenosis and/or regurgitation, and in its later stages aortic stenosis, cause left atrial dilatation leading to AF. Rheumatic heart disease is now relatively rare in developed nations. In the Framingham Study, patients with rheumatic heart disease and AF had a 17-fold increase in stroke risk compared with age-matched controls.[25]

Non-valvular AF

AF occurring in the absence of rheumatic mitral stenosis or a prosthetic heart valve is termed *non-valvular AF*,[18] which can then be further subdivided as follows.

With associated cardiovascular disease

Hypertension (see Chapter 3, Hypertension), diabetes requiring medical treatment, heart failure (see Chapter 8, Heart Failure), cardiomyopathies, coronary artery disease (Chapter 7, Ischaemic Heart Disease) and congenital heart defects such as atrial septal defect are commonly associated with AF. Of these, heart failure carries the highest predictive risk for the development of AF.[26] Hypertension is identified as a risk factor for AF and related complications such stroke and thromboembolism.

Hypertension, when associated with left ventricular hypertrophy by electrical criteria on the ECG, strengthens its contribution towards predicting development of AF. Coronary artery disease can be both a reversible risk factor (ongoing ischaemia or infarction) or irreversible (scar formation from prior infarction).

Other causes

Other identifiable and potentially reversible causes include obesity and obstructive sleep apnoea, electrolyte disturbance, sepsis, stress, hyperthyroidism, pulmonary disease, hypoxia and alcohol binge drinking. These factors need to be considered both in a first detected episode of AF and for the patient with a recent compromise in rate control.

Lone AF

Patients with a structurally normal heart in whom no identifiable cause can be found for their AF are denoted as having lone AF. This is probably rare in the elderly population since almost all patients will have a degree of underlying heart disease by this stage and such a diagnosis of exclusion should only be made with caution in elderly people. In a small number of younger patients, sympathetic or vagal overstimulation may trigger AF and could influence the choice of anti-arrhythmic medication.

Consequences of AF

AF independently increases the mortality by twofold and is associated with stroke, other systemic thromboembolic disease, heart failure and related morbidity, leading to poor quality of life. Only antithrombotic treatment has been shown to reduce AF-related mortality.[27]

Atrial remodelling

It is a common finding for patients presenting with PAF to cardiovert spontaneously to sinus rhythm within 24 h of its onset.

The success of electrical or chemical cardioversion and the subsequent maintenance of sinus rhythm are generally higher with AF of a shorter duration. These observations are consistent with the concept that AF itself is capable of inducing an electrical remodelling of the atria, which in turn sustains the arrhythmia. Electrophysiological artificial maintenance of AF in animal models has been shown to induce reversible atrial changes (shortened atrial refractoriness) that lead to the perpetuation of AF[28] and eventually to histological (cellular dedifferentiation, fibrosis) and gross structural changes (atrial dilatation).

Haemodynamic function

With the chaotic activation inherent in AF, synchronous atrial mechanical function is not possible. The left ventricle in AF can only fill passively in the absence of the late diastolic contribution from atrial contraction. This in turn can lead to a 5–15% decrease in cardiac output, an effect that is more pronounced in patients with reduced ventricular compliance (e.g. hypertensives) in whom ventricular filling is significantly reliant on the atrial contribution. Further deterioration in haemodynamic function results from high ventricular rates due to shortening of the diastolic filling time and additionally tachycardia-related myopathy (tachycardiomyopathy) at rates persistently above 120–130 bpm. Restoration of atrial mechanical function after successful ventricular rate control or cardioversion leads to quantifiable improvements in left ventricular function.[29] However, the return of atrial contraction may be delayed or insufficient if AF has been present for a substantial period of time.

Thromboembolism

The risk of stroke in non-rheumatic AF patients is 5.6 times greater than in age-matched controls with an identical blood pressure distribution.[25] Thrombus formation, often in the left atrial appendage (LAA), is responsible for embolic stroke and systemic embolism in the context of

AF. Stroke risk consistently and significantly increases with age from 6.7% in those aged 50–59 years to 36.2% for those aged 80–89 years.[30] Asymptomatic cerebral infarction based on computed tomography (CT) findings has been found in 14.7–48% of AF patients.[31–33] The large variation in incidence is probably due to the use of different radiological definitions of infarction and study size. The two largest studies[31,32] showed statistically significant associations of silent infarction with increasing age. Compared with non-AF strokes, those occurring in the context of AF have a greater mortality and survivors are more likely to suffer a recurrence and greater disability.[34] Asymptomatic AF carries the same thromboembolic risk as symptomatic AF. PAF has been shown also to have similar rates of ischaemic stroke and predictors as sustained AF.[35,36]

Multivariate analysis from antithrombotic trials in AF have demonstrated several clinical risk factors for stroke in non-rheumatic AF: increasing age, history of hypertension, previous stroke or TIA and diabetes.[37] A pooled analysis of echocardiographic data from three of these trials demonstrated that left ventricular systolic dysfunction (as defined by global or regional wall motion abnormalities shown on 2D transthoracic echo) is an independent risk factor for stroke in AF.[38] Recent 2010 ESC guidance additionally suggests vascular disease and sex category (female) as additional important risk factors (CHA_2-DS_2-VASc scoring system; see below). Moreover, increased left atrial diameter (measured by m-mode echocardiography) is an independent predictor of thromboembolism.[39] The presence of thrombus in the LAA and its precursor, the appearance of spontaneous echo contrast, are also associated with thromboembolism.[40] Therefore, patients with AF can be risk stratified for stroke on the basis of clinical and echocardiographic data.

Clinical manifestations

AF can have a diverse clinical presentation, whether symptomatic or asymptomatic. Patients may report experiencing palpitations, dyspnoea or chest pain. Release of atrial natriuretic peptide (ANP) can be associated with polyuria, although this is relatively uncommon in elderly people. Patients may only present with the consequences of disease: thromboembolic complications, heart failure secondary to the tachycardia-induced cardiomyopathy or symptoms secondary to reduced cardiac output (light-headedness, fatigue). Cognitive impairment secondary to cerebral hypoperfusion or recurrent thromboembolism is important to distinguish as this would identify a potentially treatable cause of impairment. Syncope is not a common presentation of AF and generally indicates additional pathology such as conduction system disease or aortic stenosis.

History and examination

There needs to be a focused work-up concentrating on the following points.

Confirmation of arrhythmia

The clinician should elucidate any prior history of palpitations and associated symptoms. A review of medication past and present, for warfarin or anti-arrhythmics, should be undertaken and response/tolerance to these agents noted. On examination, there is an irregularly irregular pulse and variation in loudness of the first heart sound. There is good evidence that manual pulse check with ECG follow-up of an irregular pulse is a sensitive screening method.[41] A 12-lead ECG is essential, as this can provide evidence of prior myocardial infarction, left ventricular hypertrophy and AV node or bundle branch conduction disease.

Aetiology of arrhythmia

It is essential to identify any possible reversible triggers that may be responsible for a new episode of AF or deterioration in previously well-controlled disease. An assessment of associated cardiovascular disease should also be made both for aetiology and stroke risk assessment.

Effect of arrhythmia on the patient

It is important to identify a clear pattern of symptoms attributable to the arrhythmia and any indication of cardiovascular compromise. Evidence of end-organ effects such as heart failure or stroke should also be sought, as this may influence treatment decisions such as anticoagulation.

Patient assessment for management options

A balanced decision regarding rate versus rhythm control and the risks and benefits of anticoagulation should be made. It is imperative that any potential bleeding risks (such as previous haemorrhage or history of falls) are identified. A social history (emphasizing exercise tolerance, living conditions, access to support and cognitive function) is important. A review of medication will establish potential risks of drug interactions and polypharmacy. Issues of non-compliance should be explored as medication, particularly warfarin, will require stable and consistent administration.

Imaging

Transthoracic echocardiography (TTE) is an essential investigation in any patient with AF, regardless of age. It provides an assessment of the left atrium, mitral valve and left ventricular function and dimensions, thus providing information regarding aetiology and stroke risk assessment. TTE has its limitations since it cannot reliably exclude the presence of thrombus in the LAA. Transoesophageal echocardiography (TOE) is the imaging of choice to examine the LAA for thrombus or its precursor spontaneous echo contrast. Its role in cardioversion is discussed below.

Other tests

A chest X-ray and lung function tests are required when lung disease is suspected. A CT head scan is indicated if there is any evidence of cerebrovascular disease which may be important in making a decision regarding anticoagulation. Relevant blood and urine tests include those to rule out infection or inflammatory disorders, liver and renal functions, thyroid functions, full blood count and coagulation profile.

Management

There are two aims in the management of AF: to prevent thromboembolism and to control the arrhythmia (rate or rhythm control). The classification of AF into paroxysmal, persistent, long-standing persistent and permanent is clinically useful as it gives a clear guide to a management strategy for each patient. In PAF, the aim is to maintain sinus rhythm and control the ventricular rate when AF does occur. For a patient with permanent AF, the decision has been made to accept the arrhythmia and instead symptomatic improvement is attained with ventricular rate control. Persistent AF may present the clinician with a dilemma: standard practice has been to strive for sinus rhythm by electrical or pharmacological means with symptom control, improved haemodynamics and reduced risk of thromboembolism being the proposed rationale. However, rhythm control medication could pose the problem of pro-arrhythmia and randomized controlled trials[42–47] have not shown superiority of rhythm control over rate control; these are summarized in Table 5.3.

The conclusion to draw from these trials is that for relatively asymptomatic elderly patients with persistent AF, rate control is generally no worse an option than rhythm control. In a first detected episode of AF, one should consider an attempt at rhythm control, cardioversion being the first-line therapy for acute haemodynamic compromise related to AF. However, in elderly patients who are tolerating the arrhythmia, accepting rate control should not be viewed as a failure. Acceptable methods of rate and rhythm control for elderly people are described in the following section. Anticoagulation to prevent thromboembolism needs to be considered whichever strategy is chosen. How a patient is anticoagulated will depend upon the options available, duration of anticoagulation and a risk–benefit analysis for each patient.

Table 5.3 Randomized controlled trials of rate versus rhythm control in AF.

Trial[a]	No. of patients	Mean age (years)	Follow-up (years)	Outcome
AFIRM AF + risk factor for stroke	4060	69.7	3.5	No difference on overall mortality or quality of life Increased hospitalization in rhythm control group
PIAF Persistent AF + symptoms	252	61	1	No difference in symptoms or quality of life Increased hospitalization in rhythm control group Increased walking distance in rhythm control group
RACE Persistent AF or flutter post-cardioversion	522	68	2.3	No difference in composite end-points (cardiovascular death, heart failure, thromboembolism, bleeding, severe drug adverse effects, pacemaker implantation)
STAF Persistent AF + symptoms + LVEF <45%	200	65	1.6	No difference in composite end-points (death, cerebrovascular event, systemic embolization, cardiopulmonary resuscitation) Increased hospitalization in rhythm control group
HOT-CAFÉ First clinically overt persistent AF	205	60.8	1.7	No difference in composite end-points of death, thromboembolic events, intracranial or major haemorrhage
AF–CHF AF + symptoms of heart failure + LVEF ≤ 35%	1376	66	3.1	No difference in cardiovascular deaths

[a]AFFIRM, Atrial Fibrillation Follow-up Investigation of Rhythm Management;[43] PIAF, Pharmacological Intervention in Atrial Fibrillation;[42] RACE, Rate Control versus Electrical Cardioversion for Persistent Atrial Fibrillation;[44] STAF, Strategies of Treatment of Atrial Fibrillation;[45] HOT-CAFÉ, How to Treat Chronic Atrial Fibrillation;[46] AF-CHF, Atrial Fibrillation-Congestive Heart Failure;[47] LVEF, left ventricular ejection fraction.

Rate control

As has already been discussed, bradycardia is not a normal finding for elderly people and similarly a slow ventricular rate in an elderly patient with untreated AF implies underlying conduction system disease.[48] The aim of rate control is to maintain a patient's heart rate at what is physiologically appropriate for the level of exertion. This must not be at the expense of symptomatic pauses or bradycardia. Therapy must be tailored to the individual, but rates of 60–80 bpm at rest and 90–115 bpm during moderate exercise have been suggested as a target.[49] This can be achieved through medication and/or non-pharmacological methods, although not infrequently no specific rate control therapy is needed in elderly people. The recent RACE II trial[50] showed that in patients with fast ventricular rates, but without severe symptoms, stringent rate control (resting heart rate <80 bpm) conferred no symptomatic benefit over lenient rate control (resting heart rate <110 bpm).

Digoxin

Digoxin, a muscarinic agonist, slows AV nodal conduction. This is sufficient to produce adequate rate control for elderly patients with low levels of exertion. This action can be overwhelmed when faced with high sympathetic stimulation, which explains why digoxin is less effective during exercise and why patients with previously well-controlled AF present with inadequate rate control in the context of an acute illness.[51] Although digoxin can be considered as first-line therapy for an inactive elderly patient, it should not be solely relied upon in the presence of high sympathetic tone (i.e. sepsis, pain, β-agonist medication). Digoxin also blocks the sodium/potassium ATPase exchange pump by occupying the potassium binding site (hence digoxin toxicity is potentiated in hypokalaemia) and can act as a mild positive ionotrope (although probably not in the context of AF). Digoxin has not been shown to be of prognostic benefit in heart failure[52] but it can be safely used in patients with heart failure. In comparison with beta-blockers and the non-DHP calcium channel antagonists used for rate control, digoxin has a relatively slow onset of action of the order of hours compared with minutes.[48] This is acceptable if there is no urgency for rate control to be achieved. Digoxin compared with placebo produces a small but statistically significant reduction in the frequency of symptomatic episodes of PAF,[53] probably via a significant reduction in ventricular rate, recorded during patient-activated recordings. However, 24 h ambulatory ECG monitoring during this period failed to show any reduction in frequency, duration of AF or ventricular rate. Digoxin was well tolerated by these patients and so is not believed to be detrimental in PAF, although its benefit is questionable. Concerns have been expressed regarding its use in PAF, as digoxin has been shown to augment the shortening in atrial effective refractory period that can predispose to further episodes of AF.[54] Digoxin has no role to play in cardioversion. Neither oral[55] nor intravenous[56] preparations have been shown to be more effective than placebo. Digoxin is excreted in an unchanged form via the kidneys. Serum level monitoring and dose adjustment will be required in renal dysfunction. To reduce the risk of toxicity, a lower dosage than that required in younger patients should initially be used. The dose may then be up-titrated if the response is inadequate. There is an age-related decline in glomerular filtration rate and impaired renal function can easily develop with acute illness or changes to medication, such as introduction of a diuretic.

Beta-blockers

β-Receptor antagonists block the action of catecholamines and hence are particularly useful in the context of high sympathetic drive. This may on occasion also be to their detriment as a decrease in maximum exercise tolerance has been reported,[57] as have measured reductions in $VO_{2\,max}$ and cardiac output during exercise.[58] A reduction in exercise tolerance is not universal, however, and beta-blockers remain the most effective agent for controlling ventricular rate during exertion. They should also be considered as first-line treatment in the context of hypertension, ischaemic heart disease or stable LV dysfunction, although usually more beta-blockade is needed for rate control than for heart failure and so beta-blocker monotherapy is not useful for patients with both conditions. These agents have a rapid onset of action, but their use is restricted by bronchospasm. In cases of acute pulmonary oedema, they should only be considered where there is no doubt that it is has been precipitated by decompensated AF (not an easy diagnosis to be certain of) and used in small, titrated doses.

Non-dihydropyridine calcium channel antagonists

Verapamil and diltiazem act directly on the AV node, slowing conduction. Both have a rapid onset of action similar to that of beta-blockers and are a useful alternative in the context of airways disease. These too should be used with caution in pulmonary oedema and do not have the prognostic benefits enjoyed by beta-blockers in heart disease.

Amiodarone

In cases where amiodarone fails to cardiovert AF chemically, significant improvements in ventricular rate control can occur.[59] This is clinically useful where rapid control of AF is required to relieve symptoms and effective rate control can provide a significant benefit, even if cardioversion is unsuccessful. However, for the purposes of rate control, the agents discussed above are a more practical long-term option as the use of amiodarone may be limited due to severe extracardiac side effects, including thyroid dysfunction.

Dronedarone

This is a new multichannel blocker that is used for maintaining sinus rhythm, but also has anti-adrenergic activity and is effective as a rate-controlling agent during rest as well as exercise. It can be added to other rate-controlling agents and effectively reduces heart rates in AF relapses (not currently approved for permanent AF).[60]

Combination of rate control agents

A combination of beta-blocker and non-DHP calcium channel antagonists is to be used only with caution. These are both negative ionotropes, which together can cause life-threatening hypotension or bradycardia. In addition, verapamil and diltiazem both inhibit the metabolism of propranolol and metoprolol and hence if used together can result in synergistic detrimental effects.[61] Verapamil can cause a significant and unpredictable elevation in plasma digoxin levels and should not be used together. There are, however, no significant interactions of digoxin with diltiazem,[62] making it a preferred option over verapamil. Digoxin can also be used in combination with beta-blockers, but vigilant follow-up is required for any of these combinations as the risk of conduction disease and hence the potential for bradyarrhythmias are more common in elderly patients. Amiodarone causes significant elevation in the plasma levels of digoxin, necessitating halving of the digoxin dose if used simultaneously with amiodarone.[61]

Recommendations for rate control

Monotherapy for ventricular rate control should be chosen on an individual basis: digoxin is recommended for relatively sedentary patients with low levels of exertion, beta-blockers for active patients or those with ischaemic heart disease, and calcium channel antagonists (diltiazem or verapamil) if beta-blockers are not tolerated or are contraindicated.

Combination therapy of the above may be required to achieve adequate rate control at rest and during exercise, with careful monitoring to avoid bradycardia. Amiodarone is also an effective rate-controlling agent and may be suitable for some patients when other drugs are unsuccessful. In certain situations, such as heart failure, combination of a beta-blocker with digoxin may be beneficial.

For acute rate control in patients without heart failure or hypotension, intravenous beta-blocker or calcium channel antagonist (diltiazem or verapamil) can be used. In patients where adequate rate control cannot be achieved or medication is not tolerated, non-pharmacological methods should be considered.

Non-pharmacological rate control

Permanent pacemaker

In the elderly patient, AF may be a part of wider conduction system disease ('tachy-brady syndrome', sick sinus syndrome) and adequate rate control may only be achieved at the expense of intolerant bradycardia. Implantation of a permanent pacemaker may then become necessary to allow continuation or up-titration of rate-control medication.

Ablate and pace strategy

If the ventricular response is refractory to medical rate control therapy or a patient is intolerant to drug therapy and other non-pharmacological treatments such as catheter-based or surgical ablation of AF are not indicated, the option of catheter-based ablation of AV node/bundle of His should be considered. The main benefits of this approach are a reduction in symptoms and improved quality of life.[63] This involves irreversible destruction of normal AV conduction tissue, an irreversible process that renders the patient permanently pacemaker dependent. Cardiac resynchronization therapy (biventricular pacemaker) may provide additional long-term benefit in patients with severe heart failure symptoms (NYHA functional class III or IV) and LV ejection fraction ≤35%.

Rhythm control

Urgent DC cardioversion (DCC)

Patients with acute, uncontrolled AF who become haemodynamically compromised or experience evolving myocardial ischaemia/infarction require urgent synchronized electrical DCC under short-acting general anaesthetic or conscious sedation. Unless AF duration is <48 h or if the patient is not already anticoagulated within the therapeutic range, then the procedure should be preceded by an intravenous bolus of unfractionated heparin followed by either continuous infusion or subcutaneous low molecular weight heparin (LMWH). A prospective study of 357 patients (mean age 68 years) presenting with AF of duration that was clinically estimated at <48 h and without prior anticoagulation demonstrated a low incidence of thromboembolism with cardioversion.[64] If the duration of arrhythmia is uncertain or when there is high risk of left atrial/atrial appendage thrombus, transoesophageal echocardiography can be performed prior to urgent cardioversion. Electrical cardioversion can cause temporary disruption of left atrial mechanical function, which can lead to the development of spontaneous echo contrast and thrombus formation. Therefore, despite the low incidence of thrombus formation in AF of <48 h duration, thromboembolic risk becomes evident in the period after cardioversion. The duration of risk is uncertain, especially in cases of cardioversion for acute AF. A retrospective, pooled analysis of studies of electrical cardioversion of AF of various durations demonstrated that 98% of embolic episodes occurred within 10 days of cardioversion.[65] Current recommendations are to commence oral anticoagulation with warfarin and maintain an international normalized ratio (INR) of 2–3 for at least 4 weeks after cardioversion, except when AF is of recent onset and no other thromboembolic risk factors are present.[18]

Elective DC cardioversion

Elective cardioversion should be considered for patients with AF who are stable and do not have severe underlying heart disease. At least 3 weeks of adequate anticoagulation with warfarin is mandatory prior to attempted cardioversion of AF of >48 h duration. This has been shown successfully to resolve preformed atrial thrombus and results in an 87% improvement in the incidence of thromboembolism at cardioversion.[66] Some trials have shown that an alternative strategy of transoesophageal echo-guided cardioversion to exclude the presence of LAA thrombus obviates the need for prior anticoagulation, is safe, reduces the time to cardioversion, is associated with fewer haemorrhagic events[67] and is cost-effective.[68] Timing of recovery of left atrial mechanical function is related to duration of prior AF.[29] If the patient remains in sinus rhythm at 4 weeks post-cardioversion, anticoagulation may be stopped depending on long-term thromboembolic risk. However, as discussed above, the duration of thromboembolic risk still remains uncertain. In the Rate Control versus Electrical Cardioversion trial,[44] 17% of all thromboembolic complications occurred in the rhythm control arm when warfarin therapy was ceased. Electrolyte imbalances must be excluded prior to an attempt at cardioversion. Cardioversion generally achieves high success rates,[69] but relapse rates can be high with age, hypertension, AF duration, previous recurrences, enlarged left atrium, presence of coronary disease, pulmonary or mitral valve disease and NYHA functional class III or IV predicting long-term failure of electrical cardioversion.[70] In the event of relapse, further attempts at cardioversion by pretreatment with anti-arrhythmic medication are recommended.[49] Amiodarone would be a suitable choice for the elderly patient, but consideration must be paid to the risks of such a strategy (pro-arrhythmia/systemic side effects) as compared with accepting rate control for each individual patient.

Pharmacological cardioversion and rhythm control

The risk of thromboembolism is present irrespective of the method of cardioversion employed, requiring anticoagulation use with pharmacological attempts at rhythm control. The choice of agents that can be used in elderly patients is more restricted than that for younger patients with AF. This is because of the increased comorbidity in the elderly population and the side-effect profile of medication used.

Amiodarone

This Vaughan Williams class III anti-arrhythmic, along with sotalol and dofetilide, blocks potassium channels, thereby slowing repolarization and prolonging the QT interval. It also affects calcium and sodium channels and has an extensive half-life (~50 days) due to protein binding. It has a broad side-effect profile but a practical safety profile, permitting its use in LV dysfunction and ischaemic heart disease. It is indicated for both cardioversion and maintenance of sinus rhythm. Amiodarone is metabolized by the cytochrome P450 system and so the dosage may have to be increased when used concomitantly with enzyme inducers such as rifampicin or carbamazepine. Amiodarone itself is an enzyme inhibitor, resulting in increased drug levels of phenytoin or warfarin if used in combination. It is important to consider that because of its long half-life, side effects or interactions may persist for some time, even after discontinuation of the amiodarone. Risk of drug-induced pro-arrhythmia (QT prolongation and polymorphic ventricular tachycardia), although less in comparison with other anti-arrhythmic drugs, requires regular monitoring of QT interval.

Sotalol

Another potassium channel blocker, sotalol has additional beta-blocking action (class II) that predominates over the class III action at low doses. This may limit its efficacy in the elderly population where intolerance of substantial beta-blocker action may prevent high enough dosing for the class III effect to manifest. Sotalol appears to be as effective as amiodarone in patients with ischaemic heart disease (SAFE-T study[71]) and should be used as first-line agent in these patients.

Sotalol prolongs the QT interval, which should be closely monitored and the drug stopped or reduced if the QT interval is >500 ms (Table 5.4).

Beta-blockers

Beta-blockers are only modestly effective in preventing recurrent AF, except if it is related to thyrotoxicosis or is exercise induced. The

Table 5.4 Factors which increase the risk of sotalol-induced QT prolongation and pro-arrhythmia.

- Women
- Marked left ventricular hypertrophy (>1.4 cm)
- Severe bradycardia
- Ventricular arrhythmias
- Renal dysfunction
- Hypokalaemia
- Hypomagnesaemia

'anti-arrhythmic' effect may also be due in part to better rate control during paroxysmal episodes rendering these recurrences less symptomatic or silent.

Flecainide

The class 1C anti-arrhythmic flecainide is a sodium channel blocker that delays depolarization and can lead to prolongation of the QRS width. In suitable patients with AF <24 h, intravenous flecainide has 67–92% efficacy in converting AF to sinus rhythm, but is less effective in AF of longer duration. In the light of the Cardiac Arrhythmia Suppression Trial (CAST), where flecainide in post-infarct patients was associated with increased mortality,[72] concern has been expressed regarding its safety for use in elderly people, who will generally have a degree of ischaemic heart disease. Flecainide should be avoided in patients with coronary artery disease or left ventricular impairment. The drug prolongs the QRS duration, and thereby the QT interval, and should be stopped if the QRS duration has increased by >25% of the baseline.

Dofetilide/ibutilide

These are newer class III agents that may be effective in recent-onset AF. Ibutilide is more effective in conversion of atrial flutter than AF. However, a high incidence of ventricular arrhythmias currently limits their use in elderly patients.

Dronedarone

Dronedarone is a new multichannel blocker that is less toxic than amiodarone, in terms of systemic side effects, and may be of use to maintain sinus rhythm in stable patients without structural heart disease or heart failure. In comparison with placebo, dronedarone appears to reduce significantly all-cause mortality, cardiovascular hospitalizations and stroke risk (independent of antithrombotic treatment) in patients with paroxysmal or persistent AF or flutter (ATHENA study[73]).

Similarly to sotalol and flecainide, dronedarone is less effective than amiodarone in maintaining sinus rhythm.[74] However, it may be more important from a general perspective, especially in the elderly population, to have less cardiovascular hospitalizations or stroke risk than maintenance of sinus rhythm when other relevant therapies for rate control and anticoagulation are well maintained. Dronedarone can be safely prescribed in patients with NYHA class I–II heart failure, but there is increased mortality when used in symptomatic patients with NYHA class III–IV heart failure due to worsening of heart failure (ANDROMEDA study[75]). Although studies included patients with a history of risk factors such as hypertension and coronary disease, no definitive data exist for its use in patients with LVH or in those who are asymptomatic to justify routine prescribing.

Recommendations for rhythm control

Urgent electrical cardioversion should be considered for AF resulting in haemodynamic compromise, myocardial ischaemia or heart failure. Elective electrical or pharmacological cardioversion should be considered for patients with stable AF where there is a reasonable chance of long-term maintenance of sinus rhythm. Premedication with anti-arrhythmic medication increases the success rate in maintaining sinus rhythm after electrical cardioversion. The choice of pharmacological agent for long-term control is limited in elderly people due to underlying heart disease. Beta-blockers should be considered for rhythm (plus rate) control in patients with a first episode of AF. Amiodarone is suitable for patients with left ventricular dysfunction, whereas sotalol is preferred in patients with ischaemic heart disease in the absence of significant left ventricular hypertrophy or impairment. Dronedarone use is limited to patients without significant structural heart disease, but should be considered in order to reduce cardiovascular admissions in patients with paroxysmal/persistent AF and cardiovascular risk factors.

Non-pharmacological rhythm control

A number of non-pharmacological options have been explored to control and prevent AF, with varying degrees of success. Currently these procedures are not widely suitable for an elderly population, but can be considered on an individual basis.

Ablation procedures (surgical and catheter based)

For its continuation, AF needs a critical mass of atrial tissue to allow the spread of multiple waves of depolarization.[76] The maze operation has been developed and refined whereby multiple atrial incisions are made to interrupt abnormal conduction pathways, but maintain a route for sinus impulses from the SA node to pass to the AV node. The procedure achieves maintenance of sinus rhythm at 3 months in >90% of selected patients[77] and freedom from AF for up to 15 years in 75–95%. The major drawback is the requirement for median sternotomy and the use of cardiopulmonary bypass. This has limited its use to patients who are already requiring cardiac surgery for another indication such as valve replacement. Catheter-based approaches have attempted to duplicate the maze procedure without requiring extensive surgery and procedures targeting the left atrium have had more success than those in the right atrium.[49] The potential application of catheter ablation has grown since the detection of ectopic beats originating from pulmonary veins that are capable of instigating AF. Short-term studies have shown success in the mapping and ablation of foci for PAF.[78,79] Refinements need to be made to the localization of foci and choice of energy source used (radiofrequency, laser or cryoablation). The procedure is time consuming; there is a substantial risk of pulmonary vein stenosis, thromboembolism and damage to adjacent structures,[80] but it may prove useful in selected patients with non-permanent AF. With improvements in technology and our understanding of mechanisms of AF, catheter ablation is assuming an increasing role in AF management. Recent meta-analysis found a 77% success rate for catheter ablation versus 52% for anti-arrhythmic therapy.[81]

Nevertheless, the success rates are generally higher in younger patients with relatively normal hearts. Unlike younger patients, factors that initiate and maintain AF in elderly people are not just limited to triggers found within the pulmonary veins, but also within the atrial substrate requiring more extensive ablation and repeat procedures. Currently, most of the elderly population may not benefit from catheter-based techniques. Atrial flutter commonly coexists with AF, but can be more symptomatic than AF. Catheter ablation of atrial flutter, on the other hand, is relatively safer and quicker with high success rates even in the elderly population.

Atrial pacing

It has been reported that atrial (including dual-chamber) pacing has reduced the incidence of AF versus ventricular pacing alone in patients receiving a permanent pacemaker for sick sinus syndrome. Large trials have had conflicting results with reports of reduced incidence of AF[13,15,82] and no reported differences (UKPACE[16]). No trial has yet shown a statistically significant reduction in mortality. Therefore, in those patients receiving a pacemaker for sinus node dysfunction, atrial pacing could be considered to reduce the incidence of AF. This does not translate to AF patients who do not require a pacemaker for another clinical indication. The importance of the site of atrial pacing and multisite atrial pacing is being investigated and may find a future role in patients with symptomatic, drug-refractory AF.[83]

Anticoagulation

A large body of evidence exists for the use of antithrombotic therapy in AF to prevent thromboembolic stroke. Current options for thromboprophylaxis are vitamin K antagonists (VKA) such as adjusted-dose warfarin (INR 2–3) or antiplatelet agents such as aspirin (75–325 mg daily). A recent meta-analysis demonstrated that adjusted-dose warfarin reduced the relative risk of stroke by 64%.[84] Antiplatelet therapy, aspirin being the most commonly studied agent, reduces stroke risk by 22%. Aspirin 75 mg achieves near-complete platelet inhibition and is safer than higher doses in terms of bleeding risk. The benefits are consistent for both primary and secondary prevention.

Adjusted-dose warfarin or aspirin?

A meta-analysis of nine clinical trials comparing VKA and aspirin revealed significant superiority of VKA over aspirin with a relative risk reduction (RRR) of 39%. In the Birmingham Atrial Fibrillation Treatment of the Aged study (BAFTA[85]), VKA (INR 2–3) was superior to aspirin 75 mg daily by 52% in reducing primary endpoints of ischaemic or haemorrhagic strokes or systemic embolism. There was no difference between VKA or aspirin in risk of major haemorrhage.

In the ACTIVE trials, anticoagulation was superior to combined aspirin–clopidogrel (ACTIVE-W, RRR 40%) with no difference in bleeding rates.[86] In the ACTIVE-A study (aspirin–clopidogrel versus aspirin alone), combination therapy reduced the stroke risk by 28% at the expense of a 2% increase in major bleeding events.[87a]

VKA treatment should be considered for all patients with AF or flutter, including elderly patients, with ≥1 stroke risk factors in the absence of contraindications after assessment of risk–benefits and patient preferences. It is important to note that the type of AF does not influence the decision for thromboprophylaxis. The choice between VKA and aspirin (or other antiplatelet drugs) depends on the number of risk factors for thromboembolic events present in a given patient. The $CHADS_2$ scoring system is widely used and serves as a simple tool to guide antithrombotic treatment (1 point each for ***C***ardiac failure, ***H***ypertension, ***A***ge >75 years and ***D***iabetes and 2 points for history of ***S***troke). A score of ≥2 requires use of VKA, with aspirin or VKA for score 1 and aspirin or no antithrombotic therapy for score 0. Age >75 years independently carries a worse prognosis for stroke and mortality over other risk factors. The $CHADS_2$ system can underestimate the stroke risk, placing some patients in the 0–1 category who may significantly benefit from anticoagulation. Recent AF guidelines have addressed this issue and advise a more comprehensive risk-factor-based approach using a modified scoring system (CHA_2DS_2-VASc; see Table 5.5) in patients who score 0–1 on the $CHADS_2$ system (ESC guidelines for AF[18]).

Underuse of warfarin in the elderly population

There is considerable evidence for the underuse of warfarin, especially in elderly people, due to presumed risk of bleeding. In a survey of the prevalence of AF and eligibility for anticoagulation in Newcastle, UK, only 17% of patients aged over 75 years with AF and no irreversible contraindications were receiving warfarin.[88] A prospective study of 1138

Table 5.5 CHA_2DS_2-VASc risk factor-based scoring system.

Risk factor	Score[a]
*C*ongestive cardiac failure	1
*H*ypertension	1
*A*ge >75 years	2
*D*iabetes mellitus	1
*S*troke/TIA/thromboembolism	2
*V*ascular disease (myocardial infarction/peripheral arterial disease/aortic plaques)	1
*A*ge 65–74 years	1
*S*ex category (i.e. female sex)	1

[a]Maximum score 9 as age may score 0, 1 or 2.

stroke patients admitted to a neurology unit observed that only 12% of patients with AF who suffered a recurrent stroke were receiving warfarin prior to their recurrence.[89] An American physicians' survey reported that not only was older age a deterrent to providing anticoagulation, but also a lower intensity of anticoagulation was sought.[90]

Anticoagulation issues in elderly people

Risk of bleeding and warfarin dose

Bleeding risk has inconsistently been associated with increasing age. Recent studies show considerably lower rates of intracranial haemorrhage between 0.1 and 0.6% in the elderly population on anticoagulation maintained on INR 2.0–3.0.[91] While taking warfarin, most episodes of thrombosis occur at INR levels of <2,[92] but intracranial bleeding increases significantly with INR values >3.5–4.0. The SPAF III study[93,94] investigated the efficacy of low-intensity fixed-dose warfarin (INR 1.2–1.5) plus aspirin 325 mg versus adjusted-dose warfarin. The low-dose regimen was associated with a significantly higher incidence of stroke or thromboembolism. The Primary prevention of Arterial Thromboembolism in patients with non-valvular Atrial Fibrillation (PATAF) study[95] showed no difference between aspirin 150 mg, adjusted-dose warfarin and low-dose warfarin, but excluded patients aged over 78 years from the study, so the results cannot be applied to elderly people.

The key hurdle, however, is trying to maintain a patient's INR within the range 2–3. In the SPAF III study, only 61% of INR measurements were in that range.

Practicalities of regular monitoring in elderly people

Standard monitoring of INR has taken place in the haematology-based anticoagulation clinic. Like most hospital outpatient clinics, these can be extremely busy, have inflexibility in appointment times and dates and can represent a significant challenge for the elderly patient. Where difficulties are perceived, this may even influence the decision to anticoagulate a patient with warfarin. This need not be the case and availability and ease of use can be improved by disseminating the responsibility for monitoring into the community. Reliable and portable machines for measuring prothrombin times are available[96] and dose adjustments can be made by general practitioners or non-clinicians such as pharmacists[97] at practices or visiting nursing homes.

Pharmacokinetics of warfarin in elderly patients

Cross-sectional and longitudinal[98] studies have both reported a fall in warfarin dose requirements with increasing age. Conclusive mechanisms are yet to be fully elucidated, but reduced drug clearance will play a role in elderly people. Although this does not influence the achievement of a steady state of anticoagulation, it does affect how the anticoagulation is induced. The commonly used Fennerty regimen[99] was first described in patients with a mean age of 52 years. A low-dose induction regimen has been shown to induce fewer INR measurements >4.5 and spend more time within the therapeutic range for patients aged over 75 years.[100] This was achieved at the expense of an increase in mean time to reach therapeutic INR, which although on average was less than a single day,[100] may present an unacceptable delay in discharge from hospital.

Pharmacodynamics of warfarin in elderly patients

Issues of non-compliance or inconsistencies in consumption of tablets in elderly patients with dementia are a particular concern for warfarin, a drug with considerable individual variation and a narrow therapeutic window where a greater or lesser effect both carry significant risk. In a study of long-term care facilities, those patients with AF who were also diagnosed as having dementia were less likely to receive warfarin.[101] Clearly, dementia can encompass a wide range of degrees of cognitive impairment and no one would argue that in the presence of end-stage dementia the benefits of anticoagulation for AF would outweigh the discomfort and inconvenience of regular monitoring and minor bleeding. However, in the context of multi-infarct dementia, the benefits of anticoagulation to halt the stepwise decline become more apparent. Indeed, a supervised residential facility provides an environment where compliance issues can be managed.

Risks associated with polypharmacy

Numerous interactions have been reported with warfarin. Table 5.6 lists common agents involved, but is not intended as a comprehensive list. The anticoagulant effect will be reduced by foods that are high in vitamin K

Table 5.6 Common medication which interact with warfarin.

System	Potentiate anticoagulation	Decrease anticoagulation
Cardiovascular	Amiodarone, simvastatin, fibrates	Spironolactone
Endocrine	Thyroxine, steroids	
Gastrointestinal	Cimetidine, omeprazole	Cholestyramine
Nervous	Chlorpromazine, tricyclic antidepressants	Barbiturates, carbamazepine
Malignancy	Tamoxifen	
Antimicrobials	Aminoglycosides, metronidazole, clarithromycin	Rifampicin

such as parsley, broccoli and liver. Polypharmacy and the risk of falls have to be considered with sedative medication or postural hypotension secondary to antihypertensives.

Upcoming anticoagulants

Several new oral anticoagulants are being developed which are at least as effective as VKA, with less drug interaction and better pharmacokinetics negating the need for regular INR monitoring. These include direct thrombin inhibitors (e.g. dabigatran) and factor Xa inhibitors (e.g. rivaroxaban, apixaban). In the RE-LY study, dabigatran 110 mg b.i.d. was similar to VKA in stroke prevention with lower bleeding rates. Higher dose of 150 mg b.i.d. further lowered the risk of thromboembolic stroke with similar major bleeding rates to those with VKA.[87b] AVERROES study compared apixaban against aspirin in patients unsuitable for VKA and showed significant reductions in stroke and systemic embolism with an acceptable safety profile.[102]

Non-pharmacological possibilities to prevent stroke

As LAA is the major site for development of atrial thrombus, mechanical occlusion of LAA may reduce the risk of stroke in patients with AF. Catheter-based occlusion of the LAA (WATCHMAN device) in high-risk patients who are unsuitable for VKA showed non-inferiority to VKA, but at higher rates of adverse events, mainly due to procedure-related complications.[103] More evidence is needed to allow the routine use of such devices.

Other supraventricular arrhythmias

As discussed above, the most common supraventricular arrhythmia in elderly people is atrial fibrillation. Paroxysmal atrioventricular nodal reciprocating tachycardia (AVNRT) is more common in the younger age groups than in the elderly population. AVNRT may commonly manifest at later ages in association with coronary disease, perioperatively or chest infection. AVNRT is recognized on the ECG as rapid, narrow, complex tachycardia.

Small, inverted P waves are generally seen superimposed on the terminal portion of the QRS complex. The diagnostic challenge is when a supraventricular tachycardia presents as a broad complex tachycardia due to aberrant conduction from partially blocked right or the left bundle branches, when it will need to be distinguished from a ventricular tachycardia (VT). Both arrhythmias can be asymptomatic or symptomatic and it is safer to assume all broad complex tachycardias to be ventricular in origin until proven otherwise. In general, dissociate atrial and ventricular activity (including fusion or capture beats), concordant QRS pattern in precordial leads, prominent R wave in V1, QRS morphology similar to previously noted ventricular ectopy, electrolyte disturbances and presence of acute myocardial ischaemia favour the diagnosis of VT.

Patients with SVT and haemodynamic instability require urgent DCC. In stable patients, vagal manoeuvres such as carotid massage or the valsalva manoeuvre could terminate the tachycardia, failing which intravenous beta-blockers, non-dihydropyridine calcium channel blockers (verapamil, diltiazem) or adenosine may be necessary. In patients without any history of severe asthma or obstructive airway disease, adenosine is preferred due to its short half-life and rapid onset of action. For long-term management and prevention of future recurrences, the choice generally lies between beta-blockers, verapamil and diltiazem. Amiodarone or sotalol may be considered in selected patients, but increase the risk of systemic side effects or pro-arrhythmia.

Ventricular arrhythmias

Ventricular arrhythmias are common in elderly people and the incidence increases with advancing age and the presence of structural heart disease.[104] A ventricular ectopic beat or premature ventricular contraction (PVC) is a depolarization that originates in the ventricles, has a wide QRS complex and is followed by a normal compensatory pause (Figure 5.8). Three or more consecutively occurring PVCs with a rate in excess of 120 bpm is termed *ventricular tachycardia* (VT). VT is defined as

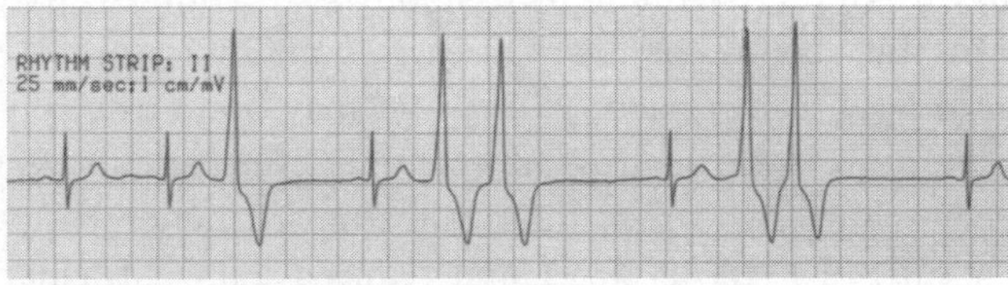

Figure 5.8 Rhythm strip showing single and paired ventricular ectopic beats followed by normal compensatory pauses.

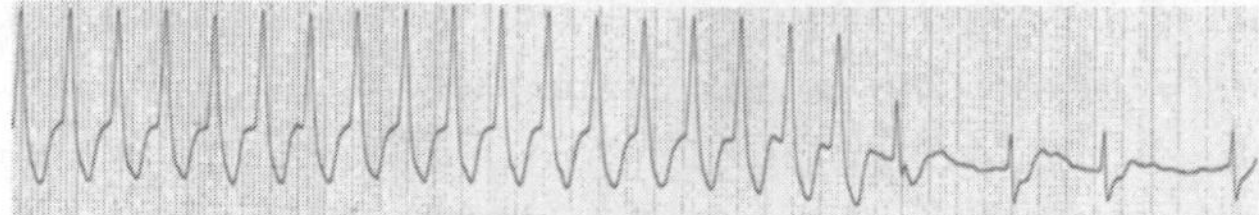

Figure 5.9 Rhythm strip showing non-sustained ventricular tachycardia.

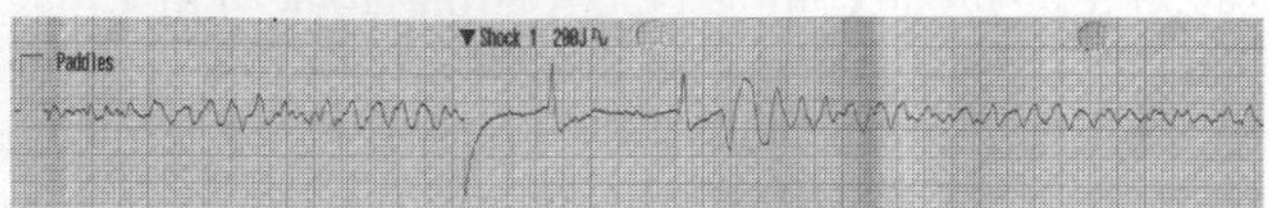

Figure 5.10 Ventricular fibrillation.

non-sustained (NSVT) if lasting <30 s (Figure 5.9) and sustained if lasting >30 s or requiring immediate cardioversion. VT is characterized by an ECG appearance of a broad, complex tachycardia with QRS duration >0.12 s (an important differential to consider is supraventricular tachycardia with aberrant conduction). VT is monomorphic if the QRS morphology remains stable or polymorphic if QRS morphology is variable (e.g. torsades de pointes – polymorphic VT with changing QRS axis). Complex ventricular arrhythmias include VT and paired, multiform or frequent PVCs. Ventricular fibrillation is rapid (>300 bpm), irregular complexes with marked variation in rate, amplitude and morphology (Figure 5.10).

Ventricular arrhythmias can be found in 70–80% of people over 60 years of age. Complex ventricular ectopy is common in elderly people, but many often remain asymptomatic. Incidence of sudden cardiac death (SCD) increases with age and 80% of SCDs from cardiac causes can be attributed to coronary heart disease, other common causes being dilated or hypertrophic cardiomyopathy and valvular heart disease. In the peri-infarction period, age >75 years appears to be independently associated with higher in-hospital cardiac arrest.[105] Channelopathies, such as congenital long QT or Brugada syndromes, are uncommon in the elderly age group.

Prognosis

PVDs and non-sustained VT in the absence of heart disease are not associated with an increase in coronary disease or mortality and do not require treatment with anti-arrhythmic medication.[106] In contrast, polymorphic VT even in the absence of heart disease is an indicator of risk. It is important to note that frequent PVCs or VT may occur as a consequence of electrolyte imbalance or drug adverse effect. In patients who have a history of previous myocardial infarction, the frequency of PVDs (>10 per hour), runs of PVDs or NSVT and reduced left ventricular ejection fraction are all independently associated with new coronary events and mortality.[107,108] Ventricular arrhythmias during first 24–48 h after acute myocardial infarction do not indicate continuing risk. In patients with non-ST elevation myocardial infarction, the long-term risk and mortality are variable and may depend on the extent of initial myocardial damage.

Pathogenesis

For a ventricular tachyarrhythmia to develop, a substrate and a triggering factor are required. The substrate can either be structural (infarcted or hypertrophic myocardium resulting in myocytes of differing refractory periods forming a potential re-entrant circuit) or electrical (the occurrence of early or delayed after-depolarizations). The triggering factor is typically a transient influence such as electrolyte imbalance, acute ischaemia or even an anti-arrhythmic medication, such as in the case of torsades de pointes.

Management

Appropriate management of ventricular arrhythmias requires not only knowledge of aetiology and mechanism of the arrhythmia, but also an understanding of other associated medical problems and the risk–benefit profile of any anti-arrhythmic therapy. The presence of reversible precipitants needs to be excluded. Treatment of heart failure, myocardial ischaemia, drug toxicity, electrolyte imbalance (e.g. hypo- or hyperkalaemia, hypomagnesaemia) can abolish or reduce the occurrences of ventricular arrhythmias. Investigations include serum electrolyte levels, 12-lead or ambulatory ECG monitoring, exercise testing to exclude cardiac ischaemia or to diagnose exercise-related arrhythmias, cardiac catheterization, echocardiography or other forms of imaging (MRI, perfusion scans) and electrophysiological testing.

The ultimate aim should be to prevent such an arrhythmia occurring in the first instance. Overall management of ventricular arrhythmias in elderly people does not differ from that recommended for the general population, but necessitates taking into account other factors such as involvement of other organ systems, presence of other comorbidities and physiological changes that occur with advancing age. These factors strongly influence the choice and appropriateness of any pharmacological or non-pharmacological management.

Drug therapy

With the exception of beta-blockers, currently available anti-arrhythmic drugs have not shown any prognostic benefit in the management of complex ventricular arrhythmias or prevention of SCD. As a general rule, anti-arrhythmic drugs are recommended as adjunctive therapy to beta-blockers due to potential pro-arrhythmic or systemic side effects. There is increased susceptibility to adverse cardiac events with advancing age, particularly in relation to class Ic anti-arrhythmic drugs (e.g. flecainide;

Vaughan Williams classification). Sotalol is less frequently used in elderly patients due to a propensity towards pro-arrhythmia by increasing the QT interval, especially in the presence of electrolyte imbalance or other major organ involvement. Treatment with flecainide[109] or d-sotalol,[110] despite successfully suppressing PVDs, both agents lead to an increased mortality in patients after myocardial infarction as compared with placebo. In survivors of cardiac arrest, amiodarone may improve prognosis.[111] A meta-analysis of 13 randomized controlled trials of prophylactic amiodarone in patients with recent myocardial infarction or congestive heart failure demonstrated a statistically significant relative risk reduction of 29% in arrhythmic/sudden death.[112] A relative risk reduction in total mortality of 13–15% was marginal, but importantly there was no increase in non-arrhythmic deaths. However, two large primary prevention trials of amiodarone post-myocardial infarction both demonstrated reductions in arrhythmic deaths, but had no effect on total mortality,[113,114] raising concerns that reductions in fatal arrhythmias are offset by increased mortality from other causes. In the Sudden Cardiac Death in Heart Failure Trial (SCD-HeFT),[115] a primary prevention study comparing placebo, amiodarone and implantable cardioverter defibrillator (ICD) in patients with NYHA functional class II or III and left ventricular ejection fraction (EF) <35%, amiodarone failed to show reduction in all-cause mortality compared with placebo.

Therefore, amiodarone, with which there is considerable clinical experience in the treatment of ventricular tachycardia, is useful in preventing arrhythmic deaths and is safe in the context of ischaemia and heart failure, but the beneficial effect on total mortality appears to be small with too little evidence to justify its routine prophylactic use.[116]

Amiodarone is associated with many side effects, particularly in elderly patients who are already on multiple drug therapy, increasing the risk of drug interaction. Systemic side effects of amiodarone include thyroid and liver dysfunction, skin sensitivity and corneal deposits.

Beta-blockers remain the mainstay of treating ventricular arrhythmias and, either alone or in combination with non-arrhythmic agents (ACE inhibitors, angiotensin receptor blockers, statins), have consistently been shown to reduce SCD and all-cause mortality in patients with heart failure or after myocardial infarction in all age groups, including the elderly population. There is also some evidence that omega-3 polyunsaturated fatty acids and statins may have anti-arrhythmic properties of their own due to a membrane-stabilizing effect.

Despite the proven efficacy of beta-blockers, these agents remain underused in the elderly population with an independent negative association with age. A retrospective analysis on use of beta-blockers after myocardial infarction in patients >65 years of age found that only 21% of 3737 patients received beta-blockers despite the absence of any contraindications. The study also found 43% lower 2-year mortality in those who had received beta-blockers.[117]

Role of implantable cardioverter defibrillator

Beyond medication, the ICD has now emerged as the most effective therapy for primary and secondary prevention of fatal ventricular tachyarrhythmias (Figures 5.11 and 5.12). The addition of an antitachycardia pacing facility can effectively terminate some tachyarrhythmias prior to shock delivery. The primary prevention Multicenter Automatic Defibrillator Implantation Trial (MADIT)[118] and Multicenter Unsustained Tachycardia Trial (MUSTT)[119] studies have both demonstrated statistically significant reductions in overall mortality as compared to anti-arrhythmic medication in patients with previous myocardial infarction (MI), reduced LV ejection fraction and non-sustained VT who were referred for electrophysiological studies (EPS). The subsequent MADIT 2 study[120] enrolled patients with prior MI and ejection fraction <30% with no requirement for the occurrence of ventricular arrhythmia or need for EPS. There was a statistically significant reduction in overall mortality as compared to conventional medical therapy alone, which persisted for both sexes in all age groups in subgroup analysis.

Two major trials have now defined the role of ICD therapy for primary prevention in patients with dilated cardiomyopathy (DCM). The SCD-HeFT consisted of 2521 patients with a mean age of 60 years. It included patients with ischaemic DCM, no history of prior sustained VT or VF, left ventricular ejection fraction <35% and NYHA functional class II

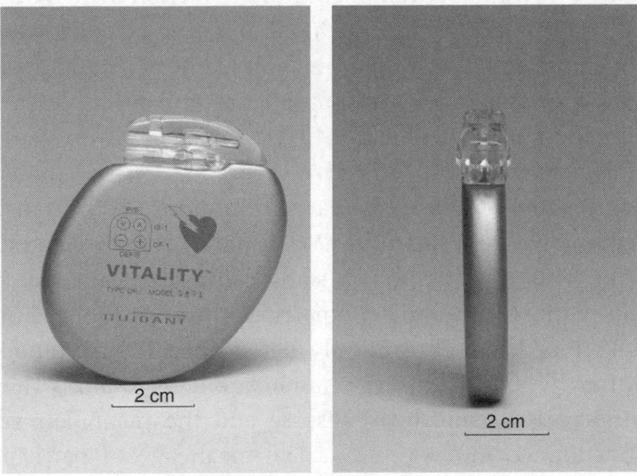

Figure 5.11 Implantable cardioverter defibrillator.

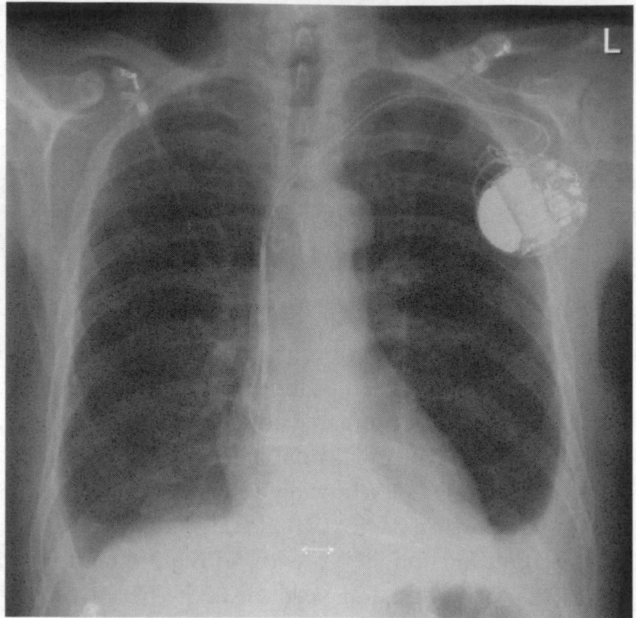

Figure 5.12 Chest X-ray of a patient with an ICD (atrial and ventricular leads).

or III on optimal medical therapy with ACE inhibitor and beta-blocker use. ICD therapy was associated with a statistically significant reduction in all-cause mortality compared with best medical therapy alone or in combination with amiodarone.[115] The Defibrillators in Nonischaemic Cardiomyopathy Treatment Evaluation (DEFINITE) consisted of patients with non-ischaemic DCM on optimal heart failure medication including ACE inhibitor and beta-blocker, but not on amiodarone therapy. ICD therapy was associated with a statistically significant reduction in arrhythmic death compared with best medical therapy alone, but only a trend towards reduction in all-cause mortality. Based on these data, ICD therapy should be considered on an individual basis for patients with severe left ventricular dysfunction and non-ischaemic DCM.[121]

There have been three prospective randomized trials comparing ICD therapy with medication for secondary prevention. The Anti-arrhythmics Versus Implantable Defibrillators (AVID) trial[122] was the largest of these and was the only one to show a statistically significant risk reduction in mortality with ICD therapy compared with medication. Patients with episodes of VF or haemodynamically significant VT were randomized to ICD or anti-arrhythmic medication (amiodarone or sotalol). The majority of patients had ischaemic heart disease and the mean left ventricular ejection fraction (LVEF) was 32%. The mean age of participants was 65 years, but subgroup analysis showed no difference in outcome for those aged over 70 years. The Canadian Implantable Defibrillator Study (CIDS) trial[123] included patients with syncope probably secondary to VT and compared ICD therapy with amiodarone. In a multivariate analysis of CIDS,[124] the patients at highest risk of cardiovascular death (age ≥70 years, LVEF ≤35% and NYHA class III or IV) were found to benefit the most from ICD therapy. The Cardiac Arrest Study Hamburg (CASH) trial[125] also had metoprolol and propafenone treatment limbs. The propafenone limb was stopped early because of excess mortality. A meta-analysis of these trials concluded a 28% relative reduction in death with ICD therapy in patients with LVEF of <35%.[126]

Implantable cardioverter defibrillators in elderly people

All major ICD trials have included a substantial number of patients >65 years of age. Subgroup analyses of these trials show equivalent benefit from ICD between younger and elderly populations and it is appropriate to consider ICD implantation irrespective of the age. Nevertheless, ICD remains an invasive treatment that may not be suitable for all. There are sparse data on the procedure-related morbidity in elderly patients. As previously discussed in the section on AF, very elderly people can present additional challenges that have to be taken into account when analysing the risk versus benefits for any given therapy. Regular follow-up at a tertiary centre clinic is vital to ensure that the device continues to function effectively and safely. Appropriate and inappropriate shocks may prove intolerable for some patients and an ICD would be unsuitable for those with significant dementia or other major comorbidities with a projected lifespan of <1 year. Any reduction in medication will be beneficial in elderly people, but anti-arrhythmics may still be required in some patients to reduce the burden of arrhythmia and hence the shock frequency. Further studies will have to be undertaken to help further risk stratify elderly patients and identify those most likely to benefit from an ICD, but age alone is not a contraindication for this therapy. There are widening indications for implantation of ICD and selected elderly patients can gain significantly from the treatment.

Key points

- Arrhythmias are common in elderly people.
- The heart is subject to both ageing and disease-related changes that predispose to arrhythmia generation and persistence.
- Atrial fibrillation is the most common sustained arrhythmia in elderly people and carries a substantial risk of morbidity and mortality from thromboembolic stroke.

- Presence or absence of non-cardiac comorbidities in elderly people play a major role, not only in the genesis of arrhythmias, but also in their specific management based on assessment of risks versus benefits for each individual patient.

References

1 Umetani K, Singer DH, McCraty R and Atkinson M. Twenty-four hour time domain heart rate variability and heart rate: relations to age and gender over nine decades. *J Am Coll Cardiol* 1998;**31**:593–601.

2 Spodick DH, Raju P, Bishop RL and Rifkin RD. Operational definition of normal sinus heart rate. *Am J Cardiol* 1992;**69**:1245–6.

3 Manolio TA, Furberg CD, Rautaharju PM *et al.* Cardiac arrhythmias on 24-h ambulatory electrocardiography in older women and men: The Cardiovascular Health Study. *J Am Coll Cardiol* 1994;**23**:916–25.

4 Camm AJ, Katritsis D and Ward DE. (1994) Clinical electrocardiography and electrophysiology in the elderly, in *Geriatric Cardiology Principles and Practice* (eds A Martin and AJ Camm), John Wiley & Sons, Ltd, Chichester, pp. 131–58.

5 Brignole M. Sick sinus syndrome. *Clin Geriatr Med* 2002;**18**:211–27.

6 Epstein AE, DiMarco JP, Ellenbogen KA *et al.* ACC/AHA/HRS 2008 Guidelines for Device-Based Therapy of Cardiac Rhythm Abnormalities. A Report of the American College of Cardiology/American Heart Association Task Force on Practice Guidelines. *Circulation* 2008;**117**:e350–408.

7 Mymin D, Mathewson FAL, Tate RB and Manfreda J. The natural history of primary first degree atrioventricular block. *N Engl J Med* 1986;**315**:1183–87.

8 Serge Barold S. Indications for permanent cardiac pacing in first degree AV block: class I, II or III? *Pacing Clin Electrophysiol* 1996;**19**:747–51.

9 Healey JS, Toff WD, Lamas GA *et al.* Cardiovascular outcomes with atrial-based pacing compared with ventricular pacing: meta-analysis of randomised trials using individual patient data. *Circulation* 2006;**114**:11–7.

10 Sulke N, Chambers J, Dritsas A *et al.* A randomised, double-blind cross-over comparison of four rate-responsive pacing modes. *J Am Coll Cardiol* 1991;**17**:696–706.

11 Ouali S, Neffeti E, Ghoul K *et al.* DDD versus VVIR pacing in patients, ages 70 and over, with complete heart block. *Pacing Clin Electrophysiol* 2010;**33**:583–9.

12 Kiviniemi MS, Pirnes MA, Eranen HJK *et al.* Complications related to permanent pacemaker therapy. *Pacing Clin Electrophysiol* 1999;**22**:711–20.

13 Connolly SJ, Kerr CR, Gent M *et al.* Effects of physiologic pacing versus ventricular pacing on the risk of stroke and death due to cardiovascular causes. *N Engl J Med* 2000;**342**:1385–91.

14 Kerr CR, Connolly SJ, Abdollah H *et al.* Canadian trial of physiologic pacing: effects of physiologic pacing during long-term follow-up. *Circulation* 2004;**109**:357–62.

15 Lamas GA, Lee KL, Sweeney MO *et al.* Ventricular or dual chamber pacing for sinus node dysfunction. *N Engl J Med* 2002;**346**:1854–62.

16 Lamas GA, Orav EJ, Stambler BS *et al.* Quality of life and clinical outcomes in elderly patients treated with ventricular pacing as compared with dual-chamber pacing. *N Engl J Med* 1998;**338**:1097–104.

17 Biblo LA, Yuan Z, Quan KJ *et al.* Risk of stroke in patients with atrial flutter. *Am J Cardiol* 2001;**87**:346–9.

18 Camm AJ, Krichhof P, Lip GY *et al.* Guidelines for the management of atrial fibrillation. The Task Force for the Management of Atrial Fibrillation of the European Society of Cardiology. *Eur Heart J* 2010;**31**:2369–429.

19 Heeringa J, van der Kuip DA, Hofman A *et al.* Prevalence, incidence and lifetime risk of developing atrial fibrillation: The Rotterdam Study. *Eur Heart J* 2006;**27**:949–53.

20 Majeed A, Moser K and Carroll K. Trends in the prevalence and management of atrial fibrillation in general practice in England and Wales 1994–1998: analysis of data from the general practice research database. *Heart* 2001;**86**:284–8.

21 Naccarelli GV, Varker H, Lin J *et al.* Increasing prevalence of atrial fibrillation and flutter in the United States. *Am J Cardiol* 2009;**104**:1534–39.

22 Camm AJ. Atrial fibrillation in the elderly – a near epidemic. *Am J Geriatr Cardiol* 2002;**11**:352.

23 Stewart S, Murphy N, Walker A *et al.* Cost of an emerging epidemic: an economic analysis of AF in the UK. *Heart* 2004;**90**:286–92.

24 Nabauer M, Gerth A, Limbourg T *et al.* The registry of the German competence NET work on atrial fibrillation: patient characteristics and initial management. *Europace* 2009;**11**:423–34.

25 Wolf PA, Dawber TR, Thomas HE Jr, *et al.* Epidemiologic assessment of chronic AF and risk of stroke: The Framingham Study. *Neurology* 1978;**28**:973–7.

26 Kannel WB, Abbott RD, Savage DD and McNamara PM. Epidemiologic features of chronic atrial fibrillation. The Framingham Study. *N Engl J Med* 1982;**306**:1018–22.

27 Hylek EM, Go AS, Chang Y *et al.* Effect of intensity of oral anticoagulation on stroke severity and mortality in atrial fibrillation. *N Engl J Med* 2003;**349**:1019–26.

28 Wijffels MCEF, Kirchhof CJHJ, Dorland R and Allessie MA. Atrial fibrillation begets atrial fibrillation: a study in awake chronically instrumented goats. *Circulation* 1995;**92**:1954–68.

29 Upshaw CB. Haemodynamic changes after cardioversion of chronic atrial fibrillation. *Arch Intern Med* 1997;**157**:1070–6.

30 Wolf PA, Abbott RD and Kannel WB. Atrial fibrillation: a major contributor to stroke in the elderly. The Framingham Study. *Arch Intern Med* 1987;**147**:1561–4.

31 Ezekowitz MD, James KE, Nazarian SM *et al.* Silent cerebral infarction in patients with non-rheumatic atrial fibrillation. *Circulation* 1995;**92**:2178–82.

32 Feinberg WM, Seeger JF, Carmody RF *et al.* Epidemiologic features of asymptomatic cerebral infarction in patients with non-valvular atrial fibrillation. *Arch Intern Med* 1990;**150**:2340–44.

33 Petersen P, Madson EB, Brun B *et al.* Silent cerebral infarction in chronic atrial fibrillation. *Stroke* 1987;**18**:1098–100.

34 Lin HJ, Wolf PA, Kelly-Hayes M *et al.* Stroke severity in AF. The Framingham Study. *Stroke* 1996;**27**:1760–64.

35 Hart RG, Pearce LA, Rothbart RM *et al.* Stroke with intermittent AF: incidence and predictors during aspirin therapy. *J Am College Cardiol* 2000;**35**:183–87.

36 Friberg L, Hammar N and Rosenqvist M. Stroke in paroxysmal atrial fibrillation: report from the Stockholm Cohort of Atrial Fibrillation. *Eur Heart J* 2010;**31**:967–75.

37 Atrial Fibrillation Investigators. Risk factors for stroke and efficacy of antithrombotic therapy in atrial fibrillation. Analysis of pooled data from five randomised controlled trials. *Arch Intern Med* 1994;**154**:1449–57.

38 Atrial Fibrillation Investigators. Echocardiographic predictors of stroke in patients with atrial fibrillation. *Arch Intern Med* 1998;**158**:1316–20.

39 Stroke Prevention in Atrial Fibrillation Investigators. Predictors of thromboembolism in atrial fibrillation: II. Echocardiographic features of patients at risk. *Ann Intern Med* 1992;**116**:6–12.

40 Stroke Prevention in Atrial Fibrillation Investigators Committee on Echocardiography. Transesophageal echocardiographic correlates of thromboembolism in high-risk patients with nonvalvular atrial fibrillation. *Ann Intern Med* 1998;**128**:639–47.

41 Fitzmaurice DA, Hobbs FDR, Jowett J *et al.* Screening versus routine practice in detection of atrial fibrillation in patients aged 65 or over; cluster randomised controlled trial. *BMJ* 2007;**335**:383–6.

42 Hohnloser SH, Kuck KH, Lilienthal J and the PIAF Investigators. Rhythm or rate control in atrial fibrillation – pharmacological intervention in atrial fibrillation (PIAF): a randomised trial. *Lancet* 2000;**356**:1789–94.

43 Wyse DG, Waldo AL, DiMarco JP *et al.* A comparison of rate control and rhythm control in patients with atrial fibrillation. *N Engl J Med* 2002;**347**:1825–33.

44 Van Gelder IC, Hagens VE, Bosker HA *et al.* A comparison of rate control and rhythm control in patients with recurrent persistent atrial fibrillation. *N Engl J Med* 2002;**347**:1834–40.

45 Carlsson J, Miketic S, Windeler J *et al.* Randomised trial of rate-control versus rhythm-control in persistent atrial fibrillation: the Strategies of Treatment of Atrial Fibrillation (STAF) study. *J Am Coll Cardiol* 2003;**41**:1073–76.

46 Opolski G, Torbicki A, Kosior DA *et al.* Rate control versus rhythm control in patients with nonvalvular persistent atrial fibrillation: results of the Polish How to Treat Chronic Atrial Fibrillation (HOT-CAFE) Study. *Chest* 2004;**126**:476–86.

47 Roy D, Talajic M, Nattel S *et al.* Rhythm control versus rate control for atrial fibrillation and heart failure. *N Engl J Med* 2008;**358**:2667–77.

48 Falk RH. Ventricular rate control in the elderly: is digoxin enough? *Am J Geriatr Cardiol* 2002;**11**:353–6.

49 Fuster V, Ryden LE, Asinger RW *et al.* ACC/AHA Practice Guidelines. ACC/AHA/ESC Guidelines for the Management of Patients with Atrial Fibrillation. Executive Summary. *Circulation* 2001;**104**:2118–50.

50 Van Gelder IC, Groenveld HF, Crijns HJ *et al.* Lenient versus strict rate control in patients with atrial fibrillation. *N Engl J Med* 2010;**362**:1363–73.

51 Dayer M and Hardman SMC. Special problems with antiarrhythmic drugs in the elderly: safety, tolerability and efficacy. *Am J Geriatr Cardiol* 2002;**11**:370–5, 379.

52 Digitalis Investigation Group. The effect of digoxin on mortality and morbidity in patients with heart failure. *N Engl J Med* 1997;**336**:5233–55.

53 Murgatroyd FD, Gibson SM, Baiyan X *et al.* Double-blind placebo-controlled trial of digoxin in symptomatic paroxysmal atrial fibrillation. *Circulation* 1999;**99**:2765–70.

54 Sticherling C, Oral H, Horrocks J *et al.* Effects of digoxin on acute, atrial fibrillation-induced changes in atrial refractoriness. *Circulation* 2000;**102**:2503–8.

55 Falk RH, Knowlton AA, Bernard SA *et al.* Digoxin for converting recent onset AF to sinus rhythm. A randomised double blind trial. *Ann Intern Med* 1987;**106**:503–6.

56 Digitalis in Acute AF (DAAF) Trial Group. Intravenous digoxin in acute atrial fibrillation. Results of a randomised, placebo controlled multicenter trial in 239 patients. *Eur Heart J* 1997;**18**:649–54.

57 Atwood JE, Sullivan M, Forbes S *et al.* Effect of beta-adrenergic blockade on exercise performance in patients with chronic atrial fibrillation. *J Am Coll Cardiol* 1987;**10**:314–20.

58 Atwood JE, Myers J, Quaglietti S *et al.* Effect of betaxolol on the hemodynamic, gas exchange and cardiac output response to exercise in chronic atrial fibrillation. *Chest* 1999;**115**:1175–80.

59 Galve E, Rius T, Ballester R *et al.* Intravenous amiodarone in treatment of recent-onset atrial fibrillation: Results of a randomised, controlled study. *J Am Coll Cardiol* 1996;**27**:1079–82.

60 Singh BN, Connolly SJ, Crijns HJ *et al.* Dronedarone for maintenance of sinus rhythm in atrial fibrillation or flutter. *N Engl J Med* 2007;**357**:987–99.

61 Karralliedde L and Henry JA. (1998) *Handbook of Drug Interactions*, 1st edn, Arnold, London.

62 Elkayam U, Parikh K, Torkan B *et al.* Effect of diltiazem on renal clearance and serum concentration of digoxin in patients with cardiac disease. *Am J Cardiol* 1985;**55**:1393–95.

63 Marshall HJ and Gamage MD. Indications and nonindications for ablation of atrioventricular conduction in the elderly: is it sensible to destroy normal tissue? *Am J Geriatr Cardiol* 2002;**11**:365–9.

64 Weigner MJ, Caulfield TA, Danias PG *et al.* Risk for clinical thromboembolism associated with conversion to sinus rhythm in patients with atrial fibrillation lasting less than 48 hours. *Ann Intern Med* 1997;**126**:615–20.

65 Berger M and Schweitzer P. Timing of thromboembolic events after electrical cardioversion of atrial fibrillation or flutter: a retrospective analysis. *Am J Cardiol* 1998;**82**:1545–7.

66 Collins LJ, Silverman DI, Douglas PS and Manning WJ. Cardioversion of non-rheumatic atrial fibrillation. Reduced thromboembolic complications with four weeks of precardioversion anticoagulation are related to atrial thrombus resolution. *Circulation* 1995;**92**:160–3.

67 Klein AL, Grimm RA, Murray RD *et al.* Use of transesophageal echo-cardiography to guide cardioversion in patients with atrial fibrillation. *N Engl J Med* 2001; **344**:1411–20.

68 Seto TB, Taira DA, Tsevat J and Manning WJ. Cost-effectiveness of transesophageal echocardiographic-guided cardioversion: a decision analytical model for patients admitted to the hospital with atrial fibrillation. *J Am Coll Cardiol* 1997;**29**:122–30.

69 Levy S, Breithardt G, Campbell RWF *et al.* Atrial fibrillation: current knowledge and recommendation for management. *Eur Heart J* 1998;**19**:1294–320.

70 Van Gelder IC, Crijns HJ, Tieleman RG *et al.* Chronic atrial fibrillation. Success of serial cardioversion therapy and safety of oral anticoagulation. *Arch Intern Med* 1996;**156**:2585–92.

71 Singh BN, Singh SN, Reda DJ *et al.* Amiodarone versus sotalol for atrial fibrillation. *N Engl J Med* 2005;**352**;1861–72.

72 Akiyama T, Pawitan Y, Greenberg H *et al.* Increased risk of death and cardiac arrest from encainide and flecainide in patients after non-Q-wave acute myocardial infarction in the Cardiac Arrhythmia Suppression Trial. *Am J Cardiol* 1991;**68**:1551–5.

73 Hohnloser SH, Crijns HJ, van Eickels M *et al.* Effect of dronedarone on cardiovascular events in atrial fibrillation. *N Engl J Med* 2009;**360**:668–78.

74 Le Heuzey J, De Ferrari GM, Radzik D *et al.* A short-term, randomised, double-blind parallel-group study to evaluate the efficacy and safety of dronedarone versus amiodarone in patients with persistent atrial fibrillation: the DIONYSOS study. *J Cardiovasc Electrophysiol* 2010;**21**:597–605.

75 Kober L, Torp-Pedersen C, McMurray JJ *et al.* Increased mortality after dronedarone therapy for severe heart failure. *N Engl J Med* 2008;**358**:2678–87.

76 Lairikyengbam SKS, Anderson MH and Davies AG. Present treatment options for atrial fibrillation. *Postgrad Med J* 2003;**79**:67–73.

77 Cox JL, Schuessler RB, Lappas DG *et al.* An 8 $^{1}/_{2}$ year experience with surgery for atrial fibrillation. *Ann Surg* 1996;**224**:267–75.

78 Haissaguerre M, Jais P, Shah DC *et al.* Spontaneous initiation of atrial fibrillation by ectopic beats originating in the pulmonary veins. *N Engl J Med* 1998;**339**:659–66.
79 Chen SA, Hsieh MH, Tai CT *et al.* Initiation of atrial fibrillation by ectopic beats originating from the pulmonary veins. Electrophysiological characteristics, pharmacological responses and effects of radiofrequency ablation. *Circulation* 1999;**100**:1879–86.
80 Wellens HJ. Pulmonary vein ablation in atrial fibrillation: hype or hope? *Circulation* 2000;**102**:2562–4.
81 Calkins H, Reynolds MR, Spector P *et al.* Treatment of atrial fibrillation with antiarrhythmic drugs or radiofrequency ablation: two systemic literature reviews and meta-analyses. *Circ Arrhythm Electrolphysiol* 2009;**2**:349–61.
82 Andersen HR, Nielsen JC, Thomsen PEB *et al.* Long-term follow-up of patients from a randomised trial of atrial versus ventricular pacing for sick sinus syndrome. *Lancet* 1997;**350**:1210–6.
83 Savelieva I and Camm AJ. Atrial pacing for the prevention and termination of atrial fibrillation. *Am J Geriatr Cardiol* 2002;**11**:380–98.
84 Hart RG, Pearce LA and Aguilar MI. Meta-analysis; antithrombotic therapy to prevent stroke in patients who have non-valvular atrial fibrillation. *Ann Intern Med* 2007;**146**:857–67.
85 Mant J, Hobbs FD, Fletcher K *et al.* Warfarin versus aspirin for stroke prevention in an elderly community population with atrial fibrillation (the Birmingham Atrial Fibrillation Treatment of the Aged study, BAFTA): a randomised-controlled trial. *Lancet* 2007;**370**;493–503.
86 Connolly SJ, Pogue J, Hart R *et al.* Clopidogrel plus aspirin versus anticoagulation for atrial fibrillation in the Atrial Fibrillation Clopidogrel Trial with Irbesartan for Prevention of Vascular Events (ACTIVE W): a randomised-controlled trial. *Lancet* 2006;**367**;1903–12.
87 (a) Connolly SJ, Pogue J, Hart R *et al.* Effect of clopidogrel added to aspirin in patients with atrial fibrillation. *N Engl J Med* 2009;360:2066–78; (b) Connolly SJ, Ezekiwitz MD, Yusuf S *et al.* Dabigatran versus warfarin in patients with atrial fibrillation. *N Engl J Med* 2009;**361**:1139–51.
88 Sudlow M, Thomson R, Thwaites B *et al.* Prevalence of atrial fibrillation and eligibility for anticoagulants in the community. *Lancet* 1998;**352**:1167–71.
89 Jorgensen HS, Nakayama H, Reith J *et al.* Stroke recurrence: predictors, severity and prognosis. The Copenhagen stroke study. *Neurology* 1997;**48**:891–5.
90 McCrory DC, Matchar DB, Samsa G *et al.* Physician attitudes about anticoagulation for nonvalvular atrial fibrillation in the elderly. *Arch Intern Med* 1995;**155**:277–81.
91 Palareti G, Hirsh J, Legnani C *et al.* Oral anticoagulation treatment in the elderly. *Arch Intern Med* 2000;**160**:470–8.
92 Hylek EM, Skates SI, Sheehan MA *et al.* An analysis of the lowest effective intensity of prophylactic anticoagulation for patients with non-rheumatic atrial fibrillation. *N Engl J Med* 1996;**335**:540–6.
93 SPAF Investigators. Adjusted-dose warfarin versus low-intensity, fixed-dose warfarin plus aspirin for high-risk patients with atrial fibrillation: Stroke Prevention in Atrial Fibrillation III randomised clinical trial. *Lancet* 1996;**348**:633–8.
94 SPAF Investigators. Bleeding during antithrombotic therapy in patients with atrial fibrillation. *Arch Intern Med* 1996;**156**:409–16.
95 Hellemons BS, Langenberg M, Lodder J *et al.* Primary prevention of arterial thromboembolism in patients with nonrheumatic atrial fibrillation in general practice (the PATAF study). *Cerebrovasc Dis* 1997;**7**(Suppl. 4):11 [abstract].

96 Fitzmaurice DA and Machin SJ. Recommendations for patients undertaking self-management of oral anticoagulation. *BMJ* 2001;**323**:985–9.

97 Chenella FC, Klotz TA, Gill MA *et al*. Comparison of physician and pharmacist management of anticoagulant therapy of inpatients. *Am J Hosp Pharm* 1983;**40**:1642–5.

98 Wynne HA, Kamali F, Edwards C *et al*. Effect of ageing upon warfarin dose requirements: a longitudinal study. *Age and Ageing* 1996;**25**:429–31.

99 Fennerty A, Dolben J, Thomas P *et al*. Flexible induction dose regimen for warfarin and prediction of maintenance dose. *BMJ* 1984;**288**:1268–70.

100 Gedge J, Orme S, Hampton KK *et al*. A comparison of a low-dose warfarin induction regimen with the modified Fennerty regimen in elderly inpatients. *Age and Ageing* 2000;**29**:31–4.

101 Gurwitz JH, Monette J, Rochon PA *et al*. Atrial fibrillation and stroke prevention with warfarin in the long-term care setting. *Arch Intern Med* 1997;**157**:978–84.

102 Connolly SJ, Eikelboom J, Joyner C *et al*. Apixaban in atrial fibrillation. *N Engl J Med* 2011;**364**:806–17.

103 Holmes DR, Reddy VK, Turi ZG *et al*. Percutaneous closure of left atrial appendage versus warfarin therapy for prevention of stroke in patients with atrial fibrillation: a randomised non-inferiority trial. *Lancet* 2009;**374**:534–42.

104 Zipes DP, Camm AJ, Borggrefe M *et al*. ACC/AHA/ESC 2006 Guidelines for Management of Patients with Ventricular Arrhythmias and Prevention of Sudden Cardiac Death. *Europace* 2006;**8**:746–837.

105 Ornato JP, Peberdy MA, Tadler SC *et al*. Factors associated with occurrence of cardiac arrest during hospitalization for acute myocardial infarction in the second national registry of myocardial infarction in the U.S. *Resuscitation* 2001;**48**:117–23.

106 Aronow WS. Management of atrial fibrillation, ventricular arrhythmias and pacemakers in older persons. *J Am Geriatr Soc* 1999;**47**:886–95.

107 Bigger JT, Fleiss JL, Kleiger R *et al*. The relationships among ventricular arrhythmias, left ventricular dysfunction and mortality in the 2 years after myocardial infarction. *Circulation* 1984;**69**:250–8.

108 Maggioni AP, Zuanetti G, Franzosi MG *et al*. Prevalence and prognostic significance of ventricular arrhythmias after acute myocardial infarction in the fibrinolytic era. *Circulation* 1993;**87**:312–22.

109 Cardiac Arrhythmia Suppression Trial (CAST) Investigators. Preliminary report: effect of encainide and flecainide on mortality in a randomised trial of arrhythmia suppression after myocardial infarction. *N Engl J Med* 1989;**321**:406–12.

110 Waldo A, Camm AJ, deRuyter H *et al*. The SWORD Investigators. Effect of d-sotalol on mortality in patients with left ventricular dysfunction after recent and remote myocardial infarction. *Lancet* 1996;**348**:7–12.

111 Sim I, McDonald KM, Lavori PW *et al*. Quantitative overview of randomised trials of amiodarone to prevent sudden cardiac death. *Circulation* 1997;**96**:2823–9.

112 Amiodarone Trials Meta-Analysis (ATMA) Investigators. Effect of prophylactic amiodarone on mortality after acute myocardial infarction and in congestive heart failure: meta-analysis of individual data from 6500 patients in randomised trials. *Lancet* 1997;**350**:1417–24.

113 Cairns JA, Connolly SJ, Robert R and Gent M. Randomised trial of outcome after myocardial infarction in patients with frequent or repetitive ventricular premature depolarisations: CAMIAT. *Lancet* 1997;**349**:675–82.

114 Julian DG, Camm AJ, Frangin G *et al*. Randomised trial effect of amiodarone on mortality in patients with left-ventricular dysfunction after recent myocardial infarction: EMIAT. *Lancet* 1997;**349**:667–74.

115 Bardy GH, Lee KL, Mark DB *et al.* Amiodarone or implantable cardioverter defibrillator for congestive heart failure. Sudden Cardiac Death in Heart Failure Trial (SCD-HeFT) study. *N Engl J Med* 2005;**352**:225–37.

116 Connolly SJ. Evidence-based analysis of amiodarone efficacy and safety. *Circulation* 1999;**100**:2025–34.

117 Soumerai SB, McLaughlin TJ, Spiegelman D *et al.* Adverse outcomes of underuse of β-blockers in elderly survivors of acute myocardial infarction. *JAMA* 1997;**277**:115–21.

118 Moss AJ, Hall WJ, Cannom DS *et al.* Improved survival with an implanted defibrillator in patients with coronary disease at high-risk for ventricular arrhythmia. *N Engl J Med* 1996;**335**:1933–40.

119 Buxton AE, Lee KL, Fisher JD *et al.* A randomised study of the prevention of sudden death in patients with coronary artery disease. *N Engl J Med* 1999;**341**:1882–90.

120 Moss AJ, Zareba W, Hall WJ *et al.* Prophylactic implantation of a defibrillator in patients with myocardial infarction and reduced ejection fraction. *N Engl J Med* 2002;**346**:877–83.

121 Kadish A, Dyer A, Daubert JP *et al.* Prophylactic defibrillator implantation in patients with nonischaemic dilated cardiomyopathy. *N Engl J Med* 2004;**350**:2151–8.

122 AVID Investigators. A comparison of antiarrhythmic drug therapy with implantable defibrillators in patients resuscitated from near-fatal ventricular arrhythmias. *N Engl J Med* 1997;**337**:1576–83.

123 Connolly SJ, Gent M, Roberts RS *et al.* A randomised trial of the implantable cardioverter defibrillator against amiodarone. *Circulation* 2000;**101**:1297–302.

124 Sheldon R, Connolly S, Krahn A *et al.* Identification of patients most likely to benefit from implantable cardioverter defibrillator therapy. The Canadian Implantable Defibrillator Study. *Circulation* 2000;**101**:1660–4.

125 Kuck KH, Cappato R, Siebels J and Ruppel R. Randomised comparison of antiarrhythmic drug therapy with implantable defibrillators in patients resuscitated from cardiac arrest: the Cardiac Arrest Study Hamburg (CASH). *Circulation* 2000;**102**:748–54.

126 Connolly SJ, Hallstrom AP, Cappato R *et al.* Meta-analysis of the implantable cardioverter defibrillator secondary prevention trials. *Eur Heart J* 2000;**21**:2071–8.

CHAPTER 6

Hypotension

Suraj Alakkassery

Saint Louis University Medical Center, St Louis, MO, USA

Introduction

Hypotension is classically defined as drop in systolic blood pressure (BP) below 90 mmHg, producing symptoms of hypoperfusion to various organs. Although generally accepted, this number is arbitrary and many people with sustained hypertension or elderly people may become symptomatic at higher BPs. The body's autoregulatory mechanism prevents a significant fall in BP so as to maintain adequate perfusion of vital organs and their proper functioning. Such compensations are very fast and individuals are generally asymptomatic. Symptoms may develop if the BP drops below the range of autoregulation or if there is a delay in initiation or disruption of the regulatory mechanism. Hypotension is significant only if associated with symptoms or in the presence of a secondary condition that, if not controlled, will worsen hypotension and produce symptoms.

Hypotension when symptomatic is never physiological and is always secondary to an underlying cause. Hypotension is associated with many conditions, such as hypovolaemia (secondary to haemorrhage, severe diarrhoea, etc.), sepsis, anaphylaxis, tachycardia, bradycardia, valvular abnormality, tamponade, myocardial ischaemia, cardiomyopathy, pulmonary embolism, pneumothorax, adrenal insufficiency or side effects/toxicity of drugs. Symptoms are related to reduced perfusion to various organs – brain (dizziness, lightheadedness, blurry vision, syncope); skin (cold extremities); heart (tachycardia, palpitations, angina); kidneys (low urine output, renal failure); or gut (nausea, vomiting) – in addition to a general feeling of lethargy and generalized weakness. Symptoms persist until the underlying causes are corrected. Although these causes can affect any age group, outcome is poorer in elderly people.

There are two conditions that classically affect the elderly population – postprandial hypotension (PPH) and orthostatic hypotension (OH) – producing a symptomatic fall in BP after eating and standing, respectively.

Cardiovascular Disease and Health in the Older Patient: Expanded from 'Pathy's Principles and Practice of Geriatric Medicine, Fifth edition', First Edition. Edited by David J. Stott and Gordon D.O. Lowe.

These are transient in nature, typically producing symptoms due to reduced cerebral perfusion – dizziness, lightheadedness, blurry vision, syncope. They rarely last long enough to produce angina or renal failure.

Post-exercise hypotension (PEH) is a transient condition usually seen in hypertensive patients after a bout of exercise.

Orthostatic hypotension

Definition

Orthostatic or postural hypotension (OH) was first described by Bradbury and Eggleston in 1925.[1] OH is diagnosed when there is a reduction of ≥20 mmHg in SBP or ≥10 mmHg in DBP within 3 min of standing or using an upright tilt table at an angle of at least 60° with or without symptoms.[2] Although the definition is based on a consensus statement and the figures are arbitrary, a more modest drop in BP associated with symptoms is equally important. Delayed orthostatic hypotension (DOH), seen in 54% of patients with OH, is defined as a sustained fall in BP occurring beyond 3 min of standing or an upright tilt table test.[3] Initial orthostatic hypotension (IOH) is defined as a transient decrease of ≥40 mmHg SBP and/or ≥20 mmHg DBP within 15 s after standing and is associated with symptoms of cerebral hypoperfusion.[4]

OH represents one end of the spectrum of disorders of cardiovascular dysregulation. The spectrum (Figure 6.1) extends from very low to very high BP. The majority of individuals with normal BP are in the middle. At the right end are hypertensive individuals who have elevated BP all the time. Labile hypertensive individuals with BP ranging from 120/80 to 140/90 occupy the borderland between hypertensive and normal population. Individuals on the right side are asymptomatic and are treated to prevent complications in the future. At the left extreme are the individuals with OH. Individuals with 'mild dysautonomias' span the region between the OH and normotensive groups and include people with postural tachycardia

OH	POTS	NMS	Normotension	Labile HBP	HBP
SYMPTOMATIC NMS – Bradycardia/hypotension POTS – Orthostatic tachycardia OH – Orthostatic hypotension				ASYMPTOMATIC	

Figure 6.1 Cardiovascular dysregulation. HBP, high blood pressure; NMS, neurally mediated syncope; OH, orthostatic hypotension; POTS, postural tachycardia syndrome. Reproduced from Robertson.[5] With kind permission of Springer Science+Business Media.

syndrome (POTS) and neurally mediated syncope (NMS). Individuals with POTS have orthostatic tachycardia whereas those with NMS have normal pressures in all postures but occasionally have 'fainting' associated with a brief period (usually less than 1 min) of hypotension and/or bradycardia. Individuals on the left side have symptoms that affect quality of life and could be dangerous.[5]

Epidemiology

OH is a transient phenomenon with a high degree of intra-individual and intra-observer variability. OH is common among elderly populations with a varied prevalence of 6–34 % in community-dwelling people over 65 years of age[6–9] and around 20% among ambulatory nursing home residents.[10] Difference in measurement techniques of BP and timing of the measurement after change in position may contribute to the wide variations noted. The prevalence of OH increases with age from 14.8% in subjects aged 65–69 years to 26% in those 85 years and older. Differences in racial distribution have been documented by some, with predominance among whites,[11] whereas others documented no such difference.[12] The incidence of hospitalization secondary to OH increases with age and peaks over the age of 75 years at 233 per 100 000 patients. The median hospital stay is 3 days and the mortality rate is 0.9%.[13] OH is an independent predictor of 4-year all-cause mortality, with an age-adjusted relative risk of 1.8 [95% confidence interval (CI), 1.22–2.65].[14]

Many drugs have been implicated in either inducing or worsening of OH. These include antidepressants (tricyclic antidepressants, older monoamine oxidase inhibitors, serotonin–norepinephrine reuptake inhibitors), antipsychotics (phenothiazines), antihypertensives including diuretics,[15] narcotics and alcohol. Many factors have been linked with increased risk of OH (Table 6.1).

Table 6.1 Factors linked with increased risk of orthostatic hypotension.

Physical and behavioural	Biochemical and humoral	Cardiovascular	Medications
Age	Hypokalaemia	Non-dipper status	Psychoactive medications
Low body mass index	Hyponatraemia	Postprandial hypotension	Vasodilators
Smoking	Changes in RAS	Supine elevated BP	Antiparkinsonians
Bed rest		Increased vascular stiffness	
		Decreased baroreceptor sensitivity	

Reproduced with permission from Hajjar.[16]

OH is highly prevalent in patients with Parkinson's disease (47%; range, 16–58%). Other neurological diseases with a high prevalence are pure autonomic failure (PAF) (33%), multiple system atrophy (MSA) (26%), idiopathic (autoimmune autonomic neuropathy) (17%) and diabetic autonomic neuropathy (14%). Among the diabetics, although the incidence of autonomic dysfunction is high (54% in type 1 and 73% in type 2), the prevalence of OH is not proportionate (8.4% in type 1 and 7.4% in type 2). OH increases the risk for coronary artery disease and all-cause mortality[17] and is associated with systolic hypertension and low body mass index,[18] stroke[19] and chronic kidney disease.[20]

Mechanism

The adoption of an upright posture by humans posed challenges for the BP regulatory system and through evolution the body developed mechanisms to accommodate the effects of gravity- and activity-mediated fluid shifts. Hormonal factors such as the renin–angiotensin–aldosterone system regulate BP over long periods. Cardiovascular regulation by the autonomic nervous system (ANS) prevents more than a 5–10 mmHg drop in SBP, increases DBP and increases the pulse rate by 10–25 bpm. Sympathetic autonomic dysfunction can result in the development of OH.

In normal individuals, upon standing, roughly 500–800 ml of blood is displaced from the upper part of body to the lower part, primarily to the abdomen and lower extremities. The drop in volume (~30%) reduces the venous return to the heart, leading to a drop in stroke volume and arterial pressure. This causes activation of two sets of pressure receptors: (a) high-pressure centres in the aortic arch and carotid sinuses and (b) low-pressure receptors in the heart and lungs. These receptors, present in both the atrium and the ventricles of the heart, produce a tonic inhibitory effect on the sympathoexcitary neurons in cardiovascular areas of the medulla. A fall in venous return diminishes the stretch, decreasing their firing rates, thus resulting in increased sympathetic outflow. This causes a rise in BP by increasing systemic vascular resistance and constriction of splanchnic capacitance vessels. The baroreceptors located in the carotid sinus at the origin of the internal carotid artery transmit the local stretch signals to the nucleus tractus solitarius along the glossopharyngeal nerve. These receptors are responsible for an immediate increase in heart rate in response to the drop in carotid arterial pressure that occurs during an upright tilt test.[5] With ageing, the baroreceptor sensitivity and cardiovascular response to sympathetic stimulation are reduced, predisposing to OH.[14]

Prolonged orthostatic stress (20–30 min of standing) causes a substantial (20% in healthy adults) transcapillary filtration of the fluid shift from the blood into the interstitial space and causes additional peripheral pooling, thus decreasing venous return to the heart with a subsequent decline in BP and cardiac output. A progressive and sustained increase in muscle sympathetic nerve activity in response to prolonged orthostatic stress, together with the renin–angiotensin–aldosterone system, release of vasopressin and attenuation of atrial natriuretic factor, maintain cardiovascular homeostasis in the upright posture. This delayed OH is a consequence of one or more of the following: (a) increased peripheral venous pooling, (b) increased fluid transudation or (c) failure of the neural and humoral mechanisms.

Initial orthostatic hypotension (IOH) differs from typical OH in being transient, occurring immediately (within 15 s) upon standing, and is associated with a much greater fall in BP (≥40 mmHg SBP and/or ≥20 mmHg DBP). This can be documented only by continuous beat-to-beat BP monitoring during active standing, hence passive tilt is of no diagnostic value. IOH is thought to be due to a mismatch between cardiac output and vascular resistance. The sudden contraction of the muscles in both the legs and the abdomen produces a compression of resistance and capacitance vessels and together with the local venoarteriolar axon reflex that constricts flow to skin muscle and adipose tissue increases the peripheral vascular resistance, thus causing an initial increase in venous return. The increase in right atrial pressure produces reflex-mediated lowering of the BP. Overcompensation drops BP to the orthostatic range. IOH explains the transient symptoms of cerebral hypoperfusion that develops after waking from an overnight sleep.[4]

Symptoms of OH occur more commonly in the mornings and after meals and is worsened by a hot bath or shower; sudden postural change, fever and alcohol consumption. It may be provoked by exercise, coughing, straining to defecate and hyperventilation. Symptoms are dependent not only on the absolute fall in BP but also on the rate of change and the ability of the cardiovasculature to autoregulate. Symptoms range from light headedness to syncope and include dizziness, weakness, blurry vision, neck pain, headache, angina, disturbed speech, confusion, impaired cognition, fall and syncope. OH is often one aspect of a more generalized disturbance in cardiovascular regulation. In the initial phase, patients tolerate the symptoms as the BP rises during the day. With progression of dysregulation, patients exhibit erratic swings of BP in response to various physiological and pharmacological stresses and develop supine hypertension by the end of the day which can cause nocturnal polyuria by pressure natriuresis.[21,22]

Causes of OH are broadly classified into acute and chronic (Table 6.2). Acute OH develops over a short duration, is more symptomatic and results from acute processes such as sepsis, dehydration or myocardial ischaemia. Chronic OH develops over a longer duration, is usually asymptomatic initially and is mostly secondary to central or peripheral nervous system diseases.[22]

Table 6.2 Classification of orthostatic hypotension.

Acute		Chronic
Neurogenic		*Non-neurogenic*
Acute pandysautonomia		Ageing
Acute paraneoplastic autonomic neuropathy		Hypertension
Autoimmune autonomic ganglionopathy (AAG)		
Bezold–Jarisch reflex activation		*Central nervous system*
Botulism		Lewy body dementia
Carotid sinus syncope		Multiple sclerosis
Drug induced/toxic acute autonomic neuropathy		Multiple system atrophy (MSA)
Guillain–Barré syndrome		Myelopathy
Micturition syncope		Olivo-ponto-cerebellar atrophy
Porphyria		Parkinson's disease
		Posterior fossa tumours
Non-neurogenic		Spinal cord tumours
Adrenal crisis	Diarrhoea	Strokes
Anaemia	Haemorrhage	Subacute combined degeneration
Arrhythmias	Mastocytosis	Syringomyelia
Arteriovenous malformation	Myocardial infarction	Transverse myelitis
	Pheochromocytoma	
Burns	Pregnancy	*Peripheral nervous system*
Carcinoid	Sepsis	Alcoholic polyneuropathy
Carditis	Vomiting	Amyloidosis
Congestive heart failure		Autoimmune autonomic neuropathy
Dialysis		
		Diabetes mellitus
		Dopamine-b-hydroxylase deficiency
Drugs		Familial dysautonomia (Riley–Day syndrome)
ACE inhibitors	Insulin	HIV/AIDS
Alpha receptor blockers	Marijuana	
Barbiturates	Monoamine oxidase inhibitors	Nutritional deficiency (vitamin B_{12}, folate)
Beta-blockers	Nitrates	Paraneoplastic syndrome
Bromocriptine	Opiates	Pure autonomic failure (PAF)
Calcium-channel blockers	Phenothiazines	Tabes dorsalis
Diuretics	Sildenafil	Uraemia
Ethanol	Tricyclic antidepressants	Wernicke–Korsakoff syndrome
Hydralazine	Tizanidine	
	Vincristine	

Evaluation and diagnosis

A detailed history and physical examination can identify the cause in about 45% of patients with OH. One must include a comprehensive neurological assessment and look for the signs of other systemic disorders causing OH.

To establish the diagnosis of OH, the first step is to determine BP and heart rate after the patient has been quietly supine for at least 5 min and again after 1 and 3 min of standing. If ambulatory BP monitoring is required, measurements before breakfast, after medication, after meals and before bed are most useful. Variations in heart rate in response to OH can provide clues to aetiology: absent or minimal cardio-acceleration (<10 bpm) suggest baroreflex impairment or defect in the autonomic nervous system, tachycardia (>20 bpm) indicates volume depletion and a drop in heart rate suggest vasovagal response.[22]

When symptoms are suggestive of OH but no obvious cause is identified, the patient's medications should be reviewed before other aetiologies are considered and potentially any causative medications should be discontinued if possible. If discontinuation of medication is not possible, consider treating OH pharmacologically. If the medication does not appear to be fully responsible for OH, check the volume status. If dehydrated, hydration may improve symptoms; if euvolaemic, look for other non-neurogenic causes. Angina, dyspnoea and oedema suggest cardiac aetiology; vomiting, diarrhoea, burns and diuretic use suggest dehydration; fever may indicate sepsis or other infections. Once medication and non-neurogenic aetiologies have been ruled out, consider neurogenic causes of OH. They are difficult to diagnose and treat and a neurology consultation may be helpful. Laboratory tests should be directed to assist clinical diagnosis and may include haemoglobin, blood urea nitrogen and a creatinine level.[23]

Anhidrosis, miosis and reduced sphincter tone point to autonomic failure. Autonomic function tests are useful to evaluate autonomic disorder and response to therapy. Heart rate variations during deep breathing accesses the function of parasympathetic effect on the heart. Arrhythmia is measured by electrocardiograph with the patient lying supine during 1 min of slow and deep breathing with 5 s inspiration and 7 s expiration. Normally the ratio of the longest expiratory to shortest inspiratory R–R interval is >1.15. The cold pressor test assesses the function of sympathetic effects on BP in response to immersion of the hands in ice-cold water (4 °C) for 1 min (Normal: rise of ≥15 mmHg in SBP or ≥10 mmHg in DBP). Age and medications may affect the response to these bedside tests. Other autonomic testing that can be performed includes the quantitative Valsalva manoeuvre, carotid sinus massage and cardiovascular sensitivity to tyramine, phenylephrine or isoproterenol. Measurement of supine and upright plasma levels of norepinephrine and vasopressin can distinguish central from peripheral causes of autonomic failure. In central causes, the supine norepinephrine level is normal but fails to increase when posture becomes upright and vasopressin is low, whereas in peripheral causes the supine norepinephrine is low and vasopressin is normal.[21,22]

Severe OH with marked supine hypertension, modest gastrointestinal impairment, very low plasma norepinephrine level and no other neurological system involvement suggests pure autonomic failure (PAF). Some, but not all, patients with Parkinson's disease and autonomic failure have OH. Patients with dementia with Lewy bodies have visual hallucinations. Multiple system atrophy (MSA), the severest of dysautonomias, involves not only the autonomic but also the cerebellar and extrapyramidal systems. Magnetic resonance imaging (MRI) shows degenerative changes in putamen. Dopamine β-hydroxylase (DBH) converts dopamine to norepinephrine and the gene is located on chromosome 9q34. DBH deficiency is an extremely rare disorder. These patients have severe OH, exercise intolerance, ptosis and retrograde ejaculation. These patients lack norepinephrine in their neurons and instead have dopamine. They respond very well to droxidopa.[5]

Orthostatic hypertension

Some individuals have orthostatic hypertension (OH), that is, an increase rather than a decrease in BP upon standing. More severely affected individuals have rare disorders such as baroreflex failure, mastocytosis, hyperadrenergic POTS or pheochromocytoma.[5]

Prevention and treatment of OH

The first step in the treatment of OH is diagnosis and management of underlying reversible causes such as anaemia and hypovolaemia. Non-pharmacological intervention is attempted before pharmacological treatment.

Non-pharmacological intervention[21,24]

1. Educating patient and family to avoid any potential aggravating factors such as heat and dehydration.
2. Increase intake of salt (10–20 g daily) and fluid (1.25–2.5 l daily) if there are no contraindications such as CHF.
3. Eat smaller and more frequent meals.
4. Avoid alcohol, prolonged standing, large meals, strenuous exercise, hyperventilation and straining during urination or defecation.
5. If possible, avoid medications known to cause OH.
6. Elevate the head end of bed while sleeping to reduce nocturia, supine hypertension and sudden pooling of blood when rising in the morning.
7. Rise slowly from supine to sitting to standing position.
8. Drinking two cups (500 ml) of water 30 min before rising will raise SBP >20 mmHg for 2 h.
9. Use compression stockings and an abdominal binder to minimize venous pooling.

10 Dorsiflex feet several times before standing.
11 For deconditioning – utilize exercise such as swimming or recumbent biking.
12 Physical counter-manoeuvres involve isometric contraction of muscles below the waist for 30 s at a time. Specific manoeuvres include toe raising, leg crossing and contraction, bending at the waist, leg elevation and slow marching in place.

Pharmacological treatment

When non-pharmacological interventions fail, medications should be tried to control the symptoms. The available medications are summarized below.

Fludrocortisone is a mineralocorticoid with minimal glucocorticoid effect. It expands blood volume by salt retention. The starting dose is 0.1 mg per day with increments of 0.1 mg every week until a maximum dose of 1 mg is reached or trace pedal oedema develops. Common side effects are headache, hypokalaemia, heart failure and supine hypertension.[22]

Midodrine (α_1-agonist), a prodrug, is converted into active desglymidodrine. It is well tolerated and increases the SBP by an average of 22 mmHg. It stimulates both arterial and venous systems without direct CNS or cardiac effects and does not increase heart rate. It is useful in PAF and diabetic neuropathy. The starting dose is 2.5 mg three times per day with increments of 2.5 mg weekly to a maximum dose of 10 mg three times per day. Side effects are piloerection, pruritus, urinary hesitancy and retention in males. This medication is contraindicated in patients with coronary heart disease, heart failure, urinary retention, thyrotoxicosis and acute renal failure.[21]

DL- and L-dihydroxyphenylserine (DOPS) are synthetic, non-physiological, norepinephrine precursors that are decarboxylated by the ubiquitous L-amino acid decarboxylase to norepinephrine. Of the four stereoisomers, only L-*threo*-DOPS is pharmacologically active. Since the conversion of DOPS to norepinephrine bypasses the dopamine β-hydroxylation step of catecholamine synthesis, DOPS is the ideal therapeutic agent for patients with dopamine β-hydroxylase deficiency since such individuals are unable to synthesize norepinephrine and epinephrine in the central and peripheral nervous system. This agent may also be of benefit in patients with familial amyloid polyneuropathy, Parkinson's disease, multiple system atrophy and pure autonomic failure.[25]

Pyridostigmine is a cholinesterase inhibitor. As it improves ganglionic neurotransmission in the sympathetic baroreflex pathway that is activated during standing, it improves OH without worsening supine hypertension. The starting dose is 30 mg two or three times per day and the maximum dose is 60 mg three times per day. Common side effects are abdominal colic and diarrhoea.[24]

Recombinant human erythropoietin increases BP by 10 mmHg and improves orthostatic tolerance, especially dizziness in patients with anaemia which often occurs in autonomic failure. The mechanism of increase in BP, although unknown, is not believed to be due to an increase in blood volume or viscosity. The dose is 25–75 U kg^{-1} subcutaneously three times per week. It is well tolerated.[21]

NSAIDs (non-steroidal anti-inflammatory drugs) are added to fludrocortisones to control smooth muscle relaxation and to increase peripheral resistance. They possibly work by inhibiting prostaglandin synthesis, particularly prostaglandin E. The indomethacin dose is 75–100 mg per day. Side effects include gastrointestinal toxicity, renal toxicity and worsening of heart failure.[26]

Indications for referral to a specialist

Geriatric consultation should be sought for frail elderly patients and those with multiple comorbid conditions. A cardiology referral is indicated for uncontrolled supine hypertension, severe heart failure and recent arrhythmia. A neurologist can be consulted for specialized autonomic testing or progressive autonomic failure.[22]

Postprandial hypotension

Definition

A postprandial fall in BP was first observed and reported in 1935 by Gladstone in a hypertensive patient and in 1953 by Smirk in patients with autonomic failure. Kjartan Seyer-Hansen in 1977 recognized postprandial hypotension as a clinical problem in a patient with Parkinson's disease.[27,28]

Epidemiology

Postprandial hypotension (PPH) is defined as a drop in systolic BP of ≥20 mmHg within 2 h after a meal or a drop of SBP from ≥100 mmHg pre-meal to below 90 mmHg within 2 h after a meal.[28]

PPH is common in elderly individuals. The prevalence of PPH varies depending on the risk group: 24–36% among nursing home residents, 50% in elderly patients with syncope and 67% in hospitalized geriatric patients. The prevalence is higher in elderly patients with autonomic failure, diabetes mellitus, hypertension, Parkinson's disease and end-stage renal disease on dialysis.[29] Hypertensive patients with PPH have a higher prevalence of asymptomatic cerebrovascular damage than those without PPH (83 vs 44%), as evidenced by a higher number of lacunae and leukoaraiosis on MRI of the brain.[30] PPH is associated with a higher incidence of falls, syncope, new coronary events, new stroke and total mortality in the elderly population.[31] PPH is not associated with OH but the two can be additive.[32]

Risk factors

Although the aetiology of PPH is poorly defined, various risk factors have been identified that influence the magnitude of a postprandial fall in BP. These include meal composition, temperature, volume and time of meal ingestion, medications and illnesses affecting autonomic nerve function.

In healthy elders, isocaloric and isovolaemic intraduodenal infusion of glucose, fat and protein reduce SBP and increase heart rate and splanchnic blood flow by similar magnitudes but the onset is earlier with glucose. The slowing of gastric emptying and the stimulation of gastrointestinal hormone release by oral fat and protein are mediated by fatty acids and amino acids, respectively. This could be the possible reason for the relative latency in the response. A warm (50 °C) meal but not cold (5 °C) reduces postprandial BP. Medications, especially psychotropic, cardiovascular and diuretic drugs, when administered with a meal can potentiate PPH.[31,33–35]

Pathophysiology

Age-related illness and unhealthy ageing cause PPH. The pathophysiology of PPH is poorly understood and is multifactorial. Factors include splanchnic blood flow, gastric distension, small intestinal nutrient delivery and neural and hormonal mechanisms.

PPH appears to be secondary to inadequate cardiovascular adjustment for the normal postprandial reduction in BP. Following a meal there is a doubling of superior mesenteric arterial flow. In healthy adults, BP is maintained by an increase in heart rate, forearm vascular resistance, cardiac index and sympathetic activity. Patients with PPH develop a postprandial decline in BP and systemic vascular resistance without a change in forearm vascular resistance, reduction in left ventricular end diastolic volume and poor sympathetic response.[36] Also, in healthy adults, gastric distension attenuates PPH by increasing BP and heart rate – 'gastrovascular reflex'. This reflex is reduced in elderly people with PPH. Muscle nerve sympathetic activity response to an oral glucose load and heart rate spectral analysis showed a blunted increase in sympathetic activity associated with the intake of a meal in elderly patients with PPH compared with young adults. A 200% increase in sympathetic activity would be needed to prevent PPH.[29]

The nitric oxide (NO) synthase inhibitor N^{G}-nitro-L-arginine methyl ester (L-NAME) attenuated PPH with minimal effect on gastric emptying, suggesting the role of NO in development of PPH.[37]

Various vasoactive peptides released from the small intestine in response to the ingestion of food have been implicated in PPH and include calcitonin gene-related peptide (CGRP) and glucagon-like peptide-1 (GLP-1). CGRP levels increase following a meal and this increase is associated with the reduction of BP and pathogenesis of postprandial hypotension.[38] GLP-1 released from 'L-cells' in the small intestine is associated with acarbose in attenuation of hypotensive response to sucrose and slows gastric emptying.[39] Failure of intravenous glucose, a potent stimulus to insulin secretion, to affect BP in elderly people, and that PPH occurs in patients with type 1 diabetes, who are by definition insulin deficient, argue against the major role of insulin in PPH. Plasma levels of VIP and substance-P, known vasodilators, are not affected by oral glucose.

Clinical features and diagnosis

Symptoms of PPH are due to cerebral hypoperfusion and manifest as dizziness, light-headedness, weakness, fall or syncope after a meal. Patients may sometimes present with chest pain or dyspnoea. PPH is suspected in any elderly person presenting with the above complaints especially in patients with autonomic failure, diabetes mellitus, Parkinson's disease or end-stage renal disease. Ambulatory BP can be monitored to include a major meal along with continued BP monitoring for at least 2 h after the meal. In admitted patients, measuring BP every 10 min starting 15 min before until 60 min after finishing breakfast utilizing a sphygmomanometer can detect about 70% of patients with PPH. This has been suggested by some as a practical and patient-friendly way to diagnose PPH.[40]

Treatment

Non-pharmacological interventions

1 Education of patients about the risk of falling after meals.
2 Lie recumbent and avoid a prolonged sitting or standing posture after meals.
3 Discontinue potential medication.
4 Drink water before meals.
5 Reduce carbohydrate consumption.
6 Eat smaller, more frequent meals.
7 Liberal salt and water intake.
8 Avoid alcoholic beverages.

Pharmacological treatment[28,29,39,41]

Acarbose, caffeine, guar and octreotide are the most frequently used medications for PPH.

Caffeine, an adenosine receptor antagonist, may ameliorate PPH. Dosage is individualized and can be titrated from 60 to 200 mg orally before meals.

Guar gum is derived from the guar bean and acts as a bulking agent. It prevents PPH by slowing glucose absorption. The dose is 4 g orally before meals. Side effects include abdominal pain, diarrhoea and flatulence.

Octreotide, a somatostatin analogue, reduces PPH most likely by increasing splanchnic and peripheral vascular resistance. The dose is a 50 μg subcutaneous injection 30 min before meals. Side effects include abdominal pain, QT prolongation and pain at injection site.

Other medications that have been evaluated for treatment include the combination of denopamine (a β_1-agonist) and midodrine (but not as monotherapy); vasopressin and indomethacin for attenuation of PPH. Cimetidine, dihydroergotamine and diphenhydramine failed to show an effect on PPH.

α-Glucosidase inhibitors such as acarbose, voglibose and miglitol act by inhibiting carbohydrate digestion at the level of the brush border in the small intestine. Their effect is secondary to alterations in circulating vasodilators and gut peptides secretion. Specifically, an increase in glucagon-like peptide I is thought to slow gastric emptying, thus inhibiting PPH. The dose is 100 mg of acarbose or 200 μg of voglibose orally before meals. Miglitol can be used at 25 mg with the first bite of the meal. Side effects include diarrhoea and flatulence.

Post-exercise hypotension (PEH)

In 1897, Hill documented PEH during the 90 min following a 400 yard dash.[42] In 1971, Groom reported a consistent decrease in systolic and diastolic BP in runners immediately after running at an estimated speed of 6 mph for more than 4 h.[43] It was only after Fitzgerald's report in 1981 of a personal observation that jogging for 25 min decreased labile pressure to near normal levels which lasted for several hours[44] that the phenomenon of PEH gained importance as a clinical entity.

Definition

Post-exercise hypotension (PEH) is a term used to describe the transient reduction in BP following an acute bout of exercise. There are no defined criteria for the magnitude and duration of this decrease in BP post-exercise to diagnose PEH. Eliciting the phenomenon of PEH by electrical stimulation of muscles instead of actual exercise is called post-stimulation hypotension (PSH).[45]

Epidemiology

PEH has been observed in young and middle-aged normotensive people and with patients with borderline and established essential hypertension. PEH lacks gender specificity and occurs in both men and women. PEH does not appear to be correlated with exercise intensity or duration or the amount of exercising muscle mass. The nadir of the PEH response generally occurs within the first 60–70 min of recovery. The average drop in BP in patients with essential hypertension varied from (systolic/diastolic)

11/4 mmHg in 30–90 min post-exercise to 9/4 mmHg between 2 and 3 h to an average of 2.8/1.7 mmHg over 24 h. The average drop in borderline hypertensive patients was 14/9 mmHg and in normotensive patients it was 8/9 mmHg.[45–47] Diurnal variations have been observed in PEH, which is less marked in the morning, probably because the exercise-mediated decrease in peripheral resistance is not as apparent at this time of day.[48]

Although PEH occurs in both normotensive and hypertensive individuals after either resistance or endurance exercise, it is more predictive in hypertensive individuals.[46] In the healthy normotensive population, chronic exercise leads to structural vascular changes that include increased arterial luminal diameter and compliance. Older hypertensive individuals are resistant to alteration due to replacement of elastic fibres by collagen and calcium. PEH also occurs in endurance-trained individuals, probably due to reduced cardiac output. In sedentary men PEH is secondary to vasodilatation, suggesting that exercise training may alter the mechanism but not the magnitude of PEH. As PEH is a function of baseline BP, the magnitude of the fall is expected to be more in hypertensive individuals. The magnitude diminishes with exercise-induced reduction in baseline BP. About 25% of hypertensive individuals called 'non-responders' do not appear to sustain BP reductions after endurance training, suggesting a genetic role in PEH. Meta-analysis of longitudinal studies showed no influence of frequency or intensity of exercise training programmes on the BP-lowering effect.[49]

PEH and initial OH are not predictors of syncope post-exercise even though the inability to maintain BP is a crucial factor.

Syncope post-exercise is a phenomenon seen exclusively after prolonged exercise (~4 h). PEH is seen even after short bouts of exercise and the magnitude is unrelated to the duration of exercise, thus indicating the role of other factors involved in post-exercise syncope.[50]

Clinical implications

If PEH is of sufficient magnitude, it could be sustained and evoked under conditions of normal daily living. Then regular periodic exercise can potentially become a non-pharmacological tool in the management of hypertension. Although some studies have shown a sufficient drop in BP and sustained effect, many others are contradictory. Further studies are needed to determine the dose, timing and type of exercise required for a sustained hypertensive effect.

Key points

- Hypotension is a major problem in older persons, leading to dizziness, falls, syncope, stroke, myocardial infarction and death.

- Orthostatic hypotension can occur immediately on standing or after a few minutes.
- Postprandial hypotension is due to an increase in the vasodilatory peptide calcitonin gene-related peptide.
- Postprandial hypotension can be treated with α_1-glucosidase inhibitors, which increase glucagon-like peptide-1.

References

1 Laufer ST. Orthostatic hypotension (report of a case). *Can Med Assoc J* 1942;**46**:160–4.

2 The Consensus Committee of the American Autonomic Society and the American Academy of Neurology. Consensus statement on the definition of orthostatic hypotension, pure autonomic failure and multiple system atrophy. *Neurology* 1996;**46**:1470–1.

3 Gibbons CH and Freeman R. Delayed orthostatic hypotension: a frequent cause of orthostatic intolerance. *Neurology* 2006;**67**:28–32.

4 Wieling W, Krediet CT, van Dijk N *et al.* Initial orthostatic hypotension: review of a forgotten condition. *Clin Sci* 2007;**112**:157–65.

5 Robertson D. The pathophysiology and diagnosis of orthostatic hypotension. *Clin Auton Res* 2008;**18**(Suppl. 1):2–7.

6 Mader SL, Josephson KR and Rubenstein LZ. Low prevalence of postural hypotension among community-dwelling elderly. *JAMA* 1987;**258**:1511–4.

7 Rutan GH, Hermanson B, Bild DE *et al.* Orthostatic hypotension in older adults. The Cardiovascular Health Study. CHS Collaborative Research Group. *Hypertension* 1992;**19**:508–19.

8 Wu JS, Yang YC, Lu FH *et al.* Population-based study on the prevalence and correlates of orthostatic hypotension/hypertension and orthostatic dizziness. *Hypertens Res* 2008;**31**:897–904.

9 Hiitola P, Enlund H, Kettunen R *et al.* Postural changes in blood pressure and the prevalence of orthostatic hypotension among home-dwelling elderly aged 75 years or older. *J Hum Hypertens* 2009;**23**:33–9.

10 Si M, Rodstein M, Neufeld RR *et al.* Orthostatic change in blood pressure in non-demented, ambulatory nursing home patients. *Arch Gerontol Geriatr* 1992;**14**:123–9.

11 Strogatz DS, Keenan NL, Barnett EM and Wagner EH. Correlates of postural hypotension in a community sample of elderly blacks and whites. *J Am Geriatr Soc* 1991;**39**:562–6.

12 Parmer RJ, Cervenka JH, Stone RA and O'Connor DT. Autonomic function in hypertension. Are there racial differences? *Circulation* 1990;**81**:1305–11.

13 Shibao C, Grijalva CG, Raj SR *et al.* Orthostatic hypotension-related hospitalizations in the United States. *Am J Med* 2007;**120**:975–80.

14 Masaki KH, Schatz IJ, Burchfiel CM *et al.* Orthostatic hypotension predicts mortality in elderly men: the Honolulu Heart Program. *Circulation* 1998;**98**:2290–5.

15 Low PA. Prevalence of orthostatic hypotension. *Clin Auton Res* 2008;**18**(Suppl. 1): 8–13.

16 Hajjar I. Postural blood pressure changes and orthostatic hypotension in the elderly patient: impact of antihypertensive medications. *Drugs Ageing* 2005;**22**:55–68.

17 Verwoert GC, Mattace-Raso FU, Hofman A *et al.* Orthostatic hypotension and risk of cardiovascular disease in elderly people: the Rotterdam study. *J Am Geriatr Soc* 2008;**56**:1816–20.

18 Applegate WB, Davis BR, Black HR *et al.* Prevalence of postural hypotension at baseline in the Systolic Hypertension in the Elderly Program (SHEP) cohort. *J Am Geriatr Soc* 1991;**39**:1057–64.

19 Eigenbrodt ML, Rose KM, Couper DJ *et al.* Orthostatic hypotension as a risk factor for stroke: the Atherosclerosis Risk in Communities (ARIC) Study, 1987–1996. *Stroke* 2000;**31**:2307–13.

20 Franceschini N, Rose KM, Astor BC *et al.* Orthostatic hypotension and incident chronic kidney disease: the Atherosclerosis Risk in Communities Study. *Hypertension* 2010;**56**:1054–9.

21 Medow MS, Stewart JM, Sanyal S *et al.* Pathophysiology, diagnosis and treatment of orthostatic hypotension and vasovagal syncope. *Cardiol Rev* 2008;**16**:4–20.

22 Gupta V and Lipsitz LA. Orthostatic hypotension in the elderly: diagnosis and treatment. *Am J Med* 2007;**120**:841–7.

23 Bradley JG and Davis KA. Orthostatic hypotension. *Am Fam Physician* 2003;**68**:2393–8.

24 Figueroa JJ, Basford JR and Low PA. Preventing and treating orthostatic hypotension: as easy as A, B, C. *Cleve Clin J Med* 2010;**77**:298–306.

25 Freeman R and Landsberg L. The treatment of orthostatic hypotension with dihydroxyphenylserine. *Clin Neuropharmacol* 1991;**14**:296–304.

26 Iwanczyk L, Weintraub NT and Rubenstein LZ. Orthostatic hypotension in the nursing home setting. *J Am Med Dir Assoc* javascript:AL_get(this, 'jour', 'J Am Med Dir Assoc.');2006;**7**:163–7.

27 Seyer-Hansen K. Postprandial hypotension. *BMJ* 1977;**ii**:1262.

28 Jansen RW and Lipsitz LA. Postprandial hypotension: epidemiology, pathophysiology and clinical management. *Ann Intern Med* 1995;**122**:286–95.

29 Luciano GL, Brennan MJ and Rothberg MB. Postprandial hypotension. *Am J Med* 2010;123:281.e1–6.

30 Kohara K, Jiang Y, Igase M *et al.* Postprandial hypotension is associated with asymptomatic cerebrovascular damage in essential hypertensive patients. *Hypertension* 1999;**33**:565–8.

31 Aronow WS and Ahn C. Association of postprandial hypotension with incidence of falls, syncope, coronary events, stroke and total mortality at 29-month follow-up in 499 older nursing home residents. *J Am Geriatr Soc* 1997;**45**:1051–3.

32 Maurer MS, Karmally W, Rivadeneira H *et al.* Upright posture and postprandial hypotension in elderly persons. *Ann Intern Med* 2000;**133**:533–6.

33 Potter JF, Heseltine D, Hartley G *et al.* Effects of meal composition on the postprandial blood pressure, catecholamine and insulin changes in elderly subjects. *Clin Sci* 1989;**77**:265–72.

34 Kuipers HM, Jansen RW, Peters TL and Hoefnagels WH. The influence of food temperature on postprandial blood pressure reduction and its relation to substance-P in healthy elderly subjects. *J Am Geriatr Soc* 1991;**39**:181–4.

35 Gentilcore D, Jones KL, O'Donovan DG and Horowitz M. Postprandial hypotension – novel insights into pathophysiology and therapeutic implications. *Curr Vasc Pharmacol* 2006;**4**:161–71.

36 Lipsitz LA, Ryan SM, Parker JA *et al.* Hemodynamic and autonomic nervous system responses to mixed meal ingestion in healthy young and old subjects and dysautonomic patients with postprandial hypotension. *Circulation* 1993;**87**:391–400.

37 Gentilcore D, Visvanathan R, Russo A *et al.* Role of nitric oxide mechanisms in gastric emptying of, and the blood pressure and glycemic responses to, oral glucose in healthy older subjects. *Am J Physiol Gastrointest Liver Physiol* 2005;**288**:G1227–32.
38 Edwards BJ, Perry HM III,, Kaiser FE *et al.* Relationship of age and calcitonin gene-related peptide to postprandial hypotension. *Mech Ageing Dev* 1996;**87**:61–73.
39 Gentilcore D, Bryant B, Wishart JM *et al.* Acarbose attenuates the hypotensive response to sucrose and slows gastric emptying in the elderly. *Am J Med* 2005;118:1289.e5–11.
40 Van Orshoven NP, Jansen PA, Oudejans I *et al.* Postprandial hypotension in clinical geriatric patients and healthy elderly: prevalence related to patient selection and diagnostic criteria. *J Ageing Res* 2010;**30**:2437–52.
41 Hirayama M, Watanabe H, Koike Y *et al.* Treatment of postprandial hypotension with selective alpha 1 and beta 1 adrenergic agonists. *J Auton Nerv Syst* 1993;**45**:149–54.
42 Hill LJ. Arterial pressure in man while sleeping, resting, working and bathing. *J Physiol (Lond)* 1897;**22**:xxvi–xxix.
43 Groom D. Cardiovascular observations on Tarahumara Indian runners – the modern Spartans. *Am Heart J* 1971;**81**:304–14.
44 Fitzgerald W. Labile hypertension and jogging: new diagnostic tool or spurious discovery? *BMJ* 1981;**282**:542–4.
45 MacDonald JR. Potential causes, mechanisms and implications of post exercise hypotension. *J Hum Hypertens* 2002;**16**:225–36.
46 Kenney MJ and Seals DR. Postexercise hypotension. Key features, mechanisms and clinical significance. *Hypertension* 1993;**22**:653–64.
47 Haapanen N, Miilunpalo S, Vuori I *et al.* Association of leisure time physical activity with the risk of coronary heart disease, hypertension and diabetes in middle-aged men and women. *Int J Epidemiol* 1997;**26**:739–47.
48 Jones H, Pritchard C, George K *et al.* The acute post-exercise response of blood pressure varies with time of day. *Eur J Appl Physiol* 2008;**104**:481–9.
49 Hamer M. The anti-hypertensive effects of exercise: integrating acute and chronic mechanisms. *Sports Med* 2006;**36**:109–16.
50 Murrell CJ, Cotter JD, George K *et al.* Syncope is unrelated to supine and postural hypotension following prolonged exercise. *Eur J Appl Physiol* 2011;**111**:469–76.

CHAPTER 7
Ischaemic Heart Disease

Wilbert S. Aronow
New York Medical College, Valhalla, NY, USA

Introduction

The most common cause of death in elderly persons is ischaemic heart disease (IHD). Coronary atherosclerosis is very common in elderly people, with autopsy studies demonstrating a prevalence of at least 70% in persons older than 70 years. The prevalence of IHD is similar in elderly women and men.[1] In one study, clinical IHD was present in 502 of 1160 men (43%), mean age 80 years, and in 1019 of 2464 women (41%), mean age 81 years. At 46-month follow-up, the incidence of new coronary events (myocardial infarction or sudden cardiac death) was 46% in the elderly men and 44% in the elderly women.[1]

IHD is diagnosed in elderly persons if they have either coronary angiographic evidence of significant IHD, a documented acute coronary syndrome – unstable angina or myocardial infarction (MI), a typical history of stable angina pectoris with myocardial ischaemia diagnosed by stress testing, or sudden cardiac death. The incidence of sudden cardiac death as the first clinical manifestation of IHD increases with age.

Clinical manifestations

Dyspnoea on exertion is a more common clinical manifestation of IHD in elderly persons than is the typical chest pain of angina pectoris. The dyspnoea is usually exertional and is related to a transient rise in left ventricular (LV) end-diastolic pressure caused by ischaemia superimposed on decreased LV compliance. Because elderly persons are more limited in their activities, angina pectoris in elderly persons is less often associated with exertion. Elderly persons with angina pectoris are less likely to have substernal chest pain, and they describe their anginal pain as less severe

Cardiovascular Disease and Health in the Older Patient: Expanded from 'Pathy's Principles and Practice of Geriatric Medicine, Fifth edition', First Edition. Edited by David J. Stott and Gordon D.O. Lowe.

and of shorter duration than do younger persons. Angina pectoris in elderly persons may occur as a burning postprandial epigastric pain or as pain in the back or shoulders. Acute pulmonary oedema unassociated with an acute MI may be a clinical manifestation of unstable angina pectoris due to extensive IHD in elderly persons.

Myocardial ischaemia, appearing as shoulder or back pain in elderly persons, may be misdiagnosed as degenerative joint disease. Myocardial ischaemia, appearing as epigastric pain, may be misdiagnosed as peptic ulcer disease. Nocturnal or postprandial epigastric discomfort that is burning in quality may be misdiagnosed as hiatus hernia or oesophageal reflux instead of myocardial ischaemia due to IHD. The presence of comorbid conditions in elderly persons may also lead to misdiagnosis of symptoms due to myocardial ischaemia.

Elderly persons with IHD may have silent or asymptomatic myocardial ischaemia. In a prospective study, 133 of 195 men (34%), mean age 80 years, with IHD and 256 of 771 women (33%), mean age 81 years, with IHD had silent myocardial ischaemia detected by 24-hour ambulatory electrocardiograms (ECGs). At 45-month follow-up, the incidence of new coronary events in elderly men with IHD was 90% in men with silent myocardial ischaemia versus 44% in men without silent ischaemia. At 47-month follow-up, the incidence of new coronary events in elderly women with IHD was 88% in women with silent ischaemia versus 43% in women without silent ischaemia.[2]

Recognized and unrecognized MI

Pathy demonstrated in 387 elderly patients with acute MI that 19% had chest pain, 56% had dyspnoea or neurological symptoms or gastrointestinal symptoms, 8% had sudden death, and 17% had other symptoms.[3] Another study showed in 110 elderly patients with acute MI that 21% had no symptoms, 22% had chest pain, 35% had dyspnoea, 18% had neurological symptoms, and 4% had gastrointestinal symptoms (Table 7.1).[3] Other studies have also shown a high prevalence of dyspnoea and neurological symptoms in elderly patients with acute MI.[3] In these studies, dyspnoea was present in 22% of 87 patients, in 42% of 777 patients, and in 57% of 96 patients. Neurological symptoms were present in 16% of 87 patients, in 30% of 777 patients, and in 34% of 96 patients.

As with myocardial ischaemia, some patients with acute MI may be completely asymptomatic or the symptoms may be so vague that they are unrecognized by the patient or physician as an acute MI. Studies have reported that 21–68% of MIs in elderly patients are unrecognized or silent.[3] These studies also demonstrated that the incidence of new

Table 7.1 Presenting symptoms in 110 elderly patients with acute myocardial infarction.

Dyspnoea was present in 35% of patients
Chest pain was present in 22% of patients
Neurological symptoms were present in 18% of patients
Gastrointestinal symptoms were present in 4% of patients
No symptoms were present in 21% of patients

Source: Paper by Aronow WS discussed in Aronow and Fleg, 2008.[3]

coronary events including recurrent myocardial infarction, ventricular fibrillation and sudden death in patients with unrecognized MI, is similar to that in patients with recognized MI.

Diagnostic techniques

Resting ECG

In addition to diagnosing recent or prior MI, the resting ECG may show ischaemic ST-segment depression, arrhythmias, conduction defects and LV hypertrophy that are related to subsequent coronary events. At 37-month mean follow-up, elderly patients with ischaemic ST-segment depression 1 mm or greater on the resting ECG were 3.1 times more likely to develop new coronary events than were elderly patients with no significant ST-segment depression.[3] Elderly patients with ischaemic ST-segment depression 0.5 to 0.9 mm on the resting ECG were 1.9 times more likely to develop new coronary events during 37-month follow-up than were elderly patients with no significant ST-segment depression. At 45-month mean follow-up, pacemaker rhythm, atrial fibrillation, premature ventricular complexes, left bundle branch block, intraventricular conduction defect and type II second-degree atrioventricular block were associated with a higher incidence of new coronary events in patients.[3] Numerous studies have also documented that elderly patients with ECG LV hypertrophy have an increased incidence of new coronary events.[3]

Many studies have shown that complex ventricular arrhythmias in elderly persons with IHD are associated with an increased incidence of new coronary events including sudden cardiac death.[3] The incidence of new coronary events is especially increased in elderly persons with complex ventricular arrhythmias and abnormal LV ejection fraction or LV hypertrophy. At 45-month follow-up of 395 men, mean age 80 years, with IHD, complex ventricular arrhythmias detected by 24-hour ambulatory ECGs increased the incidence of new coronary events 2.4 times.[4] At 47-month follow-up of 771 women, mean age 81 years, with IHD, complex ventricular arrhythmias detected by 24-hour ambulatory ECGs increased the incidence of new coronary events 2.5 times.[4]

Exercise stress testing

Hlatky *et al.* found the exercise ECG to have a sensitivity of 84% and a specificity of 70% for the diagnosis of IHD in persons older than 60 years of age.[3] Newman and Phillips found a sensitivity of 85%, a specificity of 56%, and a positive predictive value of 86% for the exercise ECG in diagnosing IHD.[3] The increased sensitivity of the exercise ECG with increasing age found in these two treadmill exercise studies was probably due to the increased prevalence and severity of IHD in elderly persons.

Exercise stress testing also has prognostic value in elderly patients with IHD. Deckers *et al.*[3] showed that the one-year mortality was 4% for 48 patients 65 years of age or older who were able to do an exercise stress test after acute MI and 37% for the 63 elderly patients unable to do the exercise stress test after acute MI.

Exercise stress testing using thallium perfusion scintigraphy, radionuclide ventriculography, and echocardiography are also useful in the diagnosis and prognosis of CHD. Iskandirian *et al.*[3] showed that exercise thallium-201 imaging can be used for risk stratification of elderly patients with IHD. The risk for cardiac death or non-fatal MI at 25-month follow-up in 449 patients 60 years of age or older was less than 1% in patients with normal images, 5% in patients with single-vessel thallium-201 abnormality, and 13% in patients with multivessel thallium-201 abnormality.

Pharmacological stress testing

Intravenous dipyridamole-thallium imaging may be used to determine the presence of IHD in elderly patients who are unable to undergo treadmill or bicycle exercise stress testing. In patients 70 years of age or older, the sensitivity of intravenous dipyridamole-thallium imaging for diagnosing significant IHD was 86% , and the specificity was 75%.[3] In 120 patients older than 70 years, adenosine echocardiography had a 66% sensitivity and a 90% specificity in diagnosing IHD.[3] An abnormal adenosine echocardiogram predicted a threefold risk of future coronary events, independent of coronary risk factors.[3] In 120 patients older than 70 years, dobutamine echocardiography had a 87% sensitivity and a 84% specificity in diagnosing IHD.[3] An abnormal dobutamine echocardiogram predicted a 7.3-fold risk of future coronary events.[3]

Signal-averaged electrocardiography

Signal-averaged electrocardiography (SAECG) was performed in 121 elderly post-infarction patients with asymptomatic complex ventricular arrhythmias detected by 24-hour ambulatory ECGs and a LV ejection fraction of 40% or higher.[3] At 29-month follow-up, the sensitivity, specificity, positive predictive value and negative predictive value for predicting sudden cardiac death were 52%, 68%, 32% and 83%, respectively for a positive SAECG; 63%, 70%, 38% and 87%, respectively for non-sustained ventricular tachycardia; and 26%, 89%, 41% and 81%, respectively for a positive SAECG plus non-sustained ventricular tachycardia.[3]

Coronary risk factors

Cigarette smoking

The Cardiovascular Health Study demonstrated in 5201 men and women 65 years of age or older that >50 pack-years of smoking increased 5-year mortality 1.6 times.[5] The Systolic Hypertension in the Elderly Program pilot project showed that smoking was a predictor of first cardiovascular event and MI/sudden death.[5] At 5-year follow-up of 7178 persons ≥65 years of age in three communities, the relative risk for CVD mortality was 2.0 for male smokers and 1.6 for female smokers.[5] The incidence of CVD mortality in former smokers was similar to those who had never smoked.[5] At 40-month follow-up of 664 men, mean age 80 years, and at 48-month follow-up of 1488 women, mean age 82 years, current cigarette smoking increased the relative risk of new coronary events 2.2 times in men and 2.0 times in women.[6] At 6-year follow-up of older men and women in the Coronary Artery Surgery Study registry, the relative risk of MI or death was 1.5 for persons 65–69 years of age and 2.9 for persons 70 years of age and older who continued smoking compared with quitters during the year before study enrolment.[5]

Elderly men and women who smoke cigarettes should be strongly encouraged to stop smoking to reduce the development of IHD. Smoking cessation will decrease mortality from IHD, other cardiovascular disease and all-cause mortality in elderly men and women. A smoking cessation programme should strongly be recommended (see Chapter 1).

Hypertension

Systolic hypertension in elderly persons is diagnosed if the systolic blood pressure (SBP) is 140 mmHg or higher from two or more readings on two or more visits.[7] Diastolic hypertension in elderly persons is similarly diagnosed if the diastolic blood pressure (DBP) is 90 mmHg or higher. In a study of 1819 persons, mean age 80 years, living in the community, the prevalence of hypertension was 71% in elderly African Americans, 64% in elderly Asians, 62% in elderly Hispanics and 52% in elderly whites.[5] Isolated systolic hypertension in elderly persons is diagnosed if the SBP is 140 mmHg or higher with a DBP of less than 90 mmHg. Approximately two-thirds of elderly persons with hypertension have isolated systolic hypertension.

Isolated systolic hypertension and diastolic hypertension are both associated with increased IHD morbidity and mortality in elderly persons.[5] Increased SBP is a greater risk factor for IHD morbidity and mortality than is increased DBP. The higher the systolic or diastolic BP, the greater the morbidity and mortality from IHD in elderly women and men. The Cardiovascular Health Study demonstrated in 5202 elderly men and women that a brachial SBP >169 mmHg was associated with a 2.4-fold greater 5-year mortality.[5]

At 30-year follow-up of persons 65 years of age and older in the Framingham Heart Study, systolic hypertension was related to a greater incidence of IHD in elderly men and women.[5] Diastolic hypertension correlated with the incidence of IHD in elderly men but not in elderly women. At 40-month follow-up of 664 elderly men and 48-month follow-up of 1488 elderly women, systolic or diastolic hypertension was associated with a relative risk of new coronary events of 2.0 in men and 1.6 in women.[6] Data from Framingham also suggests the importance of increased pulse pressure, a measure of large artery stiffness. Among 1924 men and women aged 50–79 years, at any given level of SBP of 120 mmHg or greater, the risk of IHD over 20 years rose with lower DBP, suggesting that higher pulse pressure was an important component of risk.[5] Among 1061 men and women aged 60–79 years in the Framingham Heart Study, the strongest predictor of IHD risk was pulse pressure [hazard ratio(HR) = 1.24].

Elderly persons with hypertension should be treated with salt restriction, weight reduction if necessary, discontinuation of drugs that increase blood pressure, avoidance of alcohol and tobacco, increase in physical activity, decrease of dietary saturated fat and cholesterol, and maintenance of adequate dietary potassium, calcium and magnesium intake.[7] In addition, antihypertensive drugs have been shown to reduce IHD events in elderly men and in elderly women with hypertension.[7,8]

Despite multiple large randomized trials, treatment of hypertension in patients aged 80 years or older remained controversial until the publication of HYVET.[8] In HYVET, 3845 persons aged 80 years and older (mean age 83.6 years) with a sustained SBP of 160 mmHg or higher were randomized to indapamide (sustained-release 1.5 mg) or matching placebo. Perindopril 2 mg or 4 mg, or matching placebo, was added if needed to achieve the target blood pressure of 150/80 mmHg. The study was terminated early after a median follow-up of 1.8 years.

Antihypertensive drug treatment reduced the incidence of the primary endpoint (fatal or non-fatal stroke) by 30%, fatal stroke by 39%, all-cause mortality by 21%, death from cardiovascular causes by 23%, and heart failure by 64%. The significant 21% reduction in all-cause mortality by antihypertensive drug treatment was unexpected. The benefits of antihypertensive drug treatment appeared during the first year of follow-up.

The prevalence of cardiovascular disease was only 12% at baseline in HYVET patients (i.e. much lower than generally reported in community-based samples of octogenarians). For example, in a cohort of patients with hypertension, mean age 80 years, in a university geriatrics practice, 70% had cardiovascular disease, target organ damage or diabetes mellitus.[5] The absolute reduction in cardiovascular events resulting from antihypertensive drug therapy in an elderly population with a high prevalence of cardiovascular disease could be much greater than observed in HYVET.

Elderly persons with IHD should have their blood pressure reduced to <140/90 mm and to less than 130/80 mmHg if diabetes mellitus or chronic renal disease is present.[7] Most patients with hypertension will require two or more antihypertensive drugs to achieve this blood pressure goal.[7] The drugs of choice for treating IHD with hypertension are beta-blockers and calcium antagonists (angina pectoris) or beta-blockers, ACE inhibitors, aldosterone antagonists or angiotensin receptor blockers (post myocardial infarction).[7]

Left ventricular hypertrophy

Elderly men and women with ECG LV hypertrophy and echocardiographic LV hypertrophy have an increased risk of developing new coronary events.[5] At 4-year follow-up of 406 elderly men and 735 elderly women in the Framingham study, echocardiographic LV hypertrophy was 15.3 times more sensitive in predicting new coronary events in elderly men and 4.3 times more sensitive in predicting new coronary events in elderly women than was electrocardiographic LV hypertrophy.[5] At 37-month follow-up of 360 men and women, mean age 82 years, with hypertension or IHD, echocardiographic LV hypertrophy was 4.3 times more sensitive in predicting new coronary events than was electrocardiographic LV hypertrophy.[5]

Physicians should try to prevent LV hypertrophy from developing or progressing in elderly men and women with IHD. A meta-analysis of 109 treatment studies found that ACE inhibitors were more effective than other antihypertensive drugs in decreasing LV mass.[5]

Dyslipidaemia

Numerous studies have demonstrated that a high serum total cholesterol is a risk factor for new or recurrent coronary events in elderly men and women.[5] At 40-month follow-up of 664 elderly men and at 48-month follow-up of 1488 elderly women, an increment of 10 mg dl^{-1} of serum total cholesterol was associated with an increase in the relative risk of 1.12 for new coronary events in both men and in women.[6]

A low serum high-density lipoprotein (HDL) cholesterol is a risk factor for new coronary events in elderly men and women.[5] In the Framingham study, in the Established Populations for Epidemiologic Studies of the Elderly study, and in a large cohort of convalescent home patients,[5] a low serum HDL cholesterol was a more powerful predictor of new coronary events than was serum total cholesterol. At 40-month follow-up of 664 elderly men and at 48-month follow-up of 1488 elderly women, a decrement of 10 mg dl^{-1} of serum HDL cholesterol increased the relative risk of new coronary events 1.70 times in men and 1.95 times in women.[6]

Hypertriglyceridaemia is a risk factor for new coronary events in elderly women but not in elderly men.[5] At 40-month follow-up of elderly men and at 48-month follow-up of elderly women, the level of serum triglycerides was not a risk factor for new coronary events in men and was a very weak risk factor for new coronary events in women.[6]

Numerous studies have demonstrated that statins reduce new coronary events in elderly men and in elderly women with IHD.[9] The absolute reduction in new coronary events in these studies is greater for elderly persons than for younger persons. In an observational prospective study of 488 men and 922 women, mean age 81 years, with prior MI and a serum low-density lipoprotein (LDL) cholesterol of 125 mg dl^{-1} or higher, 48% of persons were treated with statins.[10] At 3-year follow-up, statins reduced new coronary events by 50%. The lower the LDL cholesterol achieved by statin therapy, the greater the reduction in coronary events in elderly patients with prior MI.[10]

Recent guidelines recommend lipid-lowering therapy in elderly men and women with IHD to reduce their serum LDL cholesterol to less than 70 mg dl^{-1} (1.8 mmol l^{-1}).[11,12] Data from the Cholesterol Trialists' Collaboration suggest that elderly men and women with (or without) IHD should be treated intensively with statins regardless of initial levels of serum lipids.[13] (See also Chapter 4.)

Diabetes mellitus

Diabetes mellitus is a risk factor for new coronary events in elderly men and women.[5] In the Cardiovascular Health Study, an elevated fasting glucose level (>130 mg dl^{-1}) increased 5-year mortality 1.9 times.[5] At 40-month follow-up of 664 elderly men and at 48-month follow-up of 1488 elderly women, diabetes mellitus increased the relative risk of new coronary events 1.9 times in men and 1.8 times in women.[6] Elderly diabetics without IHD have a higher incidence of new coronary events than elderly non-diabetics with IHD.[5]

Persons with diabetes mellitus are more often obese and have higher serum LDL cholesterol and triglyceride levels and lower serum HDL cholesterol levels than do non-diabetics. Diabetics also have a higher prevalence of hypertension and LV hypertrophy than do non-diabetics. These risk factors contribute to the increased incidence of new IHD events in diabetics compared to non-diabetics. Increased age can further amplify these risk factor differences and contribute to greater IHD risk.

Elderly persons with diabetes mellitus should be treated with dietary therapy, weight reduction if necessary, and appropriate drugs if necessary to control hyperglycaemia. The HbA1c level should be maintained at less than 7%.[5,12] Other risk factors such as smoking, hypertension, dyslipidemia, obesity and physical inactivity should be controlled. The serum LDL cholesterol level should be reduced to less than 70 mg dl^{-1}.[9,11,12] The blood pressure should be reduced to less than 140/90 mmHg. Sulfonylureas should be avoided in persons with IHD.[5]

Obesity

Obesity was an independent risk factor for new IHD events in elderly men and women in the Framingham Heart Study.[5] Disproportionate distribution of fat to the abdomen assessed by the waist:hip circumference ratio has also been shown to be a risk factor for cardiovascular disease, mortality from CHD and total mortality in elderly men and women.[5]

Obese men and women with IHD must undergo weight reduction. Weight reduction is also a first approach to controlling mild hypertension, hyperglycaemia and dyslipidaemia. Regular aerobic exercise should be used in addition to diet to treat obesity.

Physical inactivity

Physical inactivity is associated with obesity, hypertension, hyperglycaemia and dyslipidaemia. At 12-year follow-up in the Honolulu Heart Program, physically active men 65 years of age or older had a relative risk of 0.43 for IHD compared with inactive men.[5] Lack of moderate or vigorous exercise increased 5-year mortality in elderly men and women in the Cardiovascular Heart Study.[5]

Moderate exercise programmes suitable for elderly persons include walking, climbing stairs, swimming or bicycling. However, care must be taken in prescribing any exercise programme because of the high risk of injury in this age group. Group or supervised sessions, including aerobic classes, offered by senior healthcare plans are especially appealing. Exercise training programmes are not only beneficial in preventing CHD but have also been found to improve endurance and functional capacity in elderly persons after MI.[5] (See also Chapter 10.)

Therapy of stable angina

Nitroglycerin is used for relief of the acute anginal attack. It is given either as a sublingual tablet or as a sublingual spray.[14] Long-acting nitrates prevent recurrent anginal attacks, improve exercise time until the onset of angina, and reduce exercise-induced ischaemic ST-segment depression. To prevent nitrate tolerance, it is recommended that a 12- to 14-hour nitrate-free interval be established when using long-acting nitrate preparations. During the nitrate-free interval, the use of another anti-anginal drug will be necessary.

Beta-blockers prevent recurrent anginal attacks and are the drug of choice to prevent new coronary events.[14] Beta-blockers also improve exercise time until the onset of angina and reduce exercise-induced ischaemic ST-segment depression. Beta-blockers should be administered along with long-acting nitrates to all patients with angina unless there are contraindications to the use of these drugs. Antiplatelet drugs such as aspirin or clopidogrel should also be administered to all patients with angina to reduce new coronary events.[11,14,15]

There are no class I indications for the use of calcium channel blockers in the treatment of patients with IHD.[12] However, if angina pectoris persists despite the use of beta-blockers and nitrates, long-acting calcium channel blockers such as diltiazem or verapamil should be used in elderly patients with IHD and normal LV systolic function and amlodipine or felodipine in patients with IHD and abnormal LV systolic function as anti-anginal agents.

If angina persists despite intensive medical management, coronary revascularization with either coronary angioplasty or coronary artery bypass surgery should be considered.[16,17] (See Chapter 9.) The use of other approaches to manage angina that persists despite anti-anginal drugs and coronary revascularization is discussed elsewhere.[14]

Acute coronary syndromes

Unstable angina pectoris is a transitory syndrome that results from disruption of a coronary atherosclerotic plaque that critically decreases coronary blood flow causing new onset angina pectoris or exacerbation of angina pectoris. Transient episodes of coronary artery occlusion or near occlusion by thrombus at the site of plaque injury may occur and cause angina pectoris at rest. The thrombus may be labile and cause temporary obstruction to flow. Release of vasoconstriction substances by platelets and vasoconstriction due to endothelial vasodilator dysfunction contribute to a further reduction in coronary blood flow, and in some patients, myocardial necrosis with non-ST-elevation myocardial infarction (NSTEMI) or ST-elevation myocardial infarction (STEMI) occurs. Elevation of serum cardiospecific troponin I or T or creatine kinase-MB levels occur in patients with NSTEMI and STEMI, but not in patients with unstable angina.

Older patients with acute coronary syndromes should be hospitalized, and depending on their risk stratification, may need monitoring in an intensive or coronary care unit. In a prospective study of 177 consecutive unselected patients hospitalized for an acute coronary syndrome (91 women and 86 men) aged 70–94 years, unstable angina was diagnosed in 54%, NSTEMI in 34% and STEMI in 12%.[18] Obstructive IHD was diagnosed by coronary angiography in 94% of elderly men and in 80% of elderly women.

Therapy of unstable angina pectoris/NSTEMI

Treatment of patients with unstable angina pectoris/NSTEMI should be initiated in the emergency department.[14] Reversible factors precipitating unstable angina pectoris should be identified and corrected. Oxygen should be administered to patients who have cyanosis, respiratory distress, congestive heart failure or high-risk features. Oxygen therapy should be guided by arterial oxygen saturation and should not be given if the arterial oxygen saturation is more than 94%. Morphine sulphate should be administered intravenously when anginal chest pain is not immediately relieved with nitroglycerin or when acute pulmonary congestion and/or severe agitation is present.

Aspirin should be administered to all patients with unstable angina pectoris/NSTEMI as soon as possible after hospital presentation, unless contraindicated, and continued indefinitely. The first dose of aspirin should be chewed rather than swallowed to ensure rapid absorption. Clopidogrel should be given if aspirin is contraindicated

The American College of Cardiology (ACC)/American Heart Association (AHA) 2011 guidelines update states that dual antiplatelet therapy clopidogrel (aspirin plus an IV GP IIb/IIIa inhibitor, or prasugrel) should be administered to patients at high risk.[19]

Nitrates should be administered immediately in the emergency department to patients with unstable angina/NSTEMI.[14] Patients whose symptoms are not fully relieved with three 0.4 mg sublingual nitroglycerin tablets or spray taken five minutes apart and the initiation of an intravenous beta-blocker should be treated with continuous intravenous nitroglycerin. Topical or oral nitrates are alternatives for patients without ongoing refractory symptoms.

Beta-blockers should be administered intravenously in the emergency department unless there are contraindications to their use followed by oral administration and continued indefinitely.[14,19] Metoprolol may be given intravenously in 5 mg increments over 1 to 2 minutes and repeated every

5 minutes until 15 mg has been given followed by oral metoprolol 100 mg twice daily. The target resting heart rate is 50 to 60 beats per minute.

An oral ACE inhibitor should also be given unless there are contraindications to its use and continued indefinitely.[19] In patients with continuing or frequently recurring myocardial ischaemia despite nitrates and beta-blockers, verapamil or diltiazem should be added to their therapeutic regimen in the absence of LV systolic dysfunction (class IIa indication). The benefit of calcium channel blockers in the treatment of unstable angina pectoris is limited to symptom control. Intra-aortic balloon pump counterpulsation should be used for severe myocardial ischaemia that is continuing or occurs frequently despite intensive medical therapy or for haemodynamic instability in patients before or after coronary angiography.

Intravenous thrombolytic therapy is not recommended for the treatment of unstable angina/NSTEMI. Prompt coronary angiography should be performed without non-invasive risk stratification in patients who fail to stabilize with intensive medical treatment. Coronary revascularization should be performed in patients with high-risk features to reduce coronary events and mortality.[14,19]

On the basis of the available data, the ACC/AHA 2011 guidelines recommend the use of statins in patients with acute coronary syndromes and a serum LDL cholesterol of $100\,\mathrm{mg\,dl^{-1}}$ or higher 24 to 96 hours after hospitalization.[12] Statins should be continued indefinitely after hospital discharge.

Patients should be discharged on aspirin plus clopidogrel, (see Chapter 9) beta-blockers, and on ACE inhibitors in the absence of contraindications. Nitrates should be given for ischaemic symptoms. A long-acting non-dihydropyridine calcium channel blocker may be given for ischaemic symptoms that occur despite treatment with nitrates plus beta-blockers. Hormonal therapy should not be administered to postmenopausal women.

Therapy of STEMI

Chest pain due to acute STEMI should be treated with morphine, nitroglycerin and beta-blockers.[20] If arterial saturation is lower than 94%, oxygen should be administered. Aspirin should be given on day 1 of an acute STEMI; subsequent antiplatelet therapy depends on the use of percutaneous catheter intervention (PCI)[21] (see also Chapter 9). The first dose of aspirin should be chewed rather than swallowed. Early intravenous beta-blockade should be used during acute STEMI and oral beta-blockers continued indefinitely to reduce coronary events and mortality. ACE inhibitors should be given within 24 hours of acute STEMI and continued indefinitely to reduce coronary events and mortality. Statins should be given to patients with acute STEMI and should be continued indefinitely after hospital discharge to reduce coronary events and mortality.[12,21]

Primary PCI is currently recommended over thrombolysis in STEMI patients who present early; thrombolysis is an alternative for patients who cannot undergo early PCI, unless contraindicated.[21–23]

The ACC/AHA guidelines recommend using intravenous heparin in persons with acute STEMI undergoing primary coronary interventions or surgical coronary revascularization and in persons with acute STEMI at high risk for systemic embolization such as persons with a large or anterior MI, atrial fibrillation, history of pulmonary or systemic embolus, or LV thrombus.[21,22] In persons with acute MI not receiving intravenous heparin, the ACC/AHA guidelines recommend using subcutaneous heparin 7500 U twice daily for 24 to 48 hours to decrease the incidence of deep venous thrombosis.[21,22]

Therapy after MI

Elderly persons after MI should have their modifiable coronary risk factors intensively treated as discussed previously in this chapter.[21] Aspirin or clopidogrel, and statins, should be given indefinitely to reduce new coronary events and mortality.[12,15,22,24] The ACC/AHA guidelines recommend as class I indications for long-term oral anticoagulant therapy after MI: (1) secondary prevention of MI in post-MI patients unable to tolerate daily aspirin or clopidogrel; (2) post-MI patients with persistent atrial fibrillation; and (3) post-MI patients with LV thrombus.[21,22] Long-term warfarin should be given in a dose to achieve an INR between 2.0 and 3.0.

Beta-blockers (Table 7.2) and ACE inhibitors (or ARBs in patients intolerant of ACE inhibitors) (Table 7.3) should be given indefinitely unless contraindications exist to the use of these drugs to reduce new coronary events and mortality.[12,21,22,24] Long-acting nitrates are effective anti-anginal and anti-ischaemic drugs.[24]

There are no class I indications for the use of calcium channel blockers after MI.[21] Teo *et al.* analysed randomized controlled trials comprising 20 342 persons that investigated the use of calcium channel blockers after MI.[24,25] Mortality was 4% insignificantly higher in persons treated with calcium channel blockers. In this study, beta-blockers significantly reduced mortality by 19% in 53 268 persons. In another study, elderly persons who were treated with beta-blockers after MI had a 43% decrease in 2-year mortality and a 22% decrease in 2-year cardiac hospital readmissions than elderly persons who were not treated with beta-blockers.[24] Use of a calcium channel blocker instead of a beta-blocker after MI doubled the risk of mortality.[24]

Table 7.2 Effect of beta-blockers on mortality in older patients after myocardial infarction.

Study	Follow-up	Results
Goteborg Trial	90 days	Compared with placebo, metoprolol caused a 45% significant decrease in mortality in patients aged 65–74 years
Norwegian Multicentre Study	17 months (up to 33 months)	Compared with placebo, timolol caused a 43% significant reduction in mortality in patients aged 65–74 years
Norwegian Multicentre Study	61 months (up to 72 months)	Compared with placebo, timolol caused a 19% significant decrease in mortality in patients aged 65–74 years
Beta-Blocker Heart Attack Trial	25 months (up to 36 months)	Compared with placebo, propranolol caused a 33% significant reduction in mortality in patients aged 60–69 years
Carvedilol Post-Infarct Survival Control in Left Ventricular Dysfunction Trial	1.3 years	Compared with placebo, carvedilol caused a 23% significant reduction in mortality, a 24% significant reduction in cardiovascular mortality, a 40% significant reduction in non-fatal myocardial infarction, and a 30% significant reduction in all-cause mortality or non-fatal myocardial infarction in patients, mean age 63 years

Source: The studies are discussed in Aronow, 2008.[24]

Anti-arrhythmic therapy after MI

A meta-analysis of 59 randomized controlled trials comprising 23 229 persons that investigated the use of class I anti-arrhythmic drugs after MI showed that mortality was 14% significantly higher in persons receiving class I anti-arrhythmic drugs than in persons receiving no anti-arrhythmic drugs.[25] None of the 59 studies showed a reduction in mortality by class I anti-arrhythmic drugs.

In the Cardiac Arrhythmia Suppression Trials I and II, older age also increased the likelihood of adverse effects including death in persons after MI receiving encainide, flecainide, or moricizine.[24,26] Compared with no anti-arrhythmic drug, quinidine or procainamide did not reduce mortality in elderly persons with CAD, normal or abnormal LVEF, and presence versus absence of ventricular tachycardia.[26]

Compared with placebo, d,l-sotalol did not reduce mortality in post-MI persons followed for one year.[26] Mortality was also significantly higher at 148-day follow-up in persons treated with d-sotalol (5.0%) than in persons treated with placebo. On the basis of the available data, persons after MI should not receive class I anti-arrhythmic drugs or sotalol.

Table 7.3 Effect of angiotensin-converting-enzyme inhibitors on mortality in older patients after myocardial infarction.

Study	Follow-up	Results
Survival and Ventricular Enlargement Trial	42 months (up to 60 months)	In patients with MI and LVEF ≤40%, compared with placebo, captopril reduced mortality 25% in patients aged ≥65 years
Acute Infarction Ramipril Efficacy Study	15 months	In patients with MI and clinical evidence of CHF, compared with placebo, ramipril decreased mortality 36% in patients aged ≥65 years
Survival of Myocardial Infarction Long-Term Evaluation Trial	1 year	In patients with anterior MI, compared with placebo, zofenopril reduced mortality or severe CHF 39% in patients aged ≥65 years
Trandolapril Cardiac Evaluation Study	24 to 50 months	In patients, mean age 68 years, with LVEF ≤35%, compared with placebo, trandolapril reduced mortality 33% in patients with anterior MI and 14% in patients without anterior MI
Heart Outcomes Prevention Evaluation Study	4.5 years (up to 6 years)	In patients aged ≥55 years with MI (53%), cardiovascular disease (88%), or diabetes (38%) but no CHF or abnormal LVEF, ramipril reduced MI, stroke, and cardiovascular death 22%
European trial on reduction of cardiac events with perindopril in patients with stable coronary artery disease	4.2 years	In patients, mean age 60 years, with coronary artery disease and no CHF, compared with placebo, perindopril reduced cardiovascular death, MI, or cardiac arrest 20%

CHF, congestive heart failure; LVEF, left ventricular ejection fraction; MI, myocardial infarction
Source: The studies are discussed in Aronow, 2008.[24]

In the European Myocardial Infarction Amiodarone Trial, 1486 survivors of MI with a LV ejection fraction of 40% or less were randomized to amiodarone (743 patients) or to placebo (743 patients).[24] At 2-year follow-up, 103 patients treated with amiodarone and 102 patients treated with placebo had died. In the Canadian Amiodarone Myocardial Infarction Arrhythmia Trial, 1202 survivors of MI with non-sustained ventricular tachycardia or complex ventricular arrhythmias were randomized to amiodarone or to placebo.[24,26] Amiodarone was very effective in suppressing ventricular tachycardia and complex ventricular arrhythmias. However, the mortality rate at 1.8-year follow-up was not significantly different in the persons treated with amiodarone or placebo. In addition, early permanent discontinuation of drug for reasons other than outcome events occurred in 36% of persons taking amiodarone.

In the Cardiac Arrest in Seattle: Conventional Versus Amiodarone Drug Evaluation Study, the incidence of pulmonary toxicity was 10% at two years in persons receiving amiodarone in a mean dose of 158 mg daily.[24,26] The incidence of adverse effects for amiodarone also approaches 90% after five years of treatment. On the basis of the available data, amiodarone should not be used in the treatment of persons after MI.

However, beta-blockers have been shown to reduce mortality in persons with non-sustained ventricular tachycardia or complex ventricular arrhythmias after MI in patients with normal or abnormal LV ejection fraction.[24,26] On the basis of the available data, beta-blockers should be used in the treatment of elderly persons after MI, especially if non-sustained ventricular tachycardia or complex ventricular arrhythmias are present, unless there are specific contraindications to their use.

In the Antiarrhythmics Versus Implantable Defibrillators (AVID) trial, 1016 persons, mean age 65 years, with a history of ventricular fibrillation or serious sustained ventricular tachycardia were randomized to an automatic implantable cardioverter defibrillator (AICD) or to drug therapy with amiodarone or d,l-sotalol.[26] Persons treated with an AICD had a 39% reduction in mortality at one year, a 27% reduction in mortality at two years, and a 31% reduction in mortality at three years. If persons after MI have life-threatening ventricular tachycardia or ventricular fibrillation, an AICD should be inserted.

The Multicenter Automatic Defibrillator Implantation Trial (MADIT) II randomized 1232 persons, mean age 64 years, with a prior MI and a LVEF of 30% or less to an AICD or to conventional medical therapy.[27] At 20-month follow-up, compared with conventional medical therapy, the AICD significantly decreased all-cause mortality 31% from 19.8% to 14.2%. The effect of AICD therapy in improving survival was similar in persons stratified according to age, sex, LV ejection fraction, New York Heart Association class, and QRS interval. These data favour considering the prophylactic implantation of an AICD in post-MI persons with a LVEF of 30% or lower.

Hormone replacement therapy

The Heart Estrogen/Progestin Replacement Study (HERS) investigated in 2763 women with documented IHD the effect of hormonal therapy versus double-blind placebo on coronary events.[28] At 4.1-year follow-up, there were no significant differences between hormonal therapy and placebo in the primary outcome (non-fatal MI or IHD death) or in any of the secondary cardiovascular outcomes. However, there was a 52% significantly higher incidence of non-fatal MI or death from IHD in the first year in persons treated with hormonal therapy than in persons treated with placebo. Women on hormonal therapy had a 289% significantly higher incidence of venous thromboembolic events and a 38% significantly higher incidence of gallbladder disease requiring surgery than women on placebo.

At 6.8-year follow-up in the HERS trial, hormonal therapy did not reduce the risk of cardiovascular events in women with IHD.[29] The investigators concluded that hormonal therapy should not be used to decrease the risk of coronary events in women with IHD. At 6.8-year follow-up in the HERS trial, all-cause mortality was non-significantly increased 10% by hormonal therapy. The overall incidence of venous thromboembolism at 6.8-year follow-up was significantly increased 208% by hormonal therapy. At 6.8-year follow-up, the overall incidence of biliary tract surgery was significantly increased 48%, the overall incidence for any cancer was insignificantly increased 19%, and the overall incidence for any fracture was insignificantly increased 4%.

Revascularization

Medical therapy alone is the preferred treatment in elderly persons after MI (Table 7.4). The two indications for revascularization in elderly persons after MI are prolongation of life and relief of unacceptable symptoms despite optimal medical management. In a prospective study of 305 patients aged 75 years and older with chest pain refractory to at least

Table 7.4 Overall medical approach to older patients after myocardial infarction.

Stop cigarette smoking and refer to smoking cessation programme.
Treat hypertension with beta-blockers and angiotensin-converting enzyme (ACE) inhibitors; the blood pressure should be reduced to <140/90 mm Hg.
The serum low-density lipoprotein cholesterol should be reduced to <70 mg dl^{-1} with statins if necessary and at least 30–40%.
Diabetes, obesity, and physical inactivity should be treated.
Aspirin or clopidogrel, beta-blockers, and ACE inhibitors should be given indefinitely unless contraindications exist to the use of these drugs.
Long-acting nitrates are effective anti-anginal and anti-ischaemic drugs.
There are no class I indications for the use of calcium-channel blockers after myocardial infarction (MI).
Post-infarction patients should not receive class I anti-arrhythmic drugs, sotalol, or amiodarone.
An automatic implantable cardioverter-defibrillator should be implanted in post-infarction patients at very high risk for sudden cardiac death.
Hormone replacement therapy should not be administered to postmenopausal women after MI.
The two indications for coronary revascularization in elderly persons after MI are prolongation of life and relief of unacceptable symptoms despite optimal medical management.

two anti-anginal drugs, 150 patients were randomized to optimal medical therapy and 155 patients to invasive therapy.[30] In the invasive group, 74% had coronary revascularization (54% coronary angioplasty and 20% coronary artery bypass surgery). During the 6-month follow-up, one-third of the medically treated group needed coronary revascularization for uncontrollable symptoms. At 6-month follow-up, death, non-fatal MI, or hospital admission for an acute coronary syndrome was significantly higher in the medically treated group (49%) than in the invasive group (19%). Revascularization by coronary angioplasty[16] or by coronary artery bypass surgery[17] in elderly persons is extensively discussed elsewhere. If coronary revascularization is performed, aggressive medical therapy must be continued. (See also Chapter 9.)

Key points

- Coronary risk factors should be intensively treated in elderly persons with IHD.
- Elderly persons with IHD should be treated indefinitely with antiplatelet drugs, beta-blockers, ACE inhibitors and statins unless contraindications to the use of these drugs exist.
- The data favour the use of early primary percutaneous coronary intervention in eligible patients younger and older than 75 years with acute STEMI to reduce coronary events and mortality.
- Hormone replacement therapy should not be administered to elderly women with IHD.
- The two indications for revascularization in elderly persons with IHD are prolongation of life and relief of unacceptable symptoms despite optimal medical management.

References

1 Aronow WS, Ahn C and Gutstein H. Prevalence and incidence of cardiovascular disease in 1160 older men and 2464 older women in a long-term health care facility. *J Gerontol Med Sci* 2002;**57A**:M45–6.

2 Aronow WS, Ahn C, Mercando AD *et al*. Prevalence of and association between silent myocardial ischemia and new coronary events in older men and women with and without cardiovascular disease. *J Am Geriatr Soc* 2002;**50**:1075–8.

3 Aronow WS and Fleg JL. (2008) Diagnosis of coronary artery disease in the elderly, in *Cardiovascular Disease in the Elderly*, 4th (eds WS Aronow, JL Fleg and MW Rich), New York City, Informa Healthcare, pp. 351–85.

4 Aronow WS, Ahn C, Mercando A *et al*. Prevalence and association of ventricular tachycardia and complex ventricular arrhythmias with new coronary events in older men and women with and without cardiovascular disease. *J Gerontol Med Sci* 2002;**57A**:M178–80.

5 Aronow WS. (2005) Seniors, in *Preventive Cardiology*, 2nd (eds ND Wong, HR Black and JM Gardin), New York City , McGraw-Hill , Inc., pp. 399–414.
6 Aronow WS and Ahn C. Risk factors for new coronary events in a large cohort of very elderly patients with and without coronary artery disease. *Am J Cardiol* 1996;**77**:864–6.
7 Aronow WS, Fleg JL, Pepine CJ *et al*. ACCF/AHI 2011 expert consensus document on hypertension in the elderly: a report of the American College of Cardiology Foundation Task Force on Clinical Expert Consensus Documents. *Circulation* 2011;**123**:2434–500.
8 Beckett NS, Peters R, Fletcher AE *et al*. Treatment of hypertension in patients years of age or older. *N Engl J Med* 2008;**358**:1887–98.
9 Aronow WS and Frishman WH. Management of hypercholesterolemia in older persons. *Cardiol Rev* 2010;**18**:132–40.
10 Aronow WS and Ahn C. Incidence of new coronary events in older persons with prior myocardial infarction and serum low-density lipoprotein cholesterol ≥125 mg/dL treated with statins versus no lipid-lowering drug. *Am J Cardiol* 2002;**89**:67–9.
11 Grundy SM, Cleeman JI, Merz CN *et al*. Implications of recent clinical trials for the National Cholesterol Education Program Adult Treatment Panel III guidelines. *Circulation* 2004;**110**:227–239.
12 Smith SC Jr, Benjamin EJ, Bonow RO *et al*.; World Heart Federation and the Preventive Cardiovascular Nurses Association. AHA/ACCF Secondary Prevention and Risk Reduction Therapy for Patients with Coronary and other Atherosclerotic Vascular Disease: 2011 update: a guideline from the American Heart Association and American College of Cardiology Foundation. *Circulation* 2011;**124**(22):2458–73.
13 Heart Protection Study Collaborative Group. MRC/BHF Heart Protection Study of cholesterol lowering with simvastatin in 20 536 high-risk individuals: a randomised placebo-controlled trial. *Lancet* 2002;**360**:7–22.
14 Aronow WS and Frishman WH. (2008) Angina in the elderly, in *Cardiovascular Disease in the Elderly*, 4th (eds WS Aronow, JL Fleg and MW Rich), New York City, Informa Healthcare, pp. 269–92.
15 Antithrombotic Trialists' Collaboration. Collaborative meta-analysis of randomised trials of antiplatelet therapy for prevention of death, myocardial infarction, and stroke in high risk patients. *Br Med J* 2002;**324**:71–86.
16 Holmes DR Jr, and Singh M. (2008) Percutaneous coronary intervention in the elderly, in *Cardiovascular Disease in the Elderly*, 4th edn (eds WS Aronow, JL Fleg and MW Rich), New York City, Informa Healthcare, pp. 387–404.
17 Stemmer EA and Aronow WS. (2008) Surgical management of coronary artery disease in the elderly, in *Cardiovascular Disease in the Elderly*, 4th (eds WS Aronow, JL Fleg and MW Rich), New York City, Informa Healthcare, pp. 351–85.
18 Woodworth S, Nayak D, Aronow WS *et al*. Comparison of acute coronary syndromes in men versus women ≥70 years of age. *Am J Cardiol* 2002;**90**:1145–7.
19 Wright RS, Anderson JL, Adams CD *et al*. 2011 Focused Update: ACCF/AHA Guidelines for the Management of Patients with Unstable Angina/Non-ST-Segment Elevation Myocardial Infarction. A Report of the American College of Cardiology Foundation/American Heart Association Task Force on Practice Guidelines. *Circulation* 2011;**123**:2022–60.
20 Rich MW. (2008) Therapy of acute myocardial infarction, in *Cardiovascular Disease in the Elderly*, 4th edn (eds WS Aronow, JL Fleg and MW Rich), New York City, Informa Healthcare, pp. 293–325.
21 Kushner FG, Hand M, Smith SC Jr, *et al*. 2009 Focused Updates: ACC/AHA Guidelines for the Management of Patients with ST-Elevation Myocardial Infarction

and ACC/AHA/SCAI Guidelines on Percutaneous Coronary Intervention. *Circulation* 2009; **120**:2271–306.

22 Antman EM, Hand M, Armstrong PW *et al.* 2007 Focused Update: ACC/AHA Guidelines for the Management of Patients with ST-Elevation Myocardial Infarction. *Circulation* 2008; **117**:296–329.

23 Keeley EC, Boura JA and Grines CL. Primary angioplasty versus intravenous thrombolytic therapy for acute myocardial infarction: a quantitative review of 23 randomised trials. *Lancet* 2003;**361**:13–20.

24 Aronow WS. (2008) Management of the older patient after myocardial infarction, in *Cardiovascular Disease in the Elderly*, 4th (eds WS Aronow, JL Fleg and MW Rich), New York City, Informa Healthcare, pp. 327–49.

25 Teo KK, Yusuf S and Furberg CD. Effects of prophylactic antiarrhythmic drug therapy in acute myocardial infarction. An overview of results from randomized controlled trials. *JAMA* 1993;**270**:1589–95.

26 Aronow WS and Sorbera C. (2008) Ventricular arrhythmias in the elderly, in *Cardiovascular Disease in the Elderly*, 4th edn (eds WS Aronow, JL Fleg and MW Rich), New York City, Informa Healthcare, pp. 605–25.

27 Moss AJ, Zareba W, Hall WJ *et al.* Prophylactic implantation of a defibrillator in patients with myocardial infarction and reduced ejection fraction. *N Engl J Med* 2002;**346**:877–83.

28 Hulley S, Grady D, Bush T *et al.* Randomized trial of estrogen plus progestin for secondary prevention of coronary heart disease in postmenopausal women. *JAMA* 1998;**280**:605–13.

29 Grady D, Herrington D, Bittner V *et al.* Cardiovascular disease outcomes during 6.8 years of hormone therapy. Heart and Estrogen/Progestin Replacement Study follow-up (HERS II). *JAMA* 2002;**288**:49–57.

30 The TIME Investigators. Trial of invasive versus medical therapy in elderly patients with chronic symptomatic coronary artery disease (TIME): a randomised trial. *Lancet* 2001;**358**:951–7.

CHAPTER 8
Heart Failure

Michael W. Rich
Washington University School of Medicine, St Louis, MO, USA

Introduction

The combination of age-related changes in the cardiovascular system and the increasing prevalence of cardiovascular disease at older age predispose the older individual to the development of heart failure (HF). As a result, HF is predominantly a disorder of older adults, with persons over age 75 accounting for more than 50% of the over 1 million hospitalizations for HF each year in the United States, and over 60% of all HF-related deaths.[1] In addition, both the incidence and prevalence of HF are increasing, primarily due to the ageing of the population, and it is anticipated that the number of older adults with clinical HF will double over the next 25 years.

In addition to its effects on hospitalizations and mortality, HF is an important cause of chronic disability in older adults, and the functional limitations imposed by HF are often a key factor contributing to entry into a long-term care facility. HF is also one of the most common comorbid conditions in hospitalized older adults who develop delirium, and HF interacts detrimentally with every major geriatric syndrome. Thus, the societal burden attributable to HF in the ageing population is extremely high, as a consequence of which HF is one of the most costly medical illnesses in the United States today, with estimated annual expenditures in excess of $39 billion, representing approximately 5% of the total healthcare budget.[1]

Pathophysiology

Cardiovascular ageing

As discussed in Chapter 2, normal ageing is associated with extensive changes in cardiovascular structure and function. Taken together, these changes result in a marked reduction in cardiovascular reserve, so that

Cardiovascular Disease and Health in the Older Patient: Expanded from 'Pathy's Principles and Practice of Geriatric Medicine, Fifth edition', First Edition. Edited by David J. Stott and Gordon D.O. Lowe.

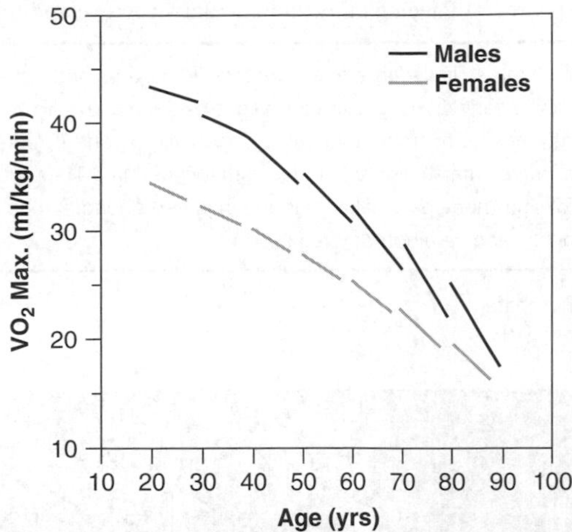

Figure 8.1 Age and VO_2max in healthy subjects: the Baltimore Longitudinal Study on Aging. Reproduced from Fleg JL *et al*. Longitudinal decline of aerobic capacity accelerates with age. *Circulation* 2000;**102**(Suppl II):II–602 [abstract], by permission of Lippincott Williams & Wilkins.

older adults are less able to maintain normal cardiac output and intracardiac pressures in response to stress, whether that stress is physiological (e.g. exercise) or pathological (e.g. ischaemia, anaemia, infection). Figure 8.1 illustrates the striking effect of normal ageing on maximum oxygen consumption (VO_2 max) in healthy men and women carefully screened to exclude occult cardiovascular disease. Note that the decline in VO_2 max with age is not simply linear, but that it actually accelerates after age 60. Moreover, normal octogenarians often have VO_2 max levels of less than 20ml O_2 min^{-1} kg^{-1}, which are similar to those typically observed in middle-aged persons with moderate HF (New York Heart Association class II). Given the normal decline in cardiovascular reserve with increasing age, it is not difficult to understand why an 85-year-old who suffers an acute myocardial infarction (MI) is substantially more prone to develop HF and cardiogenic shock than a 65-year-old who suffers an MI of equivalent size. Similarly, older patients are more likely to develop HF in response to numerous other cardiac and non-cardiac stressors, such as atrial fibrillation (AF), pneumonia, intravenous fluid administration, or any type of major surgery.

Table 8.1 summarizes the principal effects of normal ageing on cardiovascular structure and function.[2,3] Increased vascular stiffness contributes to the progressive rise in systolic blood pressure at older age, and increases impedance to left ventricular (LV) ejection (afterload). Impaired LV relaxation during early diastole (an active, energy-requiring process) and increased myocardial stiffness markedly alter the pattern of LV diastolic

Table 8.1 Principal effects of ageing on cardiovascular structure and function.

- Increased vascular 'stiffness', impedance to left ventricular ejection, and pulse wave velocity
- Impaired left ventricular early diastolic relaxation and mid-to-late diastolic compliance
- Diminished responsiveness to neurohumoral stimuli, especially β_1 and β_2 adrenergic stimulation
- Altered myocardial energy metabolism and reduced mitochondrial ATP-production capacity
- Reduced number of sinus node pacemaker cells and impaired sinoatrial function
- Endothelial dysfunction and vasomotor dysregulation

ATP, adenosine triphosphate

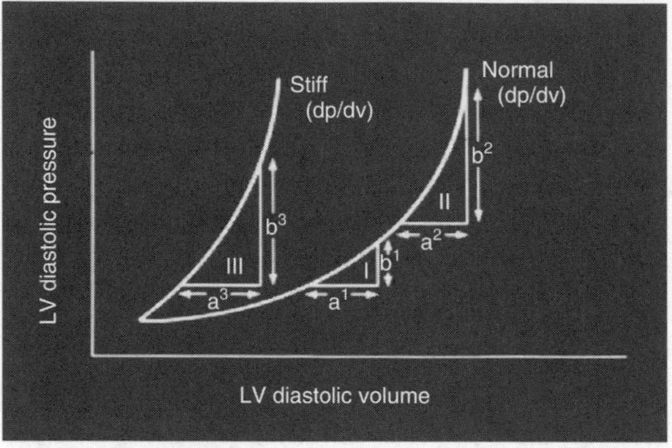

Figure 8.2 Effect of age on the left ventricular (LV) pressure-volume relationship. Note that there is a shift to the left, such that small increases in left ventricular volume are associated with greater increases in left ventricular pressure compared to younger persons. Adapted from Gaasch WH *et al.*, *Am J Cardiol* 1976;**38**:645–53.

filling (preload) and result in a shift in the LV pressure-volume relationship upwards and to the left (Figure 8.2). These changes result in an increased reliance on atrial contraction (the 'atrial kick') to optimize LV filling, and predispose the older individual to the development of HF with preserved LV ejection fraction (HFPEF) and AF. Diminished responsiveness to β-adrenergic stimulation attenuates the heart rate response to stress and also reduces peak contractility, both of which are dependent on activation of the cardiac β_1-receptors. In addition, peripheral vasodilation is impaired due to reduced responsiveness of arteriolar β_2-receptors, further increasing afterload and limiting skeletal muscle blood flow during exercise. In healthy older adults, mitochondria in the cardiac myocytes are capable of generating sufficient ATP to meet the resting energy needs of the myocardium, but they have reduced capacity to increase ATP production in response to stress, thus further limiting peak cardiac performance. There is also a reduction in the number of functioning sinus node pacemaker cells with age, giving rise to the 'sick sinus syndrome' and contributing to chronotropic incompetence; that is, the inability to increase heart rate commensurate with demands. Finally, age-related endothelial dysfunction and vasomotor dysregulation, while not affecting cardiac performance directly, limit peak coronary blood flow and contribute to the development and progression of atherosclerosis and coronary artery disease (CAD). In summary, normal cardiovascular ageing exerts deleterious effects on all four of the major determinants of cardiac output – heart rate, contractility, preload and afterload – thereby greatly reducing peak cardiac performance and cardiovascular reserve. In addition, cardiovascular ageing fosters the development of systolic hypertension and CAD, the two leading causes of HF in older adults.[1]

Other organ systems

Age-associated changes in other organ systems also contribute to the predilection of older adults to develop HF, and may affect the clinical features and response to therapy (Table 8.2). Renal function declines with age, and older adults are less able to excrete a salt and water load. Pulmonary reserve also declines with age, with decreased vital capacity and increased ventilation-perfusion mismatching resulting in more severe hypoxaemia in the setting of superimposed HF. The central nervous system is less able to maintain cerebral perfusion in response to decreased cardiac output due to impaired autoregulatory capacity, thus increasing the propensity of older HF patients to develop impaired cognition or overt delirium. Thirst is also impaired in older adults, increasing the

Table 8.2 Effects of ageing on other organ systems.

Kidneys
Decline in glomerular filtration rate (GFR), ~8 cm^3 min^{-1} per decade
Impaired water and electrolyte homeostasis
Reduced plasma renin and aldosterone activity
Impaired elimination of renally excreted drugs
Lungs
Loss of elastic recoil
Increased ventilation-perfusion (V/Q) mismatching
Reduced vital capacity and minute ventilation
Nervous system
Diminished reflex responsiveness, esp. baroreceptors
Reduced central nervous system autoregulatory capacity
Impaired thirst mechanism
Musculoskeletal system
Loss of muscle mass and strength (sarcopenia)
Loss of bone mass, esp. in women (osteopenia)
Altered pharmacokinetics and pharmacodynamics of most drugs

risk of diuretic-induced dehydration. Sarcopenia, a hallmark of ageing, contributes to impaired exercise tolerance and diminished aerobic capacity in older HF patients. Finally, age-related alterations in the alimentary tract, liver and kidneys result in substantial changes in the absorption, metabolism and excretion of virtually all medications.

Clinical features

Symptoms and signs

Exertional dyspnoea, orthopnea, lower extremity swelling and impaired exercise tolerance are the cardinal symptoms of HF at both younger and older age. However, with increasing age, which is often accompanied by a progressively more sedentary lifestyle, exertional symptoms become less prominent. Conversely, atypical symptoms, such as confusion, somnolence, irritability, fatigue, anorexia or diminished activity level, become increasingly more common manifestations of HF, especially after age 80.

Physical signs of HF include elevated jugular venous pressure, hepatojugular reflux, an S_3 gallop, pulmonary rales, hepatomegaly and dependent oedema. With the exception of rales each of these features occurs less commonly in older HF patients, in part because of the increasing prevalence of HFPEF, in which signs of right HF are a late manifestation and a third heart sound is typically absent. On the other hand, behavioural changes and altered cognition, which may range from subtle abnormalities to overt delirium, frequently accompany HF at elderly age, particularly among institutionalized or hospitalized patients.

Diagnosis

Accurate diagnosis of the HF syndrome at older age is confounded in part by the increasing prevalence of atypical symptoms and signs. In addition, exertional symptoms may be attributable to non-cardiac causes, such as pulmonary disease, anaemia, depression, physical deconditioning, or ageing itself. Likewise, peripheral oedema may be due to venous insufficiency, hepatic or renal disease, or medication side effects (e.g. calcium-channel blockers), and pulmonary crepitus may be due to atelectasis or chronic lung disease. Despite these limitations, careful clinical assessment for the presence of multiple symptoms and signs should lead to the correct diagnosis in most cases.

Chest radiography is indicated when HF is suspected, and it remains the most useful diagnostic test for determining the presence of pulmonary congestion. However, chronic lung disease, altered chest geometry (e.g. due to kyphosis), or poor inspiratory effort may confound interpretation of the chest radiograph in elderly individuals.

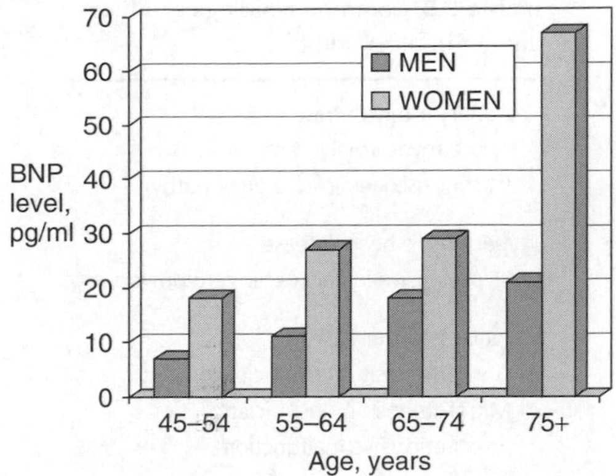

Figure 8.3 Mean B-type natriuretic peptide (BNP) levels in healthy volunteers according to age and gender. Adapted from Redfield MM *et al.*[4]

Plasma B-type natriuretic peptide (BNP) and N-terminal proBNP (NT-proBNP) levels have been shown to be a valuable aid in distinguishing dyspnoea due to HF from that related to other causes, such as pulmonary disorders. BNP and NT-proBNP levels tend to be elevated in both systolic HF and HFPEF, and they also correlate with response to therapy and prognosis. However, levels of these peptides also increase with age in healthy individuals without HF, particularly women (Figure 8.3), and as a result, the specificity and predictive accuracy of elevated levels decline with age.[4] Nonetheless, in cases of diagnostic uncertainty, a low or normal BNP or NT-proBNP level effectively excludes acute HF, whereas markedly elevated levels provide strong evidence in support of the diagnosis.

Proper management of HF is critically dependent on establishing the pathophysiology of LV dysfunction (i.e. systolic vs diastolic), determining the primary and any secondary aetiologies (Table 8.3), and identifying potentially treatable precipitating or contributory factors (Table 8.4). Differentiating systolic from diastolic dysfunction requires an assessment of LV ejection fraction by echocardiography, radionuclide ventriculography, magnetic resonance imaging or contrast angiography. Among these, echocardiography is the most widely used and clinically useful non-invasive test for evaluating systolic and diastolic function. In addition, echocardiography provides important information about LV chamber size and wall thickness, atrial size, right ventricular function, the presence and severity of valvular lesions, and pericardial disorders. For these reasons, echocardiography is recommended for all patients with newly diagnosed HF or unexplained disease progression.[5]

Other diagnostic studies that may be indicated in selected patients include an assessment of thyroid function (especially in the presence of AF), an exercise or pharmacological stress test to evaluate for the presence

Table 8.3 Common aetiologies of heart failure in older adults.

Coronary artery disease
Acute myocardial infarction
Chronic ischaemic cardiomyopathy
Hypertensive heart disease
Hypertensive hypertrophic cardiomyopathy
Valvular heart disease
Aortic stenosis or insufficiency
Mitral stenosis or insufficiency
Prosthetic valve malfunction
Infective endocarditis
Cardiomyopathy
Dilated (non-ischaemic)
Alcohol
Chemotherapeutic agents
Inflammatory myocarditis
Idiopathic
Hypertrophic
Obstructive
Non-obstructive
Restrictive (esp. amyloid)
Pericardial disease
Constrictive pericarditis
High output syndromes
Chronic anaemia
Thiamine deficiency
Hyperthyroidism
Arteriovenous shunting
Age-related diastolic dysfunction

and severity of ischaemia, and cardiac catheterization if revascularization or other corrective procedure (e.g. valve repair or replacement) is being contemplated.

Aetiology and precipitating factors

Systemic hypertension and CAD account for 70–80% of HF cases at older age.[1] Hypertension is the most common aetiology in older women, particularly those with preserved ejection fraction. In older men, HF is more often attributable to CAD. Other common aetiologies include valvular heart disease (especially aortic stenosis and mitral regurgitation) and non-ischaemic cardiomyopathy (Table 8.3). Importantly, HF in the

Table 8.4 Common precipitants of heart failure in older adults.

Myocardial ischaemia or infarction
Uncontrolled hypertension
Dietary sodium excess
Medication non-adherence
Excess fluid intake
Self-induced
Iatrogenic
Arrhythmias
Supraventricular, esp. atrial fibrillation
Ventricular
Bradycardia, esp. sick sinus syndrome
Associated medical conditions
Fever
Infections, esp. pneumonia or sepsis
Hyperthyroidism or hypothyroidism
Anaemia
Renal insufficiency
Thiamine deficiency
Pulmonary embolism
Hypoxemia due to chronic lung disease
Drugs and medications
Alcohol
Beta-adrenergic blockers (incl. ophthalmologicals)
Calcium-channel blockers
Anti-arrhythmic agents
Non-steroidal anti-inflammatory drugs
Glucocorticoids
Mineralocorticoids
Estrogen preparations
Anti-hypertensive agents (e.g. clonidine, minoxodil)

elderly population is frequently multifactorial, and it is thus essential to identify all potentially treatable causes.

In addition to determining aetiology, it is important to identify factors precipitating or contributing to HF exacerbations (Table 8.4). Non-adherence to medications and dietary restrictions is the most common cause of worsening HF, and patients should be closely questioned about their dietary and medication habits. Other common factors contributing to increased symptoms include ischaemia, volume overload due to excess fluid intake (self-inflicted or iatrogenic), tachyarrhythmias (especially AF or flutter), intercurrent infections, anaemia, thyroid disease and various medications or toxins (e.g. alcohol).

Comorbidity

A hallmark of ageing is the increasing prevalence of multiple comorbid conditions, many of which impact directly or indirectly on the diagnosis, clinical course, treatment and prognosis of HF in elderly people (Table 8.5). As noted previously, renal function declines with age, and octogenarians often have creatinine clearances of <60 cm^3 min^{-1} (i.e. stage III chronic kidney disease), despite 'normal' serum creatinine levels and in the absence of underlying renal disease. Older patients are also less able to excrete excess sodium and water, and this deficiency may contribute to volume overload. Diuretics tend to be less effective in elderly people, whereas diuretic-induced electrolyte disorders are more common, in part due to reduced capacity of the kidneys to preserve electrolyte homeostasis. Conversely, diuretics, ACE inhibitors and angiotensin receptor blockers (ARBs) can all contribute to worsening renal function, and older patients are at increased risk for this complication.

Older HF patients are at increased risk for anaemia due to comorbid chronic illnesses (renal disease, occult malignancy), inadequate dietary intake of key nutrients (iron, folate, B_{12}), and use of medications associated with gastrointestinal blood loss (aspirin, warfarin, non-steroidal anti-inflammatory drugs (NSAIDs)). Anaemia contributes to impaired tissue oxygen delivery and impaired exercise tolerance, and may exacerbate myocardial ischaemia in patients with underlying CAD. Anaemia has also

Table 8.5 Common comorbidities in older patients.

Condition	Implications
Renal dysfunction	Exacerbated by diuretics, ACE inhibitors, ARBs
Anaemia	Worsens symptoms and prognosis
Chronic lung disease	Contributes to uncertainty about diagnosis and volume status
Cognitive dysfunction	Interferes with dietary, medication and activity adherence
Depression, social isolation	Worsens prognosis, interferes with adherence
Postural hypotension, falls	Exacerbated by vasodilators, diuretics, beta-blockers
Arthritis	NSAIDs worsen heart failure, antagonize heart failure medications
Urinary incontinence	Aggravated by diuretics, ACE inhibitors (cough)
Sarcopenia, osteoporosis	Contribute to impaired exercise tolerance
Sensory deprivation	Interferes with adherence
Nutritional disorders	Exacerbated by dietary restrictions
Polypharmacy	Reduced adherence, increased drug interactions
Frailty	Exacerbated by hospitalization; increased fall risk

ACE, angiotensin-converting enzyme; ARBs, angiotensin-receptor blockers; NSAIDs, non-steroidal anti-inflammatory drugs been shown to be an independent predictor of adverse clinical outcomes in patients with HF.

Normal ageing is associated with a decline in maximum voluntary ventilation and an increase in ventilation-perfusion mismatching. In addition, chronic obstructive and restrictive lung diseases further impair pulmonary function in many older adults. Diminished pulmonary function, in turn, contributes to increased dyspnoea and exercise intolerance in older patients with HF, as the lungs are unable to compensate for impaired cardiac performance. In addition, the presence of chronic lung disease often leads to diagnostic uncertainty (is the patient's dyspnoea due to HF, pulmonary disease or a combination of both?), in part by confounding interpretation of the physical examination and chest radiograph.

Cognitive dysfunction interferes with the patient's ability to participate fully in self-care behaviours, such as weight monitoring and adherence to dietary restrictions and prescribed medications. In more severe cases, cognitive impairment substantially limits the patient's ability to provide a reliable medical history, and may prevent recognition of new or worsening symptoms. Patients with cognitive dysfunction are also at increased risk for developing delirium, which may complicate hospital management and predispose to serious adverse events (e.g. falls, aspiration, infections).

Up to 20% of elderly HF patients have clinically significant depression, which is often unrecognized. Social isolation, primarily due to the death of one's spouse, also occurs with increasing frequency at elderly age. These conditions have both been associated with adverse outcomes in elderly HF patients, including increased mortality and hospitalization rates, in part due to reduced adherence to prescribed medications and other recommended behaviours. In addition, depression has been linked with increased adrenergic tone and ventricular arrhythmias in patients with cardiovascular disease, both of which confer an increased mortality risk in HF patients.

Increased vascular stiffness and impaired baroreflex responsiveness predispose older adults to the development of postural hypotension, while age-related alterations in sinus node function increase the risk of bradyarrhythmias (sick sinus syndrome). In addition, balance and proprioception decline with age. Taken together, these factors greatly increase the risk of falls in older adults. Standard HF therapies, including diuretics, vasodilators and beta-blockers, all have the potential to further increase the risk of falls and associated morbidity.

Arthritis is the leading cause of chronic disability in older adults, and is widely treated with NSAIDs available both by prescription and over-the-counter. These agents enhance renal sodium and water reabsorption and have been associated with a significant increase in the risk of hospitalization for HF, even among patients with no prior HF history.[6] NSAIDs also antagonize the effects of diuretics and ACE inhibitors, and may inhibit the beneficial effects of aspirin in patients with CAD. In addition, NSAIDs are a common cause of gastrointestinal bleeding in older adults, thus potentiating the risk of anaemia.

The prevalence of urinary incontinence increases with age, affecting up to 35% of women and 20% of men over the age of 80. Diuretics and ACE inhibitors (ACE inhibitor cough) may aggravate incontinence in many patients. However, most patients with mild to moderate incontinence do not report the condition to their physicians unless specifically asked. Instead, they will avoid taking their medication rather than risking embarrassment, especially if they are going to be away from home without ready access to a restroom. Although the importance of urinary incontinence as a cause of medication non-adherence in elderly patients is unknown, it is likely under-appreciated, as most clinicians do not routinely inquire about this condition.

Sarcopenia contributes to muscle weakness and impaired exercise tolerance in older persons with or without HF. Osteopenia and osteoporosis compromise the structural integrity of the skeletal system (e.g. as a result of compression fractures), further reducing exercise capacity. In addition, the risk of falls and hip fractures is increased, and, as noted above, these risks may be aggravated by several of the medications used to treat HF.

Reduced visual and auditory acuity often interfere with patients' ability to comply with therapeutic recommendations, either because they did not hear the instructions properly, or because they are unable to read printed materials (e.g. medication instructions, pill bottles, nutrition labels). When coupled with social isolation, these deficits can make it particularly difficult for older patients to adhere to HF therapy.

Under-nutrition is common in older adults and is usually multifactorial, with reduced access to nutritional foods (e.g. due to loss of independence, social isolation, limited finances), diminished appetite (due to chronic illness, depression, medications), loss of enjoyment from eating (impaired sense of taste and smell, social isolation), neuromuscular conditions (stroke, Parkinsonism) and mechanical factors (poor dentition, difficulty swallowing) all playing a role. In addition, prevalent medical conditions often lead to the imposition of major dietary restrictions, including protein restriction in patients with hepatic or renal disease, carbohydrate restriction in diabetics, fat and cholesterol restriction in patients with CAD or diabetes, and sodium restriction in patients with hypertension, HF, or renal disease. Moreover, advanced HF itself is often associated with a progressive decline in lean body mass, a condition referred to as cardiac cachexia. Thus, HF *per se*, as well as its treatment (sodium restriction in almost all cases, restriction of other macronutrients in many cases due to prevalent comorbidities), may contribute to the development or progression of under-nutrition in older adults, a condition associated with immune deficiency, frailty and a poor long-term prognosis.

Polypharmacy is common in patients with HF, since drug therapy for HF alone often entails the use of three or more medications, and virtually all elderly HF patients have associated conditions for which they are receiving treatment. Apart from the high cost associated with the use of multiple medications, polypharmacy has an important role in interfering with medication adherence, since the more medications a patient is taking, the less likely it becomes that they are taking their medications correctly. In addition, there is an exponential relation between the number of medications and the risk of drug interactions, such that patients taking 10 or more medications have over a 90% probability of experiencing one or more clinically significant drug interactions.

The prevalence of frailty increases markedly with age, especially among persons over the age of 80, and the cardinal features of frailty – weight loss, weakness, slow movement, low physical activity and exhaustion – overlap significantly with the symptoms of HF.[7] Frailty confers a poor prognosis, as it tends to be associated with progressive physical and functional decline, and it is also a marker for increased risk for iatrogenic complications, such as falls related to medications. Frailty tends to worsen during hospitalization for acute illness (e.g. a HF exacerbation), and frail patients rarely return to their previous level of function following hospital discharge. Thus, HF and frailty interact in a way that is detrimental to both conditions.

Recent studies indicate that both the number and nature of non-cardiac comorbidities have a significant impact on clinical outcomes in older HF patients. In 2003, Braunstein *et al.* examined the prevalence of non-cardiac comorbidities in Medicare beneficiaries hospitalized with HF.[8] As shown in Figure 8.4, 86% of patients had two or more non-cardiac comorbidities, and more than 25% had six or more non-cardiac conditions. In addition, since common geriatric syndromes, such as dementia, depression, incontinence and frailty, are often clinically unrecognized, it is likely that the true prevalence of non-cardiac comorbidities is underestimated by Braunstein's data.

Figure 8.5 illustrates the relationship between the number of non-cardiac comorbidities and the number of hospital admissions among HF patients.[8] Overall, the proportion of patients hospitalized annually increased from about 35% among patients with no comorbidities, to over 90% among patients with nine or more comorbidities. Moreover, approximately half of all hospitalizations were considered potentially avoidable (depicted by the shaded regions in the figure), regardless of the number of comorbidities.

Several studies have examined the relationship between specific comorbidities and clinical outcomes. Chronic renal insufficiency and anaemia have both been shown to be independent predictors of mortality in elderly

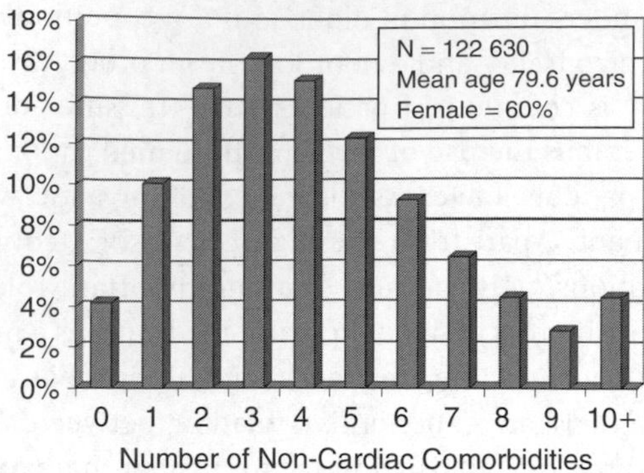

Figure 8.4 Prevalence of non-cardiac comorbidities in Medicare beneficiaries with heart failure. Adapted from Braunstein JB *et al.*[8]

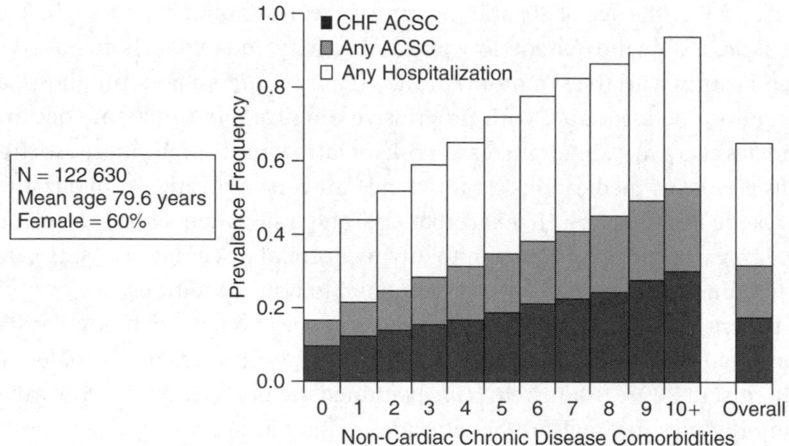

Figure 8.5 Impact of non-cardiac comorbidities on hospital admissions in Medicare beneficiaries with heart failure. ACSC, ambulatory care sensitive conditions; CHF, chronic heart failure. Reproduced from Braunstein JB *et al.*[8] Copyright 2003, with permission from Elsevier.

HF patients, and the presence of cognitive dysfunction has been associated with a striking increase in mortality among older patients hospitalized with HF. In addition, the use of NSAIDs has been associated with a 60% increase in the risk of hospitalization for HF among elderly patients with no prior history of heart disease, and a 10-fold increase among patients with pre-existing cardiac conditions.[6]

In summary, older HF patients almost invariably have one or more age-associated conditions that influence the diagnosis, clinical features and/or management of HF. Conversely, HF and its therapy often have ramifications for the clinical course and treatment of these comorbid conditions. Consideration of the interactions between HF and prevalent comorbidities is thus a critically important aspect of management in the elderly HF patient.

Management

The principal goals of HF therapy are to relieve symptoms, maintain or enhance functional capacity and quality of life, preserve independence and reduce mortality. Although it is often stated that quality of life is more important than quantity of life in the very elderly, there is wide variability in personal preferences concerning these outcomes. Furthermore, since the elderly HF population is characterized by marked heterogeneity in terms of lifestyle, comorbidity and personal goals and perspectives, management of HF in elderly patients must first and foremost be individualized and patient-centred in accordance with each patient's circumstances and needs.

The approach to HF management involves identification and treatment of the underlying aetiology and any contributing factors, implementation of an effective therapeutic regimen, and coordination of care through the use of a multidisciplinary team.

Aetiology and precipitating factors

Although HF in older adults is rarely 'curable', proper treatment of the underlying aetiology often improves symptoms and delays disease progression. Thus, hypertension should be treated aggressively, and CAD should be managed appropriately with medications and/or percutaneous or surgical revascularization. Similarly, therapy for diabetes and dyslipidaemia should be optimized, smoking should be strongly discouraged, and a suitable level of regular physical activity should be prescribed. Alcohol intake should be limited to no more than two drinks per day in men and one drink per day in women, and alcohol use should be strictly proscribed in patients with suspected alcoholic cardiomyopathy.

Severe aortic stenosis is a common cause of HF at older age, and aortic valve replacement is effective in reducing mortality and improving quality of life. Peri-operative mortality rates are acceptable (less than 10%), and long-term results are excellent, even in octogenarians. More recently, percutaneous aortic valve replacement has been shown to offer an effective alternative to valve replacement in selected patients with prohibitive operative risk.

Severe mitral regurgitation may be amenable to surgical therapy (i.e. valve repair or replacement) in selected patients, but the operative results are somewhat less favourable than for aortic valve surgery. Percutaneous approaches to reducing the severity of mitral regurgitation have recently been developed and offer an alternative to surgery in some cases. Mitral valve replacement is also effective therapy for severe mitral stenosis; rarely, percutaneous mitral balloon valvuloplasty may be feasible in older patients.

Atrial fibrillation is a common precipitant of HF in older patients, especially in the setting of diastolic dysfunction. In patients with recent onset symptomatic AF, many clinicians recommend restoration and maintenance of sinus rhythm if feasible, although the long-term benefits of this approach have not been established. In patients with chronic AF, the ventricular rate should be adequately controlled both at rest and during activity. Bradycardia is a less common cause of HF; when present, implantation of a permanent pacemaker provides definitive therapy (see section on Device therapy). Anaemia, thyroid disease and other systemic illnesses should be identified and treated accordingly.

The importance of adherence to medications and dietary restrictions, including avoidance of excessive fluid intake, cannot be overemphasized. NSAIDs are widely used by older individuals to treat arthritis and relieve chronic pain, but these agents promote sodium and water retention, interfere with the actions of ACE inhibitors and other anti-hypertensive agents, and may worsen renal function; their use should be avoided whenever possible.[6] Similarly, the use of other medications that may aggravate HF should be closely monitored.

Pharmacotherapy

The design of an effective therapeutic regimen is based in part on whether the patient has predominantly systolic HF or predominantly HFPEF. Although these two abnormalities frequently co-exist (indeed, virtually all individuals over age 70 have some degree of diastolic dysfunction), for the purposes of this discussion patients with an ejection fraction <45% (i.e. moderate or severe LV systolic dysfunction) will be considered as having systolic HF, whereas patients with an ejection fraction ≥45% will be considered as having HFPEF.

Systolic heart failure

In the past 30 years there has been considerable progress in the treatment of systolic HF. Although most studies have either excluded individuals over 75–80 years of age, or have enrolled too few elderly subjects to permit definitive conclusions, the available data indicate that the response of older patients to standard therapies is similar to that of younger patients. Therefore, current recommendations for drug treatment of systolic HF are similar in younger and older patients.[5]

ACE inhibitors

ACE inhibitors are the cornerstone of therapy for LV systolic dysfunction, whether or not clinically overt HF is present.[5] Older patients are more likely than younger patients to have potential contraindications to ACE inhibitors (e.g. renal dysfunction, renal artery stenosis, orthostatic hypotension), and they may also be at increased risk for ACE inhibitor-related side effects, such as worsening renal function, electrolyte disturbances and hypotension. Nonetheless, a trial of ACE inhibitors is indicated in virtually all older patients with documented LV systolic dysfunction.

In most cases, ACE inhibitor therapy should be initiated at a low dose (e.g. captopril 6.25–12.5 mg tid or enalapril 2.5 mg bid), and the dosage should be gradually titrated upward to the level shown to be effective in clinical trials (captopril 50 mg tid, enalapril 10 mg bid, lisinopril 20 mg qd, ramipril 10 mg qd). Once a maintenance dose has been achieved, substituting a once-daily agent (e.g. lisinopril or ramipril) at equivalent dosage may facilitate adherence. Blood pressure, renal function and serum potassium levels should be monitored closely during dose titration and periodically during maintenance therapy. In patients unable to tolerate standard ACE-inhibitor dosages due to side effects, dosage reduction is appropriate, as there is evidence that even very low doses of these agents (e.g. lisinopril 2.5–5 mg qd) provide some degree of benefit.

Angiotensin receptor blockers

Angiotensin receptor blockers (ARBs) have a somewhat more favourable side effect profile than ACE inhibitors, and the effects of ARBs on major clinical outcomes (mortality, hospitalizations) are similar to those seen with ACE inhibitors.[9] ARBs have also been shown to reduce mortality and hospitalizations in patients with systolic HF who are intolerant to ACE inhibitors due to cough or other side effects.[10] Compared with an ACE inhibitor alone, combining an ARB with an ACE inhibitor reduces HF admissions but not mortality, while increasing the risk of side effects.[9,11] Based on available evidence, ACE inhibitors are still considered first-line therapy for systolic HF, but ARBs offer an excellent alternative for patients intolerant to ACE inhibitors, and they may also be useful as adjunctive agents in selected patients with persistent symptoms despite conventional treatment.[5]

Hydralazine and isosorbide dinitrate

The combination of hydralazine 75 mg qid and isosorbide dinitrate 30–40 mg qid was associated with decreased mortality in a small trial of HF patients <75 years of age. In a more recent study that did not exclude older subjects, the combination was shown to reduce mortality in African-American patients with symptomatic systolic HF.[12] Based on this study, combination hydralazine-nitrate therapy is recommended for self-declared African-Americans with advanced systolic HF.[5] The combination also provides an alternative therapy for patients who are intolerant to ACE inhibitors and ARBs, for patients with significant renal insufficiency, and as adjunctive therapy in patients who remain highly symptomatic despite standard treatment. Side effects are common with both hydralazine and high-dose nitrates, and the combination is not available in a once-daily formulation.

Beta-blockers

Beta-blockers improve LV function and decrease mortality in a broad population of HF patients, including those with New York Heart Association (NYHA) class IV symptoms and patients up to 80 years of age, and beta-blockers are now considered standard therapy for clinically stable patients without major contraindications.[5] Use of beta-blockers in older patients may be limited by a higher prevalence of bradyarrhythmias and severe chronic lung disease, and older patients may also be more susceptible to the development of fatigue and impaired exercise tolerance during long-term beta-blocker administration.

Carvedilol, metoprolol and bisoprolol have all been shown to improve outcomes in patients with systolic HF, and one randomized trial found that carvedilol 25 mg twice daily was more effective than metoprolol 50 mg twice daily in reducing mortality.[13] In most cases, beta-blocker treatment should be initiated at low dosages in stable patients upon a background of ACE inhibitor and diuretic therapy. Recommended starting dosages are carvedilol 3.125 mg bid, metoprolol 6.25–12.5 mg bid, and bisoprolol 1.25 mg once daily. The dose should be gradually increased at 2–4 week intervals to achieve maintenance dosages of carvedilol 25–50 mg bid, metoprolol 50–100 mg bid (or, preferably, sustained release metoprolol 100–200 mg daily), or bisoprolol 5–10 mg daily. Lower dosages and a slower titration protocol may be appropriate in patients over 75 years of age. Contraindications to beta-blockade include marked sinus bradycardia (resting heart rate <45–50 bpm), PR interval ≥ 0.24 s, heart block greater than first degree, systolic blood pressure <90–100 mmHg, active bronchospastic lung disease, and severe decompensated HF.

Digoxin

Digoxin improves symptoms and reduces hospitalizations in patients with symptomatic systolic HF treated with ACE inhibitors and diuretics, but has no effect on total or cardiovascular mortality. The effects of digoxin are similar in younger and older patients, including octogenarians,[14] and digoxin is therefore a useful drug for the treatment of systolic HF in patients of all ages who have limiting symptoms despite standard therapy.

The volume of distribution and renal clearance of digoxin decline with age. In addition, the optimal therapeutic concentration for digoxin appears to be 0.5–0.9 ng ml^{-1};[15] higher concentrations are associated with increased toxicity but no greater efficacy.[15] For most older patients with preserved renal function (estimated creatinine clearance $\geq$60 cm^3 min^{-1}), digoxin 0.125 mg daily provides a therapeutic effect. Lower dosages should be used in patients with renal insufficiency. Although routine monitoring of serum digoxin levels is no longer recommended, it seems reasonable to measure the serum digoxin concentration 2–4 weeks after initiating therapy to ensure that the level does not exceed 0.9 ng ml^{-1}.In addition, a digoxin level should be obtained whenever digoxin toxicity is suspected.

Digoxin side effects include arrhythmias, heart block, gastrointestinal disturbances and altered neurological function (e.g. visual disturbances). Although older patients are often thought to be at increased risk for digitalis toxicity, this was not confirmed in an analysis from the Digitalis Investigation Group (DIG) trial.[14] On the other hand, digoxin has significant drug interactions with many medications commonly prescribed to older patients. Among these, cholestyramine and phenytoin reduce digoxin levels, whereas amiodarone, amphotericin, calcium preparations, cyclosporine, erythromycin, itraconazole, propafenone, quinidine, reserpine, tetracycline and verapamil all increase serum digoxin concentrations and the risk of digoxin toxicity.

Diuretics

Diuretics are an essential component of therapy for most patients with HF, and diuretics remain the most effective agents for relieving congestion and maintaining euvolaemia. Some patients with mild HF can be effectively controlled with a thiazide diuretic, but the majority will require a loop diuretic such as furosemide, bumetanide or torsemide. In patients with more severe HF or significant renal dysfunction (serum creatinine $\geq$2.0 mg dl^{-1}), the addition of metolazone 2.5–10 mg daily may be necessary to achieve effective diuresis.

In general, diuretic dosages should be titrated to eliminate signs of pulmonary and systemic venous congestion. Common side effects include worsening renal function (often due to over-diuresis) and electrolyte disorders. To minimize these effects, renal function and serum electrolyte levels (sodium, potassium, magnesium) should be monitored closely during the initiation and titration phase of diuretic use, and periodically thereafter.

Aldosterone antagonists

Spironolactone is a potassium-sparing diuretic that acts by antagonizing aldosterone. The addition of spironolactone 12.5–50 mg daily to standard HF therapy has been shown to reduce mortality and hospital admissions in patients with NYHA class III–IV systolic HF, with similar benefits in older and younger patients.[16] Eplerenone, a selective aldosterone antagonist, has also been shown to reduce mortality and sudden cardiac death in patients with LV systolic dysfunction following acute myocardial infarction and in patients with NYHA class II symptoms with an LV ejection fraction ≤30%.[17] Spironolactone is contraindicated in patients with severe renal insufficiency or hyperkalaemia, and up to 10% of patients develop painful gynaecomastia. In addition, older patients receiving spironolactone in combination with an ACE inhibitor or ARB may be at increased risk for hyperkalaemia, particularly in the presence of pre-existing renal insufficiency or diabetes, and at doses in excess of 25 mg per day. Combined use of an ACE inhibitor, ARB and aldosterone antagonist is not recommended.[5]

Approach to treatment

Figure 8.6 provides a suggested approach to the pharmacological treatment of systolic HF. All patients with LV systolic dysfunction, whether asymptomatic or symptomatic, should receive an ACE inhibitor (or an ARB or alternative vasodilator if ACE inhibitors are contraindicated or not tolerated). Patients with stable symptoms and no contraindications should also receive a beta-blocker, and diuretics should be administered in sufficient doses to maintain euvolaemia. Spironolactone should be used in patients with persistent NYHA class III–IV symptoms, and combination therapy with hydralazine-nitrates is indicated in black patients with symptomatic systolic HF. Digoxin and/or additional vasodilator therapy

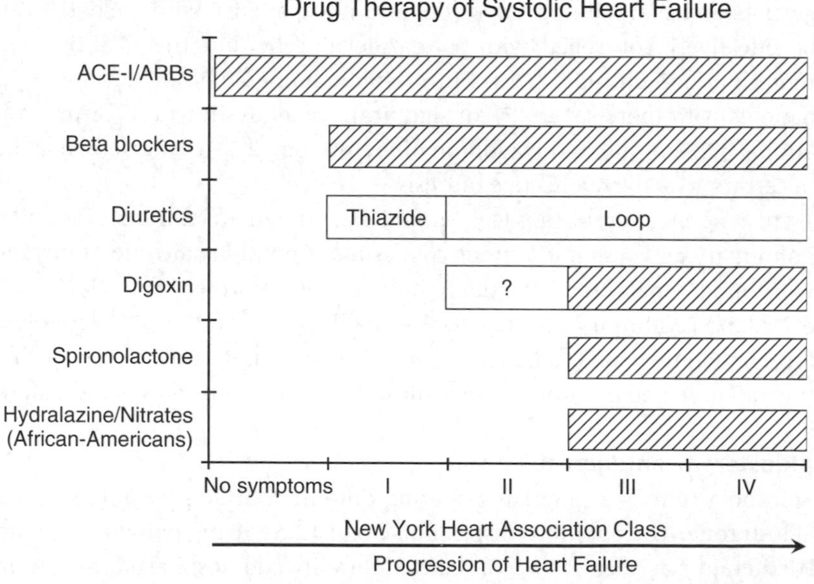

Figure 8.6 Approach to treatment of systolic heart failure; see text for details. Shaded areas refer to therapies proven to be efficacious in prospective randomized clinical trials. ACE-I, angiotensin-converting enzyme inhibitors; ARBs, angiotensin-receptor blockers.

Table 8.6 Treatment of heart failure with preserved ejection fraction: overview of randomized trials.

Trial	Agent	N	Mean age (years)	Follow-up (years)	Main findings
CHARM-Preserved[18]	candesartan	3023	67	3.1	No effect on mortality; HF admissions reduced
I-PRESERVE[19]	irbesartan	4128	72	4.1	No effect on mortality, admissions, or other endpoints
PEP-CHF[20]	perindopril	850	76	2.1	No effect on mortality; HF admissions reduced; improved NYHA class and exercise tolerance
SENIORS[21]	nebivolol	2128	76	1.8	No effect on mortality; decreased cardiovascular admissions
DIG-ancillary[22]	digoxin	988	67	3.1	No effect on mortality or cardiovascular admissions

HF, heart failure; NYHA, New York Heart Association

should be considered in patients who remain symptomatic despite the above regimen.

Heart failure with preserved ejection fraction (HFPEF)

Over 50% of elderly HF patients have preserved LV systolic function. However, although there have now been several clinical trials involving patients with HFPEF (Table 8.6), management of this condition remains largely empiric. As with systolic HF, the underlying cardiac disorder and associated contributing conditions should be treated appropriately. In particular, hypertension and CAD should be managed aggressively. Diuretics should be used judiciously to relieve congestion while avoiding over-diuresis and prerenal azotemia. Topical or oral nitrates may be beneficial in reducing pulmonary congestion and orthopnea.

In the CHARM-preserved trial (Candesartan in Heart failure: Assessment of Reduction in Mortality and morbidity), the ARB candesartan reduced HF admissions by 16% but had no effect on mortality in patients with HF and a LV ejection fraction >40%.[18] The mean age of patients in CHARM-preserved was 67 years, and 807 patients, comprising 27% of the total population, were ≥75 years of age. However, patients with substantial comorbidity were excluded, so the applicability of the study findings to older HF patients encountered in clinical practice remains unknown.

More recently, the I-PRESERVE trial (Irbesartan in Heart Failure with Preserved Systolic Function) randomized 4128 patients (mean age 72 years, 60% women) with HFPEF (LV ejection fraction ≥45%) to the ARB irbesartan or placebo and followed them for a mean of 4.1 years.[19] In this study, irbesartan failed to show a beneficial effect on the primary composite endpoint of all-cause mortality or cardiovascular hospitalization. Irbesartan also had no effect on any of the pre-specified secondary endpoints, including cardiovascular mortality and admission for HF.

In another study, PEP-CHF (Perindopril in Elderly Patients with CHF), 850 patients aged 70 years or older (mean age 76 years, 55% women) with HFPEF were randomized to the ACE-inhibitor perindopril or placebo and followed for a mean of 2.1 years.[20] Although perindopril had no effect on the primary outcome of mortality or HF admission, overall HF admissions were reduced and New York Heart Association class and 6-minute walk distance were improved at one year in patients randomized to perindopril. In subgroup analysis, perindopril appeared to have a beneficial effect on the primary outcome in patients ≤75, but not in those >75 years of age.

Although beta-blockers are of proven benefit in patients with systolic HF, there are limited data on their use in patients with HFPEF. In the SENIORS trial (Study of the Effects of Nebivolol Intervention on Outcomes and Rehospitalization in Seniors), 2128 HF patients ≥70 years of age (mean age 76 years, 35% women) were randomized to the beta-blocker nebivolol or placebo and followed for an average of 21 months.[21] Patients with either systolic HF or HFPEF were included, and the primary composite endpoint was all-cause mortality or cardiovascular hospitalization. Overall, nebivolol was associated with a significant 15% reduction in the primary endpoint. There was no effect on mortality but cardiovascular admissions were reduced, with similar findings in patients with LV ejection fraction >35% versus ≤35%.

Finally, in the DIG ancillary trial (Digitalis Investigation Group), 988 patients (mean age 67 years, 41% women) with HF and LV ejection fraction >45% were randomized to digoxin or placebo and followed for an average of 3.1 years.[22] Overall, digoxin had no effect on the primary composite endpoint of HF death or HF hospitalization; there was also no effect on all-cause mortality, cardiovascular mortality or cardiovascular hospitalizations.

In summary, despite publication of several prospective clinical trials in older patients with HFPEF, to date no pharmacological intervention has been shown to reduce mortality in this population, and, with the exception of diuretics to relieve congestion, there are currently no class I or class IIa indications for any of these agents in the treatment of HFPEF. Therefore, therapy should be individualized and guided by prevalent comorbidities and the observed response to specific therapeutic interventions.

Device therapy

Although most older HF patients can be effectively managed with behavioural interventions and medications, implantable devices are playing an increasingly important role in the management of selected subgroups of the HF population.

Cardiac pacemakers

Ageing is associated with a progressive decline in the number of functioning sinus node pacemaker cells, often leading to the 'sick sinus syndrome', which is characterized by inappropriate sinus bradycardia, sinus pauses and chronotropic incompetence (failure to adequately increase heart rate in response to increased demands). Since cardiac output is directly proportional to heart rate (Cardiac Output =Heart Rate x Stroke Volume), age-related bradyarrhythmias may contribute to HF symptoms and impaired exercise tolerance. Because there is no effective medical therapy for sick sinus syndrome, implantation of a pacemaker is appropriate in symptomatic patients. Beta-blockers may precipitate symptomatic bradyarrhythmias in elderly HF patients. However, since beta-blockers improve ventricular function and reduce mortality and hospitalizations in patients with systolic HF, placement of a pacemaker is often preferable to discontinuation of beta-blocker therapy.

Cardiac resynchronization therapy (CRT)

In the past decade, a new role has emerged for pacemakers in treating selected patients with advanced HF. Approximately 30% of HF patients have left bundle branch block or other intraventricular conduction abnormality resulting in significant prolongation of the QRS interval (≥120 ms). In these patients, LV contraction is often dyssynchronous and out of phase with right ventricular contraction. Biventricular pacing, with one lead pacing the right ventricle and a second lead pacing the left ventricle through retrograde insertion into the coronary sinus, can 'resynchronize' ventricular contraction, thus improving ejection fraction and cardiac output. The addition of atrial pacing may provide further benefit by optimizing the timing of atrial and ventricular contraction. The benefits of CRT in improving ejection fraction, reducing LV cavity size, and enhancing exercise tolerance and quality of life have now been documented in several randomized trials involving patients with advanced HF symptoms (New York Heart Association class III–IV), reduced ejection fraction and prolonged QRS duration.[23] In addition, meta-analysis indicates that CRT is associated with fewer hospitalizations and improved survival.[24] Although few older patients have been enrolled in the CRT trials, observational data suggest that CRT is associated with improved quality of life and exercise tolerance in older patients, including octogenarians.[25] Based on these findings, CRT is a reasonable option for carefully selected older patients with advanced HF symptoms despite conventional therapies.

Implantable cardioverter-defibrillators (ICDs)

Approximately 40% of all deaths in patients with HF occur suddenly, and the majority of these are attributable to ventricular tachycardia (VT) and ventricular fibrillation (VF). ICDs have the capacity to recognize VT and VF, and to restore normal rhythm either by pacing techniques (in the case of VT) or by delivering an intracardiac electrical shock (refractory VT or VF). Moreover, these devices have been shown to significantly improve survival in certain high-risk subgroups of the HF population, including those with resuscitated cardiac arrest, symptomatic sustained VT, and ischaemic or non-ischaemic cardiomyopathy with ejection fraction ≤35%.[26]

In the United States, over half of ICDs are implanted in patients 65 years of age or older, including almost 20% in patients age 80 or older. However, despite the established benefits of ICDs in appropriately selected patients, the clinical role of ICDs in elderly HF patients remains a subject of debate. Data supporting the use of ICDs in patients 80 years of age or older is limited, and a recent meta-analysis found that ICDs did not reduce mortality in women.[27] ICDs also do not improve survival during the first year following implantation, so that patients with limited life expectancy (e.g. New York Heart Association class IV HF) are not suitable candidates for an ICD.[5] In addition, the devices are expensive, and quality of life may be impaired, especially in patients who receive one or more ICD shocks. There are also ethical questions, such as how and when to turn off the device in the terminal stages of HF, or in cases where another life-threatening illness develops (e.g. stroke or cancer). In part for these reasons, many older patients who fulfil guideline criteria for an ICD may elect to forego the procedure. Although additional study is needed, it is clear that the use of ICDs in older HF patients must be individualized, especially for those 80 years of age or older, who have limited life expectancy or impaired quality of life.

Multidisciplinary care

The presence of multiple comorbid conditions, polypharmacy, dietary concerns and a host of psychosocial and financial issues frequently complicate the management of HF in older patients. Moreover, these factors often contribute to poor outcomes in older adults, including frequent hospitalizations. To address these issues, and to provide comprehensive yet individualized care for older HF patients, a coordinated multidisciplinary approach is recommended. Several randomized trials and meta-analyses have documented the efficacy of multidisciplinary HF disease management programmes in reducing hospitalizations and improving quality of life in older patients, and these interventions have also been reported to lower overall medical costs.[28]

Elements of an effective HF disease management programme include patient and caregiver education, enhancement of self-management skills, optimization of pharmacotherapy (including consideration of polypharmacy issues), and close follow-up.[5] The structure of a HF disease management team is similar to that of a multidisciplinary geriatric assessment team, and typically includes a nurse coordinator or case manager, dietician, social worker, clinical pharmacist, home health representative, primary care physician and cardiology consultant. Specific goals of disease management are to improve patient adherence to medications, diet and exercise recommendations by enhancing education and self-management skills; provide close follow-up and improved healthcare access through telephone contacts, home health visits and nurse or physician office visits; and optimize the medication regimen by promoting physician adherence to recommended HF treatment guidelines,[5] simplifying and consolidating the regimen when feasible, eliminating unnecessary medications, and minimizing the risks for drug–drug and drug–disease interactions.

Exercise

Both HF and normal ageing are associated with reduced exercise capacity, in part due to sarcopenia (loss of muscle mass) and alterations in skeletal muscle blood flow and metabolism. Regular physical activity improves exercise performance in healthy older adults, as well as in those with HF, and regular exercise is now recommended for most older HF patients. In the recently reported HF-ACTION trial (HF: A Controlled Trial Investigating Outcomes of Exercise Training), 2331 patients (mean age 59 years, 28% women) with systolic HF (mean ejection fraction 25%) were randomized to a supervised exercise programme or usual care and followed for an average of 30 months.[29] Overall, there was no difference between groups in the primary composite outcome of all-cause mortality or all-cause hospitalization. After adjusting for baseline prognostic factors, exercise was associated with a significant 11% reduction in the primary endpoint and a 15% reduction in cardiovascular mortality or HF hospitalization, with similar results in patients $\leq$70 versus >70 years of age. In addition, patients randomized to the exercise group reported modest but significant improvements in quality of life that persisted up to four years.[30]

Although supervised exercise programmes have been associated with the greatest improvements in exercise performance, such programmes are not feasible for many older patients due to lack of availability, travel concerns and cost constraints. Therefore, most older HF patients should be encouraged to engage in a self-monitored home exercise programme that includes stretching exercises, resistance exercises and aerobic activities. Stretching increases or maintains muscle flexibility and reduces the risk of injury. A daily stretching routine lasting 15–30 minutes and involving all major muscle groups is recommended. Resistance training increases muscle mass and strength and reduces the risk of falls and frailty. Older adults initiating a strength training programme should use light weights and perform 2 to 3 sets of 8 to 12 repetitions for each of 8 to 12 exercises approximately 2 to 3 times per week; as with stretching, all major muscle groups should be included in the strength training programme.

In addition to improving physical performance and quality of life, aerobic exercise may increase the likelihood that older adults will remain independent in activities of daily living. For most older adults, walking is the most suitable form of aerobic exercise, but stationary cycling and swimming are appropriate alternatives. Older adults embarking on an exercise programme should be advised to begin at a comfortable pace and exercise for a comfortable period of time. For HF patients, this may be as little as a few minutes of walking at a slow pace, but patients should not be discouraged by the fact that they are starting at a low level; indeed, data show that the greatest improvements occur in patients with the lowest baseline activity levels. Patients should exercise at least 4 to 5 days per week, gradually increasing the duration of exercise (but not the intensity) until it is possible to exercise comfortably and continuously for 20 to 30 minutes. Once this level of exercise capacity has been achieved, patients may consider further increasing the duration of exercise (e.g. up to 45 minutes) or gradually increasing the intensity. In either case, older HF patients should not exercise strenuously or to exhaustion. Additionally, patients should be instructed to stop exercising and contact their physician if they develop chest pain, undue shortness of breath, dizziness or syncope, or any other symptom that may indicate clinical instability. Finally, contraindications to exercise in elderly HF patients include decompensated HF, unstable coronary disease or arrhythmias, neurological or muscular disorders that preclude participation in an exercise programme, or any other condition that would render exercise unsafe.

End of life

The overall 5-year survival rate for older patients with established HF is less than 50%; that is, the prognosis is worse than for most forms of cancer. Clinical features portending a less favourable outcome include older age, more severe symptoms and functional impairment, lower systolic blood pressure, lower LV ejection fraction, underlying CAD, hyponatraemia, anaemia, impaired renal function and cognitive dysfunction. Older patients with advanced HF, as evidenced by NYHA class III–IV symptoms, have a 1-year mortality rate of 25–50%; for these patients, HF can properly be considered a terminal illness. In addition, all HF patients are at risk for sudden arrhythmic death, which may occur during periods of apparent clinical stability. For these reasons, it is appropriate to address end-of-life issues early in the course of HF management, and to reconsider these issues periodically as the disease progresses or when changes in clinical status occur.[5]

Although discussing end-of-life issues is often challenging for healthcare providers as well as patients and families, specific measures should be undertaken to plan for and facilitate end-of-life care.[5] These include the development of an advance directive and appointment of durable power of attorney. The advance directive should be as explicit as possible in defining circumstances under which the patient does not want to be hospitalized, placed on a respirator, subjected to other life-sustaining interventions (e.g. a feeding tube), or resuscitated. Since patients may alter their views about these issues as clinical circumstances evolve, it is important to maintain open communication throughout the disease process.

End-stage HF is frequently accompanied by considerable discomfort and anxiety, and data from the SUPPORT study indicate that most patients and families have concerns about the quality of end-of-life care.[31] A cardinal principle of end-of-life care is to provide adequate relief of pain and suffering through the judicious use of conventional therapies in conjunction with narcotics (e.g. morphine), sedatives (e.g. benzodiazepines), and other comfort measures.[32] Equally important is the provision of emotional support for the patient and family, assisted by nurses, members of the clergy, social service representatives and other qualified healthcare professionals. In some patients with terminal HF, institutional or home-based hospice care may be appropriate.[32]

Prevention

In light of the high prevalence and poor prognosis associated with HF in elderly people, it is evident that more effective means for the prevention of this disorder are needed. At present, the most effective preventive strategies involve aggressive treatment of established risk factors for the development of HF, especially hypertension and CAD. Several studies have shown that even modest declines in blood pressure are associated with substantial reductions in incident HF among elderly hypertensive patients (Table 8.7). In the HYVET study (Hypertension in the Very Elderly Trial), for example,

Table 8.7 Effect of anti-hypertensive therapy on incident heart failure in older adults.

Trial	N	Age Range (yrs)	Reduction in Heart Failure
EWPHE	840	>60	22%
Coope	884	60–79	32%
STOP-HTN	1627	70–84	51%
SHEP	4736	≥60	55%
Syst-Eur	4695	≥60	36%
STONE	1632	60–79	68%
HYVET	3845	≥80	64%

EWPHE, European Working Party on Hypertension in the Elderly; HYVET, Hypertension in the Very Elderly Trial; SHEP, Systolic Hypertension in the Elderly Program; STONE, Shanghai Trial of Nifedipine in the Elderly; STOP-HTN, Swedish Trial in Old Patients with Hypertension; Syst-Eur, Systolic Hypertension in Europe Trial

treatment of hypertension in patients 80 years of age or older was associated with a 64% reduction in incident HF over a median follow-up of 1.8 years.[33] Likewise, treatment of elevated cholesterol levels with an HMG-CoA reductase inhibitor has been shown to decrease incident HF following an acute coronary event. Similarly, it is likely that smoking cessation and effective control of diabetes will contribute to a reduction in HF.

Future directions

Current treatment of HF in the elderly population is characterized by marked under-utilization of proven therapies, insufficient evidence to guide treatment in major patient subgroups (e.g. octogenarians and beyond, nursing home residents, patients with advanced comorbidities and individuals with HFPEF), and inattention to critically important psychobehavioural issues (e.g. adherence, personal preferences and end-of-life care). Thus, there is a need for additional research aimed at developing more effective strategies for the prevention and treatment of acute and chronic HF in older adults.

As shown in Table 8.8, several new treatments for HF, both pharmacological and technological, are currently under investigation. While rigorous testing is essential for evaluating the impact of each of these new therapeutic modalities, there is hope that many of these interventions will make significant contributions towards reducing the burden of HF in our progressively ageing population.

Table 8.8 New approaches to the treatment of chronic heart failure.

Pharmacologic Agents
Neutral endopeptidase inhibitors
Endothelin receptor antagonists
Cytokine inhibitors
Calcium sensitizers
Therapeutic Angiogenesis and Anti-angiogenesis
Inhibition of Apoptosis
Gene Therapy and Pharmacogenomics
Hereditary disorders (e.g. cardiomyopathies, dyslipidaemias)
Modulation of signalling pathways
Targeted therapy based on specific genetic profile
Implantable Assist Devices
Cell Transplantation and Growth Factor Therapy
Xenotransplantation
Prevention of Cardiovascular Ageing

Key points

- Age-related changes in cardiovascular structure and function coupled with the rising prevalence of cardiovascular diseases at older age lead to progressive increases in the incidence and prevalence of heart failure with advancing age in both men and women.
- Heart failure in older adults often presents with atypical symptoms and signs, such as altered sensorium, behavioural changes, anorexia or gastrointestinal disturbances.
- Common comorbid conditions and geriatric syndromes frequently interact with heart failure leading to clinically significant alterations in the clinical manifestations and response to therapy in older patients.
- Management of heart failure with reduced ejection fraction is generally similar in older and younger patients, but treatment for heart failure with preserved ejection fraction remains largely empiric due to the lack of proven benefit from standard heart failure therapies.
- Optimal management of heart failure in older adults, especially those with multiple co-existing conditions or social isolation, is best accomplished utilizing a multidisciplinary team involving a nurse coordinator, geriatric clinical pharmacist, dietician, social worker, and one or more physicians.

References

1 Lloyd-Jones D, Adams RJ, Brown TM *et al.* Heart disease and stroke statistics – 2010 update. *Circulation* 2010;**121**:e46–e215.

2 Lakatta EG and Levy D. Arterial and cardiac aging: major shareholders in cardiovascular disease enterprises. Part I: aging arteries: a 'set up' for vascular disease. *Circulation* 2003;**107**:139–46.

3 Lakatta EG and Levy D. Arterial and cardiac aging: major shareholders in cardiovascular disease enterprises. Part II: the aging heart in health: links to heart disease. *Circulation* 2003;**107**:346–54.

4 Redfield MM, Rodeheffer RJ, Jacobsen SJ*et al.* Plasma brain natriuretic peptide concentration: impact of age and gender. *J Am Coll Cardiol* 2002;**40**:976–82.

5 Jessup M, Abraham WT, Casey DE *et al.* 2009 focused update incorporated into the ACC/AHA guidelines for the evaluation and management of heart failure in adults. *J Am Coll Cardiol* 2009;**53**:e1–e90.

6 Page J and Henry D. Consumption of NSAIDs and the development of congestive heart failure in elderly patients: an underrecognized public health problem. *Arch Intern Med* 2000;**160**:777–84.

7 Fried LP, Tangen CM, Walston J *et al.* Cardiovascular Health Study Collaborative Research Group. Frailty in older adults: evidence for a phenotype. *J Gerontol Biol Sci Med Sci* 2001;**56**:M146–56.

8 Braunstein JB, Anderson GF, Gerstenblith G *et al.* Noncardiac comorbidity increases preventable hospitalizations and mortality among medicare beneficiaries with chronic heart failure. *J Am Coll Cardiol* 2003;**42**:1226–33.

9 Jong P, Demers C, McKelvie RS and Liu PP. Angiotensin receptor blockers in heart failure: meta-analysis of randomized controlled trials. *J Am Coll Cardiol* 2002;**39**:463–70.

10 Granger CB, McMurray JJV, Yusuf S *et al.* Effects of candesartan in patients with chronic heart failure and reduced left-ventricular systolic function intolerant to angiotensin-converting-enzyme inhibitors: the CHARM-Alternative trial. *Lancet* 2003;**362**:772–6.

11 McMurray JJV, Ostergren J, Swedberg K *et al.* Effects of candesartan in patients with chronic heart failure and reduced left-ventricular systolic function taking angiotensin-converting-enzyme inhibitors: the CHARM-Added trial. *Lancet* 2003;**362**:767–71.

12 Taylor AL, Ziesche S, Yancy C *et al.* Combination of isosorbide dinitrate and hydralazine in blacks with heart failure. *New Engl J Med* 2004;**351**:2049–57.

13 Poole-Wilson PA, Swedberg K, Cleland JGF *et al.* Comparison of carvedilol and metoprolol on clinical outcomes in patients with chronic heart failure in the Carvedilol Or Metoprolol European Trial (COMET): randomised controlled trial. *Lancet* 2003;**362**:7–13.

14 Rich MW, McSherry F, Williford WO and Yusuf S, for the Digitalis Investigation Group. Effect of age on mortality, hospitalizations, and response to digoxin in patients with heart failure:The DIG Study. *J Am Coll Cardiol* 2001;**38**:806–13.

15 Ahmed A, Rich MW, Love TE *et al.* Digoxin and reduction in mortality and hospitalization in heart failure: a comprehensive post hoc analysis of the DIG trial. *Eur Heart J* 2006;**27**:178–86.

16 Pitt B, Zannad F, Remme WJ *et al.* The effect of spironolactone on morbidity and mortality in patients with severe heart failure. Randomized Aldactone Evaluation Study Investigators. *New Engl J Med* 1999;**341**:709–17.

17 Pitt B, Remme W, Zannad F *et al.* Eplerenone, a selective aldosterone blocker, in patients with left ventricular dysfunction after myocardial infarction. *New Engl J Med*2003;**348**:1309–21.

18 Yusuf S, Pfeffer MA, Swedberg K *et al.*; CHARM Investigators and Committees. Effects of candesartan in patients with chronic heart failure and preserved left-ventricular ejection fraction: the CHARM-Preserved Trial. *Lancet* 2003;**362**(9386):777–81.

19 Massie BM, Carson PE, McMurray JJ *et al.*; I-PRESERVE Investigators. Irbesartan in patients with heart failure and preserved ejection fraction. *New Engl J Med* 2008;**359**:2456–67.

20 Cleland JGF, Tendera M, Adamus J *et al.* The perindopril in elderly people with chronic heart failure (PEP-CHF) study. *Eur Heart J* 2006;**27**:2338–45.

21 Flather MD, Shibata JC, Coats AJS *et al.* Randomized trial to determine the effect of nebivolol on mortality and cardiovascular hospital admission in elderly patients with heart failure (SENIORS). *Eur Heart J* 2005;**26**:215–25.

22 Ahmed A, Rich MW, Fleg LF *et al.* Effects of digoxin on morbidity and mortality in diastolic heart failure: the ancillary Digitalis Investigation Group trial. *Circulation* 2006;**114**:397–403.

23 Bristow MR, Saxon LA, Boehmer J *et al.* Cardiac-resynchronization therapy with or without an implantable defibrillator in advanced chronic heart failure. *New Engl J Med* 2004;**350**:2140–50.

24 McAlister FA, Ezekowitz JA, Wiebe N *et al.* Systematic review: cardiac resynchronization therapy in patients with symptomatic heart failure. *Ann Intern Med* 2004;**141**:381–90.

25 Delnoy PP, Ottervanger JP, Luttikhuis HE *et al.* Clinical response of cardiac resynchronization therapy in the elderly. *Am Heart J* 2008;**155**:746–51.

26 Bardy GH, Lee KL, Mark DB *et al.* Amiodarone or an implantable cardioverter–defibrillator for congestive heart failure. *New Engl J Med* 2005;**352**:225–37.

27 Ghanbari H, Dalloul G, Hasan R *et al.* Effectiveness of implantable cardioverter-defibrillators for the primary prevention of sudden cardiac death in women with advanced heart failure: a meta-analysis of randomized controlled trials. *Arch Intern Med*2009;**169**:1500–6.

28 Phillips CO, Wright SM, Kern DE*et al.*Comprehensive discharge planning with post-discharge support for older patients with congestive heart failure. A meta-analysis. *JAMA* 2004;**291**:1358–67.

29 O'Connor CM, Whellan DJ, Lee KL *et al.* Efficacy and safely of exercise training in patients with chronic heart failure: HF-ACTION randomized controlled trial. *JAMA* 2009;**301**:1439–50.

30 Flynn KE, Pina IL, Whellan DJ *et al.* Effects of exercise training on health status in patients with chronic heart failure: HF-ACTION randomized controlled trial. *JAMA* 2009;**301**:1451–9.

31 Levenson JW, McCarthy EP, Lynn J *et al.* The last six months of life for patients with congestive heart failure. *J Am Geriatr Soc* 2000;**48**:S101–S109.

32 Adler ED, Goldfinger JZ, Kalman J*et al.*Palliative care in the treatment of advanced heart failure. *Circulation* 2009;**120**:2597–606.

33 Beckett NS, Peters R, Fletcher AE *et al.* Treatment of hypertension in patients 80 years of age or older. *New Engl J Med* 2008;**358**:1887–98.

CHAPTER 9
Cardiac Surgery

Ulrich O. von Oppell and Adam Szafranek

University Hospital of Wales, Cardiff and Vale University Health Board, University of Cardiff, Wales, UK

Introduction

The primary enabling technology that led to the exponential growth in modern cardiac surgery was the development of the heart-lung machine in 1953. Currently, Western economies' estimated needs are 1000 to 1300 cardiac operations per million population. Life expectancy in Western economies has increased significantly during the past 50 years; in Europe it is now 84 years for women and 77 years for men, and in 2008 approximately 18% of the European population were more than 65 years of age. Moreover, cardiovascular disease is the leading cause of morbidity and mortality in the elderly population,[1] and it is estimated that 25–40% of octogenarians have symptomatic cardiac disease.[2] Hence the increasing numbers of elderly patients undergoing cardiac surgery (Figure 9.1).[3]

Elderly people continue to enjoy an active lifestyle and not unexpectedly want a good quality of life, and many feel that a high operative risk, namely death on the operating table is an acceptable alternative to increasing debilitating symptoms in the last few years of life. The decision when to 'offer' or 'deny' cardiac surgery should though be answered in terms of outcome, mortality and morbidity risk in relation to the expected improvement in quality of life. Careful preoperative assessment of comorbid risk factors is also essential in elderly patients, because of competing comorbid disease mortality risks.

Cardiac surgery outcome in terms of mortality has continually improved as a result of the development of less traumatic heart-lung machines, more effective myocardial protection strategies, and improved peri-operative care. The mean age of patients undergoing cardiac surgery is progressively increasing and many octogenarians are now successfully undergoing

Cardiovascular Disease and Health in the Older Patient: Expanded from 'Pathy's Principles and Practice of Geriatric Medicine, Fifth edition', First Edition. Edited by David J. Stott and Gordon D.O. Lowe.

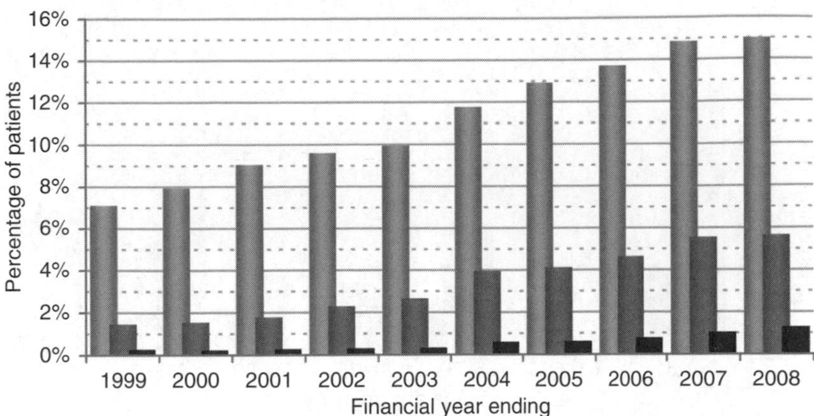

Figure 9.1 Trends in the relative proportions of older age groups by financial year, of 341 473 patients who underwent heart surgery in the United Kingdom. Age categories are, in increasing shades, 76–80 years, 81–85 years, and >85 years old. Reprinted from Bridgewater *et al.*[3] with permission from Dendrite Clinical Systems Ltd and the Society for Cardiothoracic Surgery in Great Britain & Ireland.

cardiac surgery. In the United Kingdom, 22% of patients undergoing heart surgery were over 75 years of age in 2008 compared to less than 9% in 1999 (Figure 9.1).[3]

The demographics of the octogenarian or older patient undergoing cardiac surgery differ to that of the younger patient group,[4] in that patients are more likely to be female (~45%), are less likely to have diabetes (~20%), smoke (~35%) or have chronic lung disease (~10%); these observations are possibly indicative that only in the absence of these risk factors is an individual likely to live long enough to become a nonagenarian.

Age *per se* is not a contraindication for cardiac surgery provided the elderly patient can be discharged without significant disability and loss of independence.

Cardiac surgery outcomes in the older person

Mortality

The type of cardiac surgery done is customarily grouped in terms of isolated coronary artery bypass grafting (CABG alone), CABG with concomitant valve surgery (CABG + valve), valve repair or replacement alone (valve alone), and Other procedures. Notably, the type of cardiac surgery done changes in elderly patients; isolated CABG is the more common procedure in patients under 75 years of age (64% of heart operations), whilst heart valve operations predominate in patients over the age of 85 years (69%) (Figure 9.2).[3]

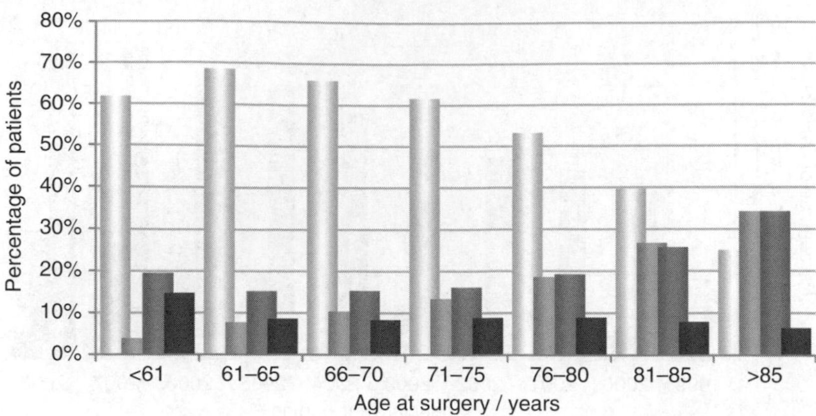

Figure 9.2 Type of cardiac surgery done in 184 461 patients undergoing heart surgery in the United Kingdom during the financial years 2004 to 2008 by patient age-group; isolated coronary artery bypass graft surgery (light shade bar), and in increasing shades combined CABG and valve surgery, valve repair or replacement surgery alone, or other procedures. Reprinted from Bridgewater *et al.*[3] with permission from Dendrite Clinical Systems Ltd and the Society for Cardiothoracic Surgery in Great Britain & Ireland.

The mortality of cardiac surgery increases with both the complexity of the required procedure as well as with increasing age. Nevertheless, the crude in-hospital mortality associated with cardiac surgery in patients older than 80 years of age has now decreased to approximately 5–9% for isolated CABG, 8–11% for combined CABG and valve surgery, and 5–7% for isolated valve surgery (Figure 9.3).[3] The lower aforementioned mortality range figures approximate that for patients electively admitted for surgery from home as opposed to patients undergoing urgent surgery because of the severity of their condition, who have a higher mortality. Nevertheless, elderly patients referred for cardiac surgery almost always have severe disease which if untreated would significantly reduce their life expectancy and result in a worse outcome than the aforementioned mortality rates.

Post-operative complications such as requirement for temporary haemodialysis (incidence: nonagenarian 9.2%, octogenarian 7.7% vs 3.5% in younger age groups), stroke and prolonged ventilation all increase with age (Figure 9.4).[1] The average length of hospital stay following cardiac surgery in patients less than 60 years of age is 9 days but this increases to more than 15 days in patients older than 85 years.[3]

Nonetheless, the expected medium-term post-cardiac surgery actuarial 5-year survival in the octogenarian is 60–75%, and with a significantly improved quality of life.[5]

Pre-existing comorbid risk factors associated with increased mortality in octogenarians undergoing open-heart operations should be taken into account when advising patients of the risk of having surgery.

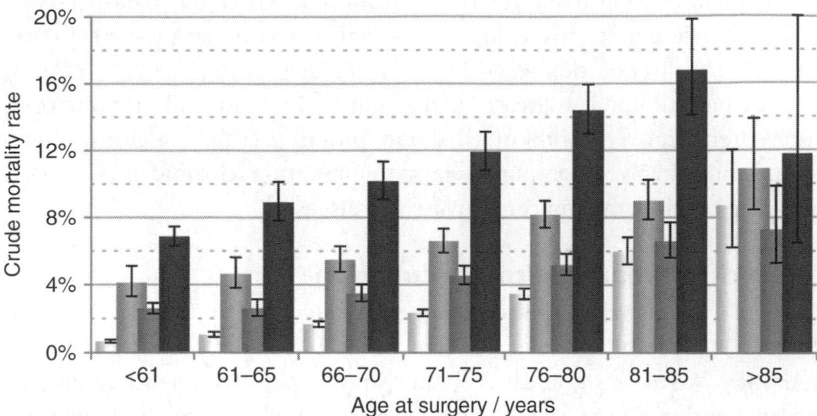

Figure 9.3 Unadjusted cardiac surgery mortality by patient age-group and procedure type in 184 461 patients undergoing cardiac surgery in the United Kingdom during the financial years 2004 to 2008; isolated coronary artery bypass graft surgery (light shade bar), and in increasing shades combined CABG and valve surgery, valve repair or replacement surgery alone, or other procedures. Reprinted from Bridgewater *et al.*[3] with permission from Dendrite Clinical Systems Ltd and the Society for Cardiothoracic Surgery in Great Britain & Ireland.

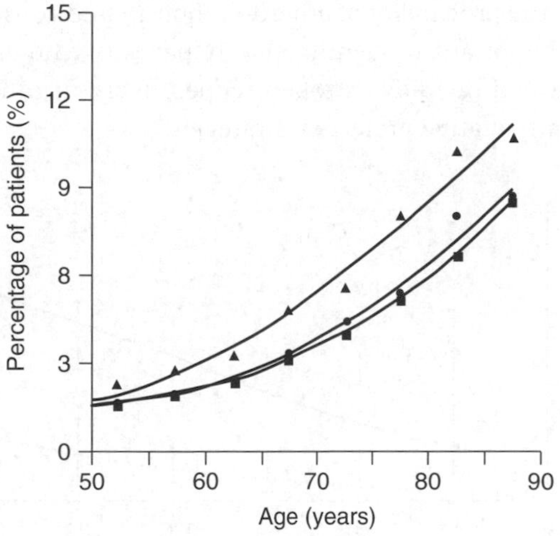

Figure 9.4 The rate of complications; in-hospital mortality (solid circles), neurological events (stroke, transient ischaemic attacks, or coma; solid triangles), and renal failure (oliguria with a creatinine >1 mg dl^{-1} or dialysis; solid boxes), by age in 64 467 patients following coronary artery bypass graft, with or without concomitant valve, surgery. Reprinted from Alexander *et al.*[1] Copyright 2000, with permission from Elsevier.

These include New York Heart Association (NYHA) dyspnoea class III or IV, female gender, previous myocardial infarction, triple-vessel coronary artery disease, depressed left ventricular ejection fraction, chronic obstructive pulmonary disease, higher left ventricular end-diastolic pressure, preoperative intra-aortic balloon pump (IABP), congestive heart failure, mitral valve operation, urgency of operation, chronic renal disease, as well as peripheral and cerebrovascular disease.[5]

Morbidity: Neurological dysfunction

The post-operative complication of greatest concern following cardiac surgery is a cerebrovascular accident (CVA), which is usually embolic in aetiology. A stroke significantly reduces post-operative quality of life and is also associated with a high late mortality following hospital discharge.

The risk of a peri-operative stroke is higher in elderly people: being 13% in octogenarian compared to 4% in younger patients. Age-related morphological and physiological changes characterized by cerebral atrophy and diminished cerebrovascular reserve capacity, subclinical degenerative brain disease and severe atherosclerosis of the aorta as well as head and neck vessels are multifactor pre-existing comorbid risks contributing to the increased risk of post-operative neurological complications in older patients (Figure 9.5).[6] Intra-operative manipulation of an atherosclerotic ascending aorta increases the probability of athero-embolism and consequent stroke. It is therefore important to identify elderly patients who are at high risk of sustaining a peri-operative stroke preoperatively in order to institute additional intra-operative protective strategies.[6]

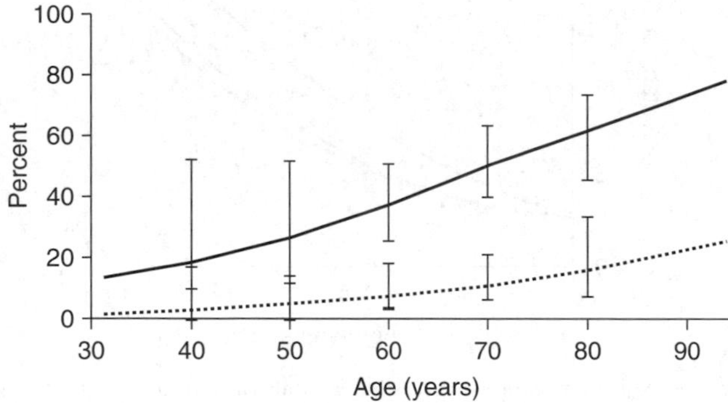

Figure 9.5 Probability of finding atheroemboli in organs, other than the heart or lungs, at 221 autopsies after cardiac operations for ischaemic or valvular heart disease, according to age and the presence of a preoperative history of peripheral vascular disease (solid line) or no history thereof (dotted line). Reprinted from Blauth *et al.*[6] Copyright 1992, with permission from Elsevier.

Table 9.1 Risk factors for internal carotid artery atheromatous disease.

- Carotid bruit
- Previous cerebrovascular accident
- Previous transient ischaemic attack
- Peripheral vascular disease
- Diabetes mellitus
- Left main stem coronary artery disease
  –If age greater than 65 years

Preoperative identification of patients with carotid artery disease is important, and our practice is to screen patients at risk for atheromatous disease with carotid duplex imaging (Table 9.1). Carotid artery disease is uncommon in the cardiac surgical patient who does not have coronary artery disease.

Patients scheduled for cardiac surgery who have coexisting symptomatic or asymptomatic carotid artery disease should then be assessed as to whether carotid artery endarterectomy is indicated either prior to or as a combined procedure with their cardiac surgery. A recent meta-analysis of combined versus staged procedure has shown that in stable cardiac patients the safer option is to perform carotid endarterectomy first followed by subsequent coronary artery bypass grafting.

The presence of severe ascending atherosclerotic plaque at the time of cardiac surgery is associated with a 10% incidence of peri-operative or late neurological events, compared to 4% in patients with normal or only mild ascending aortic atherosclerosis. Intra-operative mechanisms of identifying ascending aortic atherosclerotic plaque are therefore useful in elderly patients; either epi-aortic Doppler ultrasound or transoesophageal echocardiography. If significant atherosclerotic plaque is identified, then reducing ascending aortic manipulation such as off-pump surgery without any manipulation of the ascending aorta, cardiopulmonary bypass using single cross-clamp techniques, and the use of ascending aortic filtration devices are available techniques which can potentially reduce the risk of intra-operative athero-embolism.

More minor neurocognitive dysfunction such as memory loss and changes in visual acuity are also common after cardiac surgery and the aetiology is multifactorial. Pre-existing comorbid neurological risk factors, especially confusional states of indeterminate origin, should, however, be considered relative contraindications to cardiac surgery in older people, as undergoing open-heart surgery may aggravate them.

Assessment of the elderly patient for cardiac surgery

An improved longer term prognosis is a frequent indication for cardiac surgery in younger patients; however in elderly people, this is less of an issue. Elderly patients must be assessed individually in terms of the natural history of their disease, symptoms thereof, comorbid diseases, current quality of life, and the risk (mortality and morbidity) versus benefit (improved quality of life) of any potential surgical intervention.

Operative risk: Estimated mortality for cardiac surgery

Mortality following cardiac surgery usually refers to either in-hospital, that is, deaths occurring within the base hospital during the same admission, or 30-day mortality, that is, deaths within 30 days of surgery. In the United Kingdom, the former definition is currently more commonly used.

Crude mortality fails as a comparative measure of quality between hospitals or surgeons, if there are major variations in case mix. A mechanism of risk stratification based on preoperative factors that increase operative mortality risks, such as age, is therefore essential if referral patterns, allocation of resources and discouragement of the treatment of high-risk patients are to be avoided. Without risk stratification, surgeons and hospitals treating high-risk patients will appear, on the basis of crude mortality, to have worse results than others.[7]

The estimated risk of undergoing a given cardiac procedure is therefore determined from known preoperative risk factors and calculating the EuroScore (European System for Cardiac Operative Risk Evaluation Score), which is a weighted score that is used preoperatively to provide an estimated predicted operative mortality (Table 9.2).[7] The web site http://www.euroscore.org provides a free multilingual risk calculator for predicting cardiac surgical mortality, by both the additive and newer logistic EuroScore.

The additive EuroScore has been shown to provide a good correlation with actual observed mortality in the lower risk groups, but is less accurate and tends to underestimate operative mortality when the predicted operative mortality risk exceeds 9%. In the higher risk groups, the alternative logistic EuroScore mathematical model appears to improve prediction. Although the original simple additive model remains a useful more user-friendly clinical tool to predict immediate operative risk (Table 9.2).

In the future, procedural 1-year mortality or more will provide additional useful information for predicting 'true' outcome.

Table 9.2 Weighted risk factors relevant to a specific individual patient are added and this then provides the EuroScore predicted mortality (%) for that patient to undergo the proposed cardiac surgical procedure (range 0–42%).

Risk factors and definitions	Weighted-score
Patient-related factors	
Age (years)	
60–64	1
65–69	2
70–74	3
75–79	4
80–84	5
85–89	6
≥90	7
Gender Female	1
Chronic pulmonary disease	
Long-term use of bronchodilators or steroids for lung disease	1
Extracardiac arteriopathy (any or more of following)	
History of intermittent claudication, internal carotid occlusion greater than 50% stenosis, previous or planned abdominal aortic, limb or carotid vascular surgery	2
Neurologic dysfunction	
Severely affecting ambulation or day-to-day function	2
Previous cardiac surgery	
Requiring pericardial opening	3
Renal dysfunction	
Serum creatinine greater than 200 μmol l^{-1} prior to surgery	2
Active endocarditis	
Still under antibiotic treatment for endocarditis at time of surgery	3
Critical preoperative state (any or more of following)	
Ventricular tachycardia, ventricular fibrillation or aborted sudden death preoperative cardiac massage, preoperative inotropic or intra-aortic balloon pump support, preoperative ventilation before arrival in anesthetic room, preoperative acute renal failure (anuria or oliguria <10 ml/hour)	3
Cardiac-related factors	
Unstable angina	
Rest angina requiring intravenous nitrates preoperatively until theater	2
Left ventricular dysfunction	
Moderate (left ventricular ejection fraction 30–50%)	1
Poor (left ventricular ejection fraction <30%)	3
Recent myocardial infarct	
Within 90 days of surgery	2
Pulmonary hypertension	
Pulmonary artery systolic pressure >60 mmHg	2
Operation-related factors	
Emergency surgery	
Carried out on referral before the beginning of the next working day	2
Other than isolated CABG	
Major cardiac surgery other than or in addition to CABG	2
Surgery on thoracic aorta	
For disease of ascending, arch, or descending thoracic aorta	3
Postinfarction ischaemic ventricular septal defect	4
EuroScore Predicted Mortality (%)	
Derived by the addition of the above relevant risk factor scores for each individual patient	Σ

Source: Reprinted from Nashef *et al.*[7] Copyright 1999, with permission from Elsevier.

Benefit of surgery: Intended improved quality of life following surgery

Increased survival is not the primary benefit of cardiac surgery in the elderly patient and should therefore not necessarily be the primary outcome indicator. Nevertheless, medium-term 5-year survival for patients over the age of 80 years is remarkably good; isolated CABG ~70%, isolated AVR ~65% and isolated mitral valve repair ~72%.[3]

More important is assessing any expected improvements in quality of life intended by a proposed cardiac surgical procedure, which is difficult. A perceived improvement in the NYHA dyspnoea score is not sufficient as it does not fully address the broader aspect of quality of life and independent lifestyle.

Factors that impact on quality of life are mostly physical rather then mental conditions. The SF-36 health survey questionnaire assesses eight general health concepts: physical functioning, bodily pain, role limitation because of personal or emotional problems, emotional well-being, social functioning, energy or fatigue and general health perceptions. A study of octogenarians who had undergone cardiac surgery showed SF-36 scores equal or better than those of the general population of age greater than 65 years. Moreover, 84–94% of octogenarian operative survivors continue living on their own, and 83–98% indicated that they would in retrospect undergo cardiac surgery again because of the improvements in their lifestyle.[8]

To date preoperative quality of life assessments such as the SF-36 questionnaire have not been used to guide preoperative decision-making. An alternative simpler assessment is the EQ-5D or EuroQol, which assesses the level of mobility, self-care, usual activity, pain or discomfort and anxiety or depression, and may well assist in preoperative decision-making (Table 9.3).[9]

The elderly population more frequently have additional coexistent medical conditions, which may frequently worsen, after cardiac surgery. Coexistent medical conditions must therefore be taken into account in terms of the patient's quality of life. Diabetes mellitus with end-organ disease and renal failure are the most hazardous risk factors for a postoperative reduced quality of life. Diabetes mellitus results in decreased mobility and chronic pain, whilst renal failure directly affects survival. Care should therefore be taken when selecting patients with those comorbidities for cardiac surgery.

A confounding factor in the assessment of elderly people for cardiac surgery, however, is that suboptimal timing of surgery, namely, excessively late referral for surgery, has a significant negative impact on both operative risk and late outcome.[10] The combined effect of delay, deteriorating cardiac

Table 9.3 EuroQol questionnaire, which assesses five quality-of-life dimensions and perception of general and present health state.

EuroQol questionnaire
Mobility
I have no problem in walking about
I have some problems in walking about
I am confined to bed
Self-care
I have no problems with self-care
I have some problems washing or dressing myself
I am unable to wash or dress myself
Usual activities (work, study, housework, family, or leisure activities)
I have no problems with performing my usual activities
I have some problems with performing my usual activities
I am unable to perform my usual activities
Pain or discomfort
I have no pain or discomfort
I have moderate pain or discomfort
I have extreme pain or discomfort
Anxiety or depression
I am not anxious or depressed
I am moderately anxious or depressed
I am extremely anxious or depressed
Compared with my general level of health over the past 12 months, my health state today is:
Better
Much the same
Worse

status and exacerbating end-organ dysfunction (i.e. renal, pulmonary) may render an otherwise operable candidate beyond salvage.[8,11]

Elderly people are more sedentary, may not notice milder symptoms, or may attribute symptoms to increasing age and may thus present late. Complete assessment on initial presentation is critical, and mild symptoms in an elderly individual should not preclude further investigations such as echocardiography and coronary angiography, in order to more accurately determine the presence and extent of any underlying cardiac disease. The decision whether to operate or not should be done without delay and not on a 'wait and see how symptoms progress' basis if the best surgical outcome is to be achieved.

Coronary artery bypass graft surgery

Coronary artery bypass graft surgery forms the majority of cardiac surgery today and was introduced as a therapeutic option in the early 1960s once myocardial ischaemia (angina pectoris or myocardial infarction) was shown to be due to narrowing of the coronary arteries from atherosclerotic plaque. Prospective randomized clinical trials in coronary artery surgery defined the indications for and benefits of CABG in both relieving symptoms and improving survival. These major trials showed that CABG increases survival in patients shown to have left main stem coronary artery stenosis, triple-vessel disease, or double-vessel disease on coronary angiography and in those with impaired left ventricular function or with left ventricular aneurysms. This applies equally in the elderly population (Figure 9.6).[12]

CABG reduces the incidence of fatal myocardial infarction, relieves angina and increases exercise capacity. However, isolated CABG does not improve symptoms of congestive heart failure, especially in the absence of proven hibernating or stunned myocardium.

Care though should be taken not to use the degree of symptomatic angina as the basis to refer an elderly patient for coronary angiography, as there is a poor correlation of the degree of angina with the degree of coronary artery narrowing. Up to 42% of patients with left main stem stenosis (the cohort of ischaemic heart disease patients at greatest risk of early death with continued medical therapy) will have only mild or no angina.[13] It is therefore important to make a distinction as to the indications of referral for further investigation as opposed to those for

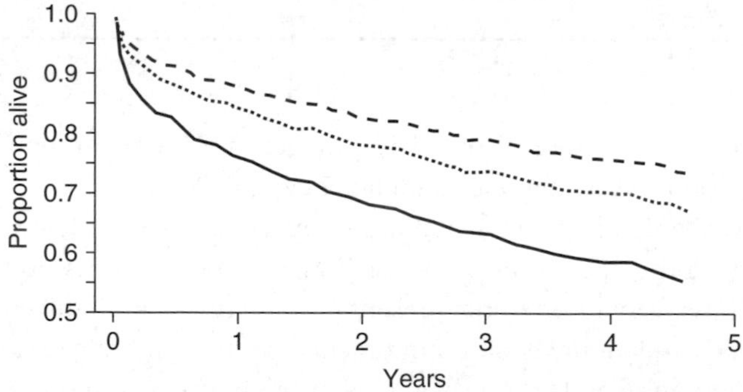

Figure 9.6 Risk-adjusted survival curves for 981 patients, 80 years of age or older, with ischaemic heart disease who underwent either revascularization by coronary artery bypass graft surgery (dashed line) or percutaneous coronary intervention (dotted line) versus continued medical therapy (solid line). Reprinted from Graham *et al.*[12] with permission from American Heart Association, Inc.

CABG surgery, which are not necessarily the same. Any recent change in angina symptoms should prompt a cardiological assessment.

Delays in referring for diagnostic coronary angiography should not occur, as this may partly account for the increased prevalence of left main stem disease in octogenarians or nonagenarians (~32%) undergoing CABG as well as need for emergent surgery.[4] Left main stem stenosis of more than 50% remains an indication for CABG in elderly patients even in the absence of severe symptoms, as less than 55% of medically treated patients 65 years or older with left main stem stenosis will survive for 3 years compared to an 87% survival for those undergoing CABG.[13]

In the United Kingdom, the operative mortality for isolated CABG in older patients (age >75 years) has progressively decreased from 7.2% in 1999 to 3.3% in 2008, representing a reduction of ~50%.[3] Preoperative risk factors associated with increased operative mortality in nonagenarians from the US Society of Thoracic Surgeons database are shown in Table 9.4.[4] Similarly, in Europe, potentially delayed surgery, that is, waiting until the patient requires emergent surgery or reaches NYHA dyspnoea class IV, are important risk factors for an increased operative mortality in octogenarians.[2,11]

A retrospective study of CABG surgery in octogenarians showed complete revascularization with CABG surgery to be more cost-effective than medical management; 3-year survival of 80% in the surgical group versus 64%, quality of life index of 84% in the surgical group (similar to an average 55-year-old in the general population) versus 61%, and lower cost per quality adjusted life-year gained in patients managed surgically.[9]

The overall outcome of CABG in the octogenarian can be improved by avoiding excessive delay prior to referral, frequently based on misperceptions that age is a contraindication for cardiac surgery.

Table 9.4 Risk factors for operative mortality in nonagenarians undergoing CABG, listed in decreasing order of discriminatory importance.

Risk factors for CABG in Nonagenarians	Operative mortality
• Emergent surgery	26.6%
• Preoperative need for an IABP	26.3%
• Renal failure (Creatinine >2.0 mg%) or dialysis	20.90%
• Peripheral or cerebrovascular disease	10.60%
• Mitral insufficiency	7.2%

[a]IABP, intra-aortic balloon pump

Source: Data derived from the Society of Thoracic Surgeons National Cardiac Database (1997–2000).[4]

Is percutaneous coronary angioplasty a better alternative in elderly patients?

Percutaneous coronary revascularization is also associated with a better survival than medical therapy in the octogenarian with significant ischaemic heart disease (Figure 9.6).[12]

Perceived increased risks of surgery in elderly people should not, however, introduce a bias to opting for 'less invasive' percutaneous coronary angioplasty as being a better option in the octogenarian. Complications of coronary angioplasty increase disproportionately in octogenarians and can be associated with a high in-hospital mortality of 8.2%. Coronary anatomy is often more suitable for bypass surgery and incomplete revascularization is an independent predictor of both in-hospital and late mortality.[12]

Elective CABG surgery as opposed to percutaneous interventions is frequently a better option in nonagenarian patients, in the absence of significant associated comorbidity.[4] Coronary artery bypass grafting provides a more favourable survivorship up to eight years after operation. Age alone should not be a deferent for aggressive treatment of coronary heart disease.

Use of the internal mammary artery as a conduit

CABG surgery was initially done using only reversed long saphenous vein as the bypass conduit between the ascending aorta and coronary artery, implanted distal to the flow limiting atherosclerotic plaque. However, the conduit that provides the best long-term patency is the internal mammary artery, and is today the conduit of choice as a pedicle graft to the left coronary system. Use of the internal mammary artery also confers an immediate survival advantage by reducing operative mortality.

Dissection of the internal mammary artery pedicle prolongs the operation time, is more technically demanding, and may be associated with increased post-operative bleeding, sternal infection in diabetics and respiratory compromise. These reasons are therefore frequently cited to justify not using this conduit in higher risk patients, such as elderly people. However, the use of an internal mammary artery has been shown to reduce mortality also in octogenarians undergoing CABG surgery (Figure 9.7).[1,14]

Newer techniques of harvesting the internal mammary artery by a skeletonized method can further reduce the risk of post-operative complications associated with its use. A high 71% use of internal mammary artery conduits in octogenarians as reported by Avery and co-workers, who also report one of the lowest operative mortalities of 2% in non-emergency octogenarian CABG, should be encouraged.[11]

The use of the internal mammary artery is beneficial in octogenarians by both reducing operative mortality and improving longer term survival. Use of bilateral mammary artery combined with off-pump surgery may in

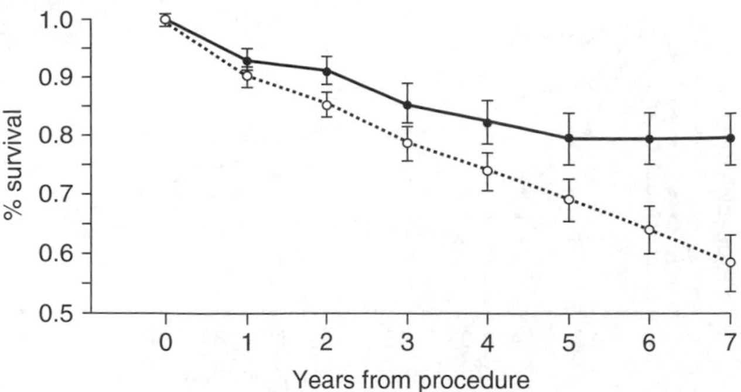

Figure 9.7 Actuarial survival rate of 487 patients 80 years of age or older who underwent coronary artery bypass graft surgery, and grouped according to whether they had received a left internal mammary artery graft to the left anterior descending coronary artery (solid line) versus those in whom only saphenous vein grafts (broken line) had been used. Reprinted from *Morris et al.*[14] Copyright 1996, with permission from Elsevier.

selected elderly patients further reduce complications related to manipulation of highly calcified aorta. Age alone should not be a contraindication to arterial revascularization in selected patients.

Antithrombotic therapy after coronary artery bypass graft surgery

Graft closure after CABG surgery is largely related to platelet aggregation and intimal hyperplasia. The current recommendation is therefore lifelong aspirin therapy at a dose of 325 mg day^{-1}. Aspirin doses of 75 mg have been suggested to be more effective than higher doses because a low dose can 'spare' prostacycline and cause less gastrointestinal toxicity. A lower dose of aspirin has also been associated with diminished risks of major bleeding in acute coronary syndrome trials and this lower dose is now frequently prescribed.[15] It is important to commence aspirin therapy immediately post-operatively as early graft patency is not improved if therapy is delayed for 48–72 hours post-operatively.

Valve surgery

The proportion of patients undergoing cardiac surgery, requiring heart valve surgery (valve or valve + CABG) as opposed to isolated CABG surgery increases with patient age and approaches 70% in patients over the age of 85 years in the United Kingdom (Figure 9.2).[3] In the elderly population though, successful cardiac surgery leads to greater improvements in perceived health status in valvular than in coronary artery disease patients.

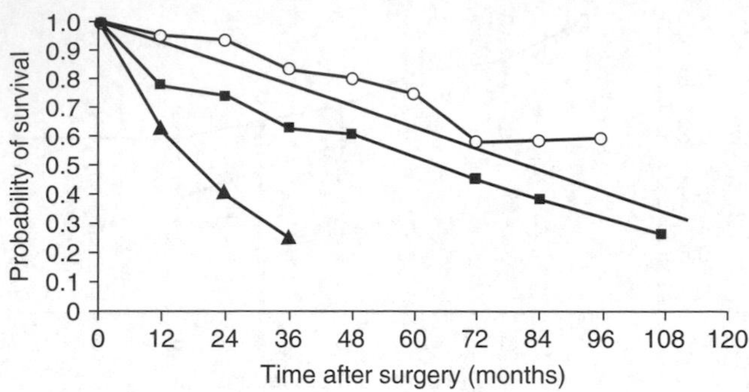

Figure 9.8 Comparative data between an unselected population of 80-year-olds in the United States (solid line), patients over 80 years of age with symptomatic aortic stenosis who did not undergo aortic valve replacement surgery (solid triangles) and 103 octogenarians with aortic stenosis who underwent aortic valve replacement with or without concomitant coronary artery bypass grafts surgery (solid squares). The survival curve of the aforementioned octogenarian patients who survived more than 30 days after surgery (open circles) is also provided. Reprinted from *Gilbert et al.*[18] with permission from the BMJ Publishing Group Ltd.

Aortic valve replacement in elderly patients

The predominant valve disease of elderly people is calcific degenerative aortic stenosis and accounts for 60–70% of the valve surgery caseload. Aortic valve cusps are calcified in 26% of adults older than 65 years and valve stenosis is observed in up to 5% of the population over the age of 75.[16] The development of symptoms (angina, syncope, or heart failure) identifies a critical point in the natural history of aortic stenosis, and symptomatic aortic stenosis without surgery is associated with only a 20% 3-year survival.[17] In contrast, survival of the elderly patient after successful aortic valve replacement (AVR) surgery is similar to that of the natural population (Figure 9.8), as well as enabling them to return to an independent active life.[18]

Operative mortality for aortic valve surgery in older people approaches that obtained in younger patients and it is not until patients reach their 80s that age alone becomes a risk factor. Early mortality in octogenarians undergoing AVR with or without associated CABG is between 5–11% in the United Kingdom.[3] Operative risk is primarily due to comorbid conditions, especially peripheral vascular disease, impaired renal function, previous cardiac surgery, poor left ventricular function and need for urgent surgery.[3,17] Once aortic valve disease is diagnosed in patients aged 80 or more, early referral for surgery should lead to the avoidance of hazardous developments (decreasing left ventricular function, loss of contractile reserve and the necessity for urgent surgery), and hence, to better post-operative outcomes.

Successful AVR surgery offers an excellent long-term outcome with long-term mortality being in most cases of non-cardiac origin. The medium-term 5-year survival of octogenarians undergoing AVR is ~65% and for AVR combined with CABG ~55% in the United Kingdom.[3]

Asymptomatic aortic stenosis

The asymptomatic state is difficult to establish in practice in elderly people, due to a gradual decrease in activity or sedentary lifestyle.[16] Nevertheless, 'asymptomatic' aortic stenotic patients who should be referred for surgery include those with severe aortic stenosis (valve area <1.0 cm^2 or an indexed aortic valve area <0.6 cm^2 m^{-2} body surface area (BSA)), an abnormal response to exercise, left ventricular systolic dysfunction (left ventricular ejection fraction less than 50%), marked left ventricular hypertrophy (≥ 15 mm wall thickness), the combination of moderate calcification and a peak jet velocity >4 m s^{-1} as well as a rapid increase in peak aortic jet velocity of ≥ 0.3 m s^{-1} within one year or patients with severe ventricular arrhythmias for which no cause other than severe aortic stenosis can be identified.[17]

Transcatheter aortic valve implantation (TAVI)

Octogenarians with symptomatic aortic stenosis who do not undergo surgery have only a 50% 1-year survival.[18] However, a number of patients referred for surgery have significant comorbidities and therefore excessively high operative risks for open heart surgery. Percutaneous balloon valvotomy of elderly calcified stenotic valves have been poor; mortality 3–10%, strokes in 10–25%, as well as a 66% incidence of restenosis within six months.[19] Less than 20% of aortic valvuloplasty patients will survive a year and most of them will not improve symptomatically.

Newer percutaneous transcatheter valve replacement techniques were developed for patients turned down for conventional surgery and first used clinically in 2002. The current prostheses used consist of porcine or bovine pericardial valves mounted in either self-expandable nitinol or balloon expandable steel stents.[20]

The majority of transcatheter techniques are done without cardiopulmonary bypass and include either percutaneous transfemoral aortic valve implantation or transapical valve implantation through a mini-thoracotomy. The transfemoral arterial approach replaces the aortic valve retrograde via the femoral artery. Femoral artery size and tortuosity, severe peripheral vascular disease with atheromatous plaque makes this approach unsuitable in some patients. The transapical valve development uses direct balloon catheter implantation from the left ventricular apex, which is accessed through a small incision in the left side of the chest. A short period of rapid ventricular pacing is used with both techniques to decrease cardiac output during deployment of the prosthesis.

Published 1-month mortality rates for TAVI range from 6–20%, cerebrovascular accidents in 2–10%, and residual paravalvular leaks in 50% of patients.[20,21] The degree of native valve insufficiency or new retrograde paravalvar leaks is though usually haemodynamically insignificant. The risk of strokes appears lower with the transapical technique by avoiding any manipulation in a calcified aortic arch, although mortality in some series has been higher with this approach.

Catheter-based aortic valve implantation is thus technically possible in elderly patients where conventional aortic valve replacement is not acceptable. However, 1-year survival is between 54–80%, and is thus relatively poor in some series.[20,21] A 1-year survival of less than 60% overlaps with that of patients treated conservatively and in addition at least one study has shown no significant improvement in quality of life 6 months post-procedure.[21]

Debilitated patients often do not return to an active existence and additional comorbid pathologies with inherent competing mortality risks contribute to outcome. The appropriateness of an intervention directed solely to correcting aortic stenosis in patients turned down for conventional surgery therefore needs very careful assessment.

Mitral valve surgery in elderly patients

Elderly people are regarded as higher risk patients for mitral valve surgery; however, higher early and late mortalities are in part due to elderly patients being referred late (more than one year after presenting with significant symptoms) and undergoing surgery later in the history of their mitral valve disease.[10] Mortality doubles in patients undergoing any form of mitral valve surgery if over the age of 70 years compared to those <60 years.[3]

The predominant pathology in the elderly population (developed economies) is either myxomatous degenerative or ischaemic-related secondary mitral valve regurgitation, and not unexpectedly in the former group, older people have significantly more associated coronary artery disease. The pathophysiology of degenerative mitral regurgitation is typically prolapse of the mitral leaflets as a result of elongated or ruptured chordae and mitral annular dilatation. In contrast, ischaemic regurgitation is usually due to restricted motion of the mitral leaflets as a result of segmental or global ventricular dilatation.

Chronic severe mitral regurgitation results in progressive and eventual irreversible left ventricular dilatation and myocardial failure (NYHA class III or IV) that is not reversed by eventual successful valve surgery (Figure 9.9).[10] Hence, early surgery (NYHA class I or II) is recommended for asymptomatic severe non-ischaemic mitral regurgitation regardless of age,

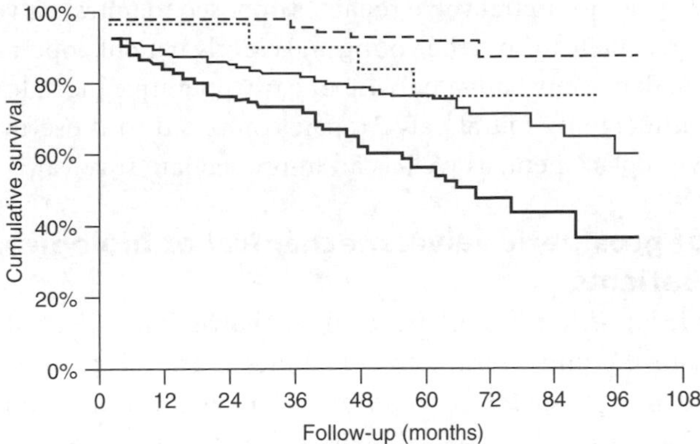

Figure 9.9 Long-term survival of 614 consecutive patients who underwent either mitral valve replacement or repair surgery, and grouped according to their preoperative NYHA dyspnoea class and age. NYHA class I or II sub-grouped according to age <70 years (dashed line) or ≥70 years (dotted line), as well as NYHA class III or IV subgrouped according to age <70 years (thin line) or ≥70 years (bold line). Reprinted from *Lee et al.*[10] with permission from ICR Publishers Ltd.

if there are signs of left ventricular dysfunction (left ventricular ejection fraction less than 60%), AF or pulmonary hypertension (pulmonary systolic pressure >50 mmHg) and preserved left ventricular function, and especially if there is a high likelihood of mitral valve repair.[16]

The survival advantage of early surgery for severe mitral regurgitation is greater in the elderly than in the younger population.[10] Seven-year freedom from all-cause death in elderly patients (≥70 yrs) undergoing mitral valve surgery early (NYHA class I or II) was 77% versus only 44% if undergoing surgery late (NYHA class III or IV). In younger patients (<70 yrs) survival was 88% and 66% respectively.

Mitral valve replacement or repair

Conservative mitral valve repair rather than valve replacement should be done whenever feasible, as this is associated with both a lower operative mortality as well as improved long-term survival, regardless of presenting symptoms. Valve repair preserves the subvalvar apparatus and left ventricular function, thereby reducing mortality from myocardial failure. In addition, late thromboembolic and haemorrhagic complications are less frequent with mitral valve repair. Advances in surgical techniques including artificial Gore-Tex chordae have now made it possible for cardiac surgeons experienced in mitral valve repair to successfully repair more than 80% of degenerative and ischaemic regurgitant mitral valves. If mitral valve repair is not feasible, then replacement with a prosthetic valve, but with preservation of the subvalvar apparatus, is the next best option.

The preference for mitral valve repair as opposed to mitral valve replacement applies equally to both the young and elderly patient populations. The UK national data show both a halving of early operative mortality in octogenarians undergoing mitral valve repair compared to those undergoing mitral valve replacement, as well as an improved late survival.[3]

Choice of prosthetic valve: mechanical or biological in elderly patients

A multitude of artificial mechanical heart valves have been developed, ranging from the initial obstructive 'ball and cage' valves to 'tilting disc' valves, and now 'bileaflet' mechanical valves made from titanium steel and pyrolytic carbon. Mechanical heart valves though have an associated lifelong thromboembolic risk from blood clots forming on the valve, which is the natural reaction of blood whenever it comes into contact with an artificial surface. This necessitates life-long anticoagulation with vitamin K antagonists (coumarin/warfarin), which in turn creates a risk of life-threatening major haemorrhage. A fine balance thus needs to be maintained for the rest of the patient's life, if mechanical prosthetic valves have been implanted; between too little anticoagulation which increases the risk of clot formation and thromboembolic ischaemic stroke, versus too much with its risk of anticoagulation-related haemorrhage and stroke (Figure 9.10).[22]

Constant lifelong monitoring and maintenance of the patient's serum international normalized ratio (INR) in the recommended range, which is discussed in more detail later in this chapter, is therefore essential in all patients receiving mechanical prosthetic valves. Contraindications to warfarin use therefore preclude the implantation of mechanical prosthetic valves (Table 9.5).[23]

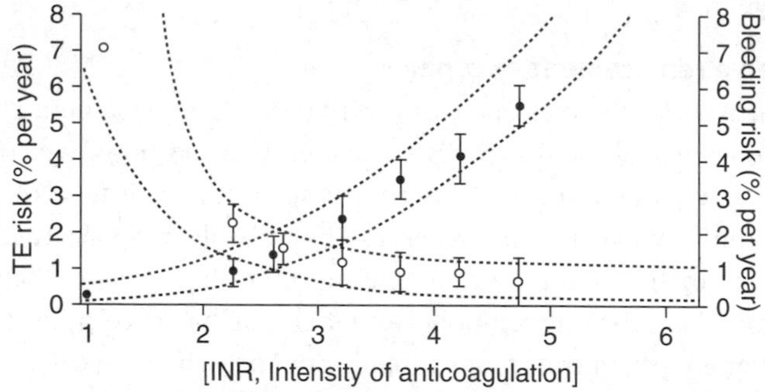

Figure 9.10 The incidence of thromboembolic (TE; open circles) and bleeding (solid circles) complications after 10-year follow-up, and grouped according to the average intensity of oral anticoagulation achieved by INR during the 10 years. The recommended target INR range was 3.0–4.5 in these patients with aortic mechanical St Jude heart valve prostheses. Reprinted from Horstkotte *et al.*[22] with permission from ICR Publishers Ltd.

Table 9.5 Contraindications to coumarin/warfarin use.

The patient
- Comorbidity; including comorbid medical conditions, falls, frailty, exposure to trauma
- Impaired cognitive function
- Possibly housebound
- Poor expected compliance

The doctor
- Poor appreciation of drug interactions
- Inefficient organization of INR monitoring

The system
- General practice versus hospital facilities; for example, remote location, poor communication, and support
- Inadequate resources and facilities available.

Source: Reprinted from Blann *et al*. ABC of antithrombotic therapy: An overview of antithrombotic therapy. *BMJ* 2002;**325**:762–5. Copyright 2002, with permission from BMJ Publishing Group Ltd.

Biological valves predominantly manufactured from bovine pericardium or porcine aortic valves have been developed as an alternative and do not require lifelong anticoagulation unless otherwise indicated. However, biological valves have a limited lifespan because of both calcium and non-calcium-related degeneration. Structural valve deterioration of bioprostheses is also higher in the mitral position than in the aortic position.[24] Fifty percent of 'first-generation' biological heart valves required replacement within 13 years of implantation. It has been thought that there is a reduced incidence of structural deterioration of bioprosthetic valves in elderly patients; however, this has been shown to not necessarily be due to improved valve survival in older people but rather due to reduced patient survival from other causes. Nevertheless, current commercial, now improved 'third-generation' biological prosthetic valves, based on animal studies, are thought to have significantly improved valve survival compared to these older 'first-generation' bioprostheses. The major advantage of bioprosthetic valves in elderly people is that, unless otherwise indicated, lifelong anticoagulation with vitamin K antagonists is not required. The elderly population (particularly >70 yrs) are at greater risk of thromboembolic and haemorrhagic complications secondary to coumarin therapy.[24]

Elderly patients would thus benefit from implantation of a biological as opposed to mechanical prosthetic valve and, therefore, either not requiring anticoagulation or alternatively at a lower therapeutic INR range if other indications for anticoagulation exist, because of the increasing comorbid pathologies associated with elderly people. Mortality from thromboembolic events and anticoagulation-related haemorrhage is three times higher in

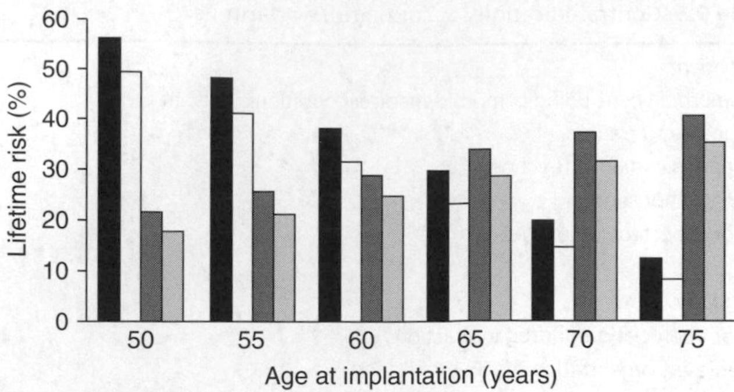

Figure 9.11 Microsimulation meta-analysis of the lifetime risk, according to the age at primary aortic valve implantation, of either structural valve degeneration of biological aortic valves without (solid bar) or with (open bar) concomitant coronary artery bypass graft surgery, or alternatively anticoagulation-related bleeding risks of mechanical aortic valves without (dark shaded bar) or with (light shaded bar) concomitant coronary artery bypass graft surgery. Reprinted from Puvimanasinghe *et al.*[26] Copyright 2003, with permission from Elsevier.

elderly patients over the age of 65 with mechanical prosthetic valves as compared to those with bioprostheses.[25]

The current recommendation is therefore to select a bioprosthetic heart valve for aortic valve replacements in patients ≥60–65 years of age, and for mitral valve replacements in patients ≥65–70 years (Figure 9.11).[24,26]

Combined coronary artery bypass graft and valve surgery in elderly patients

Previous unproven dictums such as 'do as little as possible/only what is deemed essential' are slowly being disproved in terms of the extent of cardiac surgery undertaken. In CABG surgery, incomplete revascularization is an independent predictor of both in-hospital and late mortality.[12] The survival benefit of attending to coexistent moderate or more ischaemic mitral regurgitation at the time of CABG surgery is well established.

The supporting evidence for 'prophylactic' additional aortic valve replacement for moderate aortic stenosis (aortic valve area 1–1.5 cm^2, and more so if <1.3 cm^2, valve calcification or renal failure) in older patients (aged >60–65 yrs) already accepted for CABG surgery is becoming stronger, especially when considering the extremely high operative risk of subsequent re-operative valve procedures (~30% mortality), should it become necessary in an octogenarian. The presence of either aortic valve calcification or an aortic jet velocity of 3.0–4.0 m s^{-1} would suggest the likelihood of more rapid progression of aortic stenosis and therefore justification of a concomitant 'prophylactic' aortic valve replacement at the time of the initial CABG referral.

Acceptable surgical results are being obtained with these more complex procedures in elderly patients, and should not therefore be denied to older people. Careful individual preoperative assessment as previously discussed is, however, essential.

Anticoagulation management in the elderly patient

Patients at risk for cerebral thromboembolic events include patients with mechanical prosthetic heart valves, AF, reduced left ventricular function (less than 35% ejection fraction), history of previous thromboembolism or hypercoagulable states. These patients should receive anticoagulation with vitamin K antagonists and their INR should be maintained in a range between 2.0 and 5.0.[27] Whether the target INR range is on the lower (INR 2.0–3.0), intermediate (INR 2.5–3.5), or upper (INR 3.0–4.5) side of this range will be dependent on the underlying thromboembolic risk, but will also influence the risk of anticoagulation-related haemorrhagic complications (Figure 9.10). The reason for providing a range is due to the difficulty of maintaining a 'constant' INR in any individual patient.

Warfarin, the most commonly used coumarin derivative, results in anticoagulation by inhibiting the synthesis of factors dependent on vitamin K, and has a considerable variability in its effects due to considerable pharmacokinetic and pharmacodynamic factors (Table 9.6).[23] This therefore demands frequent laboratory measurements of each individual patient's INR, and audits have shown that only 50% of patients are within their target range at any specific time point. The half-life of the vitamin K dependent factors range from 6–60 hours, thus any specific warfarin dose takes 2–3 days to produce an effect and this needs to be taken into account when managing warfarin dosage.

Patient self-management using their own 'point-of-care INR monitors' that are now available, especially in patients requiring lifelong anticoagulation, may offer the potential for both simplifying and improving oral anticoagulation management. A recently published meta-analysis of post-operative results and complications showed significant reduction in thromboembolic events, all-cause mortality and major haemorrhage in patients self-managing their INR.[28]

Anticoagulation for biological prosthetic valves

The current guidelines in patients with no other thromboembolic risk factors recommend temporary use of warfarin for only the first three months after biological valve implantation.[17] This is still controversial in

Table 9.6 This is only an illustrative list of interactive factors that influence the efficacy of warfarin.

Patient factors
Enhanced anticoagulant effect
Weight loss, increased age (>80 years), acute illness, impaired liver function, heart failure, renal failure, excess alcohol ingestion
Reduced anticoagulant effect
Weight gain, diarrhoea and vomiting, relative youth (<40 years), Asian or African-Caribbean background
Examples of some drug interactions with warfarin
Reduced protein binding
Aspirin, phenylbutazone, sulfinpyrazone, chlorpromazine
Inhibition of metabolism of warfarin
Cimetadine, erythromycin, sodium valproate
Enhanced metabolism of warfarin
Barbiturates, phenytoin, carbamazepine
Reduced synthesis of factors II, VII, IX, X
Phenytoin, salicylates
Reduced absorption of vitamin K
Broad-spectrum antibiotics, laxatives
Enhanced risk of peptic ulceration
Aspirin, non-steroidal anti-inflammatory drugs, corticosteroids
Thrombolytics
Streptokinase, tissue plasminogen activator
Antiplatelet drugs
Aspirin, non-steroidal anti-inflammatory drugs

Source: Reprinted from Blann AD *et al*. ABC of antithrombotic therapy: An overview of antithrombotic therapy. *BMJ* 2002;**325**:762–5. Copyright 2002, with permission from BMJ Publishing Group Ltd.

patients with biological aortic valves, and thus, in these patients, either a temporary low-dose anticoagulation regimen (INR target range of 2.0–3.0), or antiplatelet therapy with aspirin (acetylsalicylic acid 75–100 mg day^{-1}) in patients not having reduced left ventricular ejection fraction (<35%), NYHA class IV, preoperative AF, or a paced rhythm can be used. After the first three post-operative months and provided there are no other thromboembolic risk factors, warfarin therapy can then be discontinued and replaced with aspirin 75–100 mg day^{-1}.[17]

Anticoagulation for mechanical prosthetic valves

Mechanical prosthetic valves in the aortic position (excluding first-generation Starr-Edwards, Lillehei Kaster, Omniscience, and Björk-Shiley valves) are considered to be less thrombogenic than in the mitral position (double the risk). Hence, patients with second- or third-generation mechanical prosthetic valves (St Jude Medical bileaflet, Medtronic-Hall tilting disc, CarboMedics bileaflet) can be maintained at an INR target range of 2.5–3.0 or 3.5 for the aortic position,[17,23,27] and at a slightly higher INR range of 3.0–3.5 or 4.5 for the mitral position.[23,27] The higher top endpoint should probably be used if there are additional thromboembolic risk factors; an enlarged left atrium (>55 mm in diameter), reduced left ventricular ejection fraction (<35%), dilated left ventricle (left ventricular end-diastolic diameter greater than 70 mm), AF, or previous thromboembolic events.

Patients with mechanical prosthetic valves require lifelong constant monitoring of their INR (initially daily then at least every 1–2 weeks depending on individual variance), as diet, coexistent diseases, medication, etc. interact with the efficacy of vitamin K antagonists (Table 9.6). Inadequate anticoagulation monitoring not only increases the risk of thrombosis, but also increases the risk of stroke (3–10%), major bleeding episodes (5%), non-disabling bleeding (14%), as well as recurrent thrombosis (11%). In the event that patients have evidence of prosthetic valve obstruction or thrombosis, they should be referred for emergent reoperation.[17]

Anticoagulant management of patients with mechanical prosthetic valves undergoing non-cardiac surgery

If it is necessary to interrupt oral anticoagulant therapy in patients with mechanical prosthetic heart valves, in preparation for elective surgical procedures, it is recommended to temporarily stop oral vitamin K antagonist therapy for 4–5 days preoperatively. Once the INR is less than <2.0, then either a continuous intravenous heparin infusion (prolonging the activated partial thromboplastin time (APTT) to twice normal) or subcutaneous low-molecular-weight heparin (100 U kg^{-1} every 12 hours) should be given to prevent thromboembolism.[23,27] The advantage of low molecular-weight heparin is the ability to provide this therapy on an ambulatory basis. However, its effects are only partially neutralized by protamine because of its higher anti-Xa activity, and it should therefore in turn be temporarily stopped 12–18 hours prior to surgery. Oral anticoagulation therapy is then recommenced the day after surgery or as soon as feasible in terms of intestinal function.

The aforementioned guidelines should also be used when patients' (requiring oral anticoagulation) INRs drop below their therapeutic range.

Parenteral vitamin K is not recommended in the treatment of non-life-threatening bleeding associated with warfarin use in patients with mechanical prosthetic valves because of the potential for induced hypercoagulable states.

Anticoagulation for atrial fibrillation (AF)

The efficacy of oral anticoagulation with vitamin K antagonists for preventing stroke in patients with AF has been well documented. Targeting the lowest intensity of anticoagulation to minimize the risk of haemorrhagic complications is, however, particularly important for elderly patients with AF, and, in these patients, an INR target ranging between 2.0 and 3.0 is recommended.[23,27] The risk of anticoagulant-related haemorrhage increases with age (1–2% patients per year, if below 60 years old).[17] Hence, in AF patients more than 75 years old, a target INR range of 1.5–2.5 albeit not as effective, or only aspirin treatment (325 mg day^{-1}) may be considered if there are no other indications for coumarin anticoagulation.

Non-pharmacological curative therapy for atrial fibrillation

Atrial fibrillation is the most common serious cardiac arrhythmia and is associated with a significant risk of cerebral thromboembolism. The prevalence of AF in the general population is approximately 0.4%; however, the prevalence increases markedly with age to approximately 9% in the 80–89-year-old population group. Furthermore, the risk of stroke associated with AF also increases with age from a 1.5% risk at age 50–59 years to 23.5% risk at age 80–89 years. Anticoagulation with warfarin reduces this risk of stroke but imparts a risk of anticoagulation-related haemorrhage and reduces patients' quality of life.

The surgical Maze procedure developed by James L. Cox has been able to cure AF in up to 99% of carefully selected patients (predominantly patients with paroxysmal AF), and thereby has essentially abolished the risk of stroke associated with AF. Percutaneous transcatheter ablation of the pulmonary vein ostia, also in carefully selected patients with paroxysmal AF, now offers a less invasive approach and a success rate of approximately 75%.

Newer hyperthermic ablation devices including radiofrequency, microwave, ultrasound and laser, as well as cryoablation devices have also now been developed to allow surgeons to do more rapid reproducible modified Maze procedures concomitant with other cardiac surgical procedures. Post-operative 5-year freedom from AF in 'non-selected' patients with permanent AF of more than 1-year duration, undergoing concomitant cardiac surgery, can now be expected in 42–87% of patients depending on underlying coexistent cardiac pathology.[29]

The non-pharmacological cure of AF is currently a rapidly developing field, and clear guidelines as to patient selection are slowly being developed.

However, the elderly patient with AF who has the highest risk of stroke may potentially stand to gain the most from this emerging therapeutic option.

Thoracic aortic surgery

The incidence of thoracic aortic aneurysms and aortic dissections increases in the elderly population and is a lethal disease. The 5-year survival of patients not operated on is approximately 54%, and these patients have a 21–74% risk of acute rupture.[30]

The major factor influencing the risk of either acute rupture, dissection or death is the diameter of the aneurysm at initial presentation; aneurysms greater than or equal to 6.0 cm in diameter have an annual risk of a negative outcome of 15.6% (Figure 9.12).[30] The risk of rupture with time increases 11-fold with aortic aneurysm size of 5.0–5.9 cm, and 23-fold with size of 6.0 cm or greater.[30] This needs to be compared with the risk of surgery, which has an operative mortality of 5–9% for elective surgery, but as high as 57% for emergency operations in elderly people.

The current accepted guidelines for asymptomatic aneurysms is to operate once an ascending aortic aneurysm diameter is 5.5 cm or more, or if a descending thoracic aortic aneurysm is 6.5 cm or more. However, a smaller diameter of 4.5–5.0 cm is used in patients with Marfan's syndrome or a family history of aortic aneurysms because of the higher incidence of rupture in these subgroups. Additional operative risk factors that need

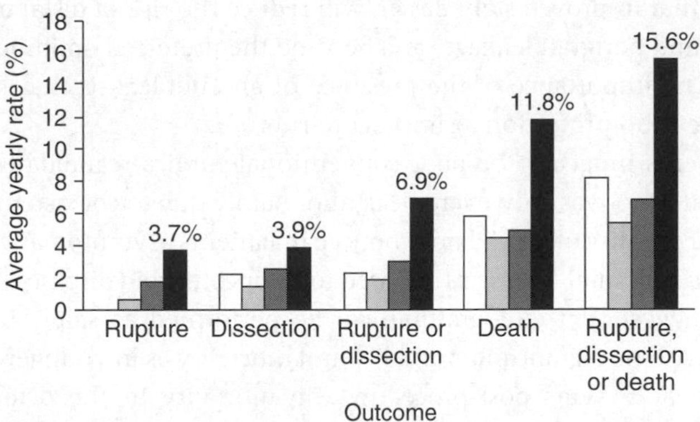

Figure 9.12 The average yearly rate (during the first five years after presentation), of negative outcomes (rupture, dissection or death) as a function of the initial thoracic aortic aneurysm (ascending, arch, descending or thoracoabdominal) size (maximal diameter); 3.5–3.9 cm (clear bar), 4.0–4.9 cm (light shade bar), 5.0–5.9 cm (medium shade bar), equal or greater than 6.0 cm (solid bar). Reprinted from Davies *et al.*[30] Copyright 2002, with permission from Elsevier.

to be taken into account when assessing a patient for surgery on the descending thoracic aorta are the risk of spinal cord injury and paraplegia of 2–8%, which is related to the extent of the aneurysm and is highest in Crawford type II thoracoabdominal aneurysms.[31]

In a large series (mean age 65 years), the risk of an adverse outcome (death, paraplegia, renal failure requiring haemodialysis or stroke) in elective thoracoabdominal aortic aneurysms was 13% and related to preoperative renal insufficiency, increasing age, type II extent and symptomatic aneurysms.[31] An important conclusion of this study was that the development of any symptoms, no matter how mild or uncharacteristic, in patients with thoracoabdominal aneurysms requires immediate evaluation. The aneurysm must be considered the cause of the symptoms until proven otherwise as it indicates progression into a subacute phase.

The main approach for these complex aortic repairs has been direct open repair, usually supported by deep hypothermic circulatory arrest. However, newer 'hybrid techniques' that combine surgical and endovascular approaches have been reported with lower morbidity and mortality.

These percutaneous inserted cloth-covered stainless steel stents were initially developed in 1969 and can now be inserted retrograde via the femoral artery into the abdominal and descending thoracic aorta, to seal off some aortic aneurysms. Current trials in appropriately selected patients have shown a procedural mortality of approximately 7% and 5-year survival of 68%. In 'good surgical candidates' 5-year survival of 78% was similar to conventional open surgical series, suggesting that cloth-covered stents are being increasingly used in patients possibly deemed unfit for conventional surgical interventions.[32] This technology is developing and it is hoped that improved stent design will reduce the risk of distal migration of stents and perigraft leakage, and become the preferred option in elderly people. The importance of the presence of an endoleak is that it implies that there is no protection against acute rupture.

In patients judged to be poor conventional surgical candidates, 5-year survival at 31% was, however, bleak and mainly due to coexistent disease. Moreover, quality of life did not improve in patients asymptomatic in terms of their aneurysmal disease as opposed to their comorbid diseases.[32] Recent studies suggest that endografting can be performed as safely in elderly patients with no significant morbidity and mortality as in younger patients. However, at 5 years post-procedure the mortality in the octogenarian group is double (31.8% vs 17.1%), although this increased mortality can be explained by the advanced age of the octogenarian who most likely died from other comorbidities. Increased age does not appear to be a risk factor for short- and mid-term morbidity and mortality for patients with stentable thoracic pathology. Older patients do as well after endostenting of the descending thoracic aorta and should be offered this less invasive approach.

Cardiac transplantation

The worldwide results of heart transplantation compiled by the International Society of Heart and Lung Transplantation Registry show that the current 1-year and 5-year survival following a heart transplant managed with modern immunosuppressive therapy is approximately 80% and 67%, respectively.[3]

A heart transplant is technically a relatively simple operation, but replaces a patient's original terminal heart disease with another disease; the disease of immunosuppression, which though is expected to carry a slightly better chance of survival. Nevertheless, constantly having to take drugs to prevent rejection of the new heart and balancing this against the risks of over-suppressing the body's defence mechanism which makes the patient prone to infection or cancer, becomes even more of an issue in the elderly patient.

In the United Kingdom, there is no prescribed age limit for acceptance onto a heart transplant programme; however, in practice, few patients above 65 years of age tend to be accepted. The international age distribution shows that less than 5% of heart transplants were in recipients aged 65 or more.[33] Availability of donor organs is the primary limiting factor for heart transplantation worldwide. Improvements in road traffic safety amongst others have resulted in a 40% reduction in the availability of cadaveric cardiothoracic donors in the United Kingdom over the past 10 years. Equitable allocation of donor hearts, an increasingly restricted national resource, is therefore necessary. In 2002–2003, only 32% of patients on an active cardiothoracic transplant waiting list (heart, lung or heart/lung) received an organ transplant.

An alternative option for patients with terminal heart disease not amenable to conventional cardiac surgery for whatever reason, which is now becoming available, is implantation of miniature blood pumps; totally implantable left ventricular assist devices. However, the current costs of these, what in the elderly population will be 'destination therapy' devices will probably preclude universal access.

Conclusions

The elderly population has and will continue to increase and up to 40% of octogenarians have symptomatic cardiac disease. In the United Kingdom, 22% of patients undergoing heart surgery were over 75 years of age in 2008 and valve procedures predominate in octogenarians. Cardiac surgery mortality and morbidity outcomes have and will continue to improve and age itself is not a contraindication for cardiac surgery. The crude operative mortality for octogenarians undergoing cardiac surgery is currently less than 5–11% with post-operative 5-year survivals of 60–75% being similar to the age-matched natural population. The major morbidity risk is that of peri-operative stroke because of the increased atherosclerotic vascular disease and can be as high as 13%.

Elderly patients must be individually assessed preoperatively in terms of the risk of the intended cardiac surgery; EuroScore-predicted mortality, versus the perceived benefit in their quality of life; EuroQol, as well as the influence of other coexistent medical conditions. Although the prime indication for cardiac surgery in elderly people continues to be 'relief of symptoms', excessively late referral has a significant negative impact on both operative risk and late outcome. Mild symptoms need to be promptly investigated, if necessary by echocardiography and angiography, in order to more accurately determine the true extent of any underlying cardiac condition.

The unadjusted operative mortality for isolated CABG in elderly people (age >75 yrs) is ~3.3% and use of the internal mammary artery as a conduit is still recommended even in the octogenarian. Percutaneous coronary stenting or incomplete revascularizations are not necessarily better alternatives in the older patient.

Aortic valve replacement accounts for the majority of valve surgery in elderly patients, and operative mortality is primarily related to comorbid conditions. Once again more complete assessment of the 'asymptomatic' patient is essential and early referral preferable. Replacement with a biological as opposed to mechanical prosthetic valve is recommended in elderly people because, unless otherwise indicated, lifelong anticoagulation is not required and the lifespan of current third-generation bioprostheses is greater than most elderly patients' projected lifespans. Percutaneous balloon aortic valvuloplasty is not considered to be a suitable alternative. However, transcatheter aortic valve replacement, usually without the use of cardiopulmonary bypass, is an emerging technique in elderly high-risk patients deemed to be unsuitable for conventional heart surgery.

Chronic severe mitral valve regurgitation results in progressive irreversible left ventricular dysfunction and the survival advantage of early surgery (NYHA dyspnoea class II) is even greater in the elderly population, especially if mitral valve reparative surgery can be confidently undertaken.

Atrial fibrillation is an increasing problem in the elderly population with an associated high risk of stroke. Developments in the non-pharmacological cure of AF are an attractive option in elderly patients, who potentially have the most to gain in reverting to normal sinus rhythm and not requiring long-term anticoagulation, especially if concomitant cardiac surgery is already indicated.

Thoracic aortic dissections and aneurysms are more prevalent in elderly people, and untreated will rupture acutely in up to 74% of patients. In principle, patients who are symptomatic or with ascending aortic aneurysms greater than 5.5 cm or descending aneurysms greater than 6.5 cm should be referred for surgery. In appropriately selected patients, percutaneous inserted cloth-covered stents are becoming the preferred technique with the descending thoracic aortic aneurysms especially in older people.

Cardiac transplantation is not a realistic option in the elderly patient with terminal heart failure. However, new miniature fully implantable blood pumps may become an option in the future.

Key points

- Age is not a contraindication for cardiac surgery in elderly patients provided they can be discharged without significant disability and loss of independence.
- Elderly patients must be assessed individually in terms of the natural history of their disease, symptoms thereof, current quality of life, and the risk (mortality and morbidity) versus benefit (improved quality of life) of any potential cardiac surgical intervention.
- Referring elderly patients at an earlier stage of the disease process even with mild symptoms can improve the outcome of cardiac surgery in older people. Advising cardiac surgery as the last option and recommending a wait-and-see policy based on symptoms results in significantly poorer outcomes.
- Aortic valve replacement surgery if indicated, offers an excellent long-term outcome in elderly patients.
- Elderly patients benefit from implantation of a biological as opposed to mechanical prosthetic valve, if valve replacement is required, as bioprostheses do not require anticoagulation or, alternatively, at a lower therapeutic INR range, if other indications for anticoagulation exist.

References

1 Alexander KP, Anstrom KJ, Muhlbaier LH *et al.* Outcomes of cardiac surgery in patients age ≥80: results from the national cardiovascular network. *J Am Coll Cardiol* 2000;**35**:731–8.

2 Kohl P, Kerzmann A, Lahaye L *et al.* Cardiac surgery in octogenarians. *Peri-operative outcome and long-term results. Eur Heart J* 2001;**22**:1235–43.

3 Bridgewater B, Keogh BE, Kinsman R and Walton P. (2009) *The Society for Cardiothoracic Surgery in Great Britain & Ireland;* Sixth National Adult Cardiac Surgical Database Report 2008: Demonstrating quality, Dendrite Clinical Systems Ltd, Henley-on-Thames.

4 Bridges CR, Edwards FH, Peterson ED *et al*. Cardiac surgery in nonagenarians and centenarians. *J Am Coll Surg* 2003;**197**:347–57.

5 Akins CW, Daggett WM, Vlahakes GJ *et al*. Cardiac operations in patients 80 years old and older. *Ann Thorac Surg* 1997;**64**:606–15.

6 Blauth CI, Cosgrove DM, Webb BW *et al*. Atheroembolism from the ascending aorta: an emerging problem in cardiac surgery. *J Thorac Cardiovasc Surg* 1992;**103**:1104–12.

7 Nashef SAM, Roques F, Michel P *et al*. European system for cardiac operative risk evaluation (EuroSCORE). *Eur J Cardiothorac Surg* 1999;**16**:9–13.

8 Hewitt TD, Santa Maria PL and Alvarez JM. Cardiac surgery in Australian octogenarians: 1996–2001. *ANZ J Surg* 2003;**73**:749–54.

9 Sollano JA, Rose EA, Williams DL *et al*. Cost-effectiveness of coronary artery bypass surgery in octogenarians. *Ann Surg* 1998;**228**:297–306.

10 Lee EM, Porter JN, Shapiro LM and Wells FC. Mitral valve surgery in the elderly. *J Heart Valve Dis* 1997;**6**:22–31.

11 Avery GJ II,, Ley SJ, Hill JD *et al*. Cardiac surgery in the octogenarian: evaluation of risk, cost and outcome. *Ann Thorac Surg* 2001;**71**:591–6.

12 Graham MM, Ghali WA, Faris PD *et al*. The Alberta Provincial Project for Outcomes Assessment in Coronary Heart Disease (APPROACH) Investigators. Survival after coronary revascularization in the elderly. *Circulation* 2002;**105**:2378–84.

13 Chaitman BR, Fisher LD, Bourassa MG *et al*. Participating CASS Medical Centers. Effect of coronary bypass surgery on survival patterns in subsets of patients with left main coronary artery disease. Report of the collaborative study in coronary artery surgery (CASS). *Am J Cardiol* 1981;**48**:765–77.

14 Morris RJ, Strong MD, Grunewald KE *et al*. Internal thoracic artery for coronary artery grafting in octogenarians. *Ann Thorac Surg* 1996;**62**:16–22.

15 Peters RJG, Mehta SR, Fox KAA *et al*. The Clopidogrel in Unstable angina to prevent Recurrent Events (CURE) Trial Investigators. Effects of aspirin dose when used alone or in combination with clopidogrel in patients with acute coronary syndromes. Observations from the clopidogrel in unstable angina to prevent recurrent events (CURE) study. *Circulation* 2003;**108**:1682–7.

16 Lung B, Gohlke-Barwolf C, Tornos P *et al*. The Working Group on Valvular Heart Disease. *Recommendations on the management of the asymptomatic patient with valvular heart disease. Eur Heart J* 2003;**23**:1253–66.

17 Bonow RO, Blase A, Carabello B *et al*. ACC/AHA 2006 Guidelines for the Management of Patients with Valvular Heart Disease: Executive Summary. A Report of the American College of Cardiology/American Heart Association Task Force on Practice Guidelines. *Circulation* 2006;**114**:450–527.

18 Gilbert T, Orr W and Banning AP. Surgery for aortic stenosis in severely symptomatic patients older than 80 years: experience in a single UK centre. *Heart* 1999;**82**:138–42.

19 Bernard Y, Etievent J, Mourand JL *et al*. Long-term results of percutaneous aortic valvoplasty compared with aortic valve replacement in patients more than 75 years old. *J Am Coll Cardiol* 1992;**20**:796–801.

20 Van Brabandt H and Neyt M. Safety of percutaneous aortic valve insertion. *A systematic review. BMC Cardiovasc Disord* 2009;**9**:45.

21 Bleiziffer S, Ruge H, Mazzitelle D *et al*. Cardiovascular results of percutaneous and transapical transcatheter aortic valve implantation performed by a surgical team. *Eur J Cardiothoracic Surg* 2009;**35**:615–21.

22 Horstkotte D, Schulte H, Bircks W and Strauer B. Unexpected findings concerning thromboembolic complications and anticoagulation after complete 10-year follow-up of patients with St. Jude Medical prostheses. *J Heart Valve Dis* 1993;**2**:291–301.

23 Lip GYH and Blann AD. (2003) *ABC of Antithrombotic Therapy*, BMJ Publishing Group, London.

24 Rahimtoola SH. Choice of prosthetic heart valve for adult patients. *J Am Coll Cardiol* 2003;**41**:893–904.

25 Holper K, Wottke M, Lewe T *et al*. Bioprosthetic and mechanical valves in the elderly: benefits and risks. *Ann Thorac Surg* 1995;**60**:443–6.

26 Puvimanasinghe JPA, Takkenberg JJM, Eijkemans MJC *et al*. Choice of a mechanical valve or a bioprosthesis for AVR: does CABG matter? *Eur J Cardiothorac Surg* 2003;**23**:688–95.

27 Hirsh J, Fuster V, Ansell J, Halperin JL *et al*. American Heart Association/American College of Cardiology Foundation guide to warfarin therapy. *Circulation* 2003;**107**:1692–1711.

28 Henegham C, Alonso-Coello P, Garcia-Alamino JM *et al*. Self-monitoring of oral anticoagulation: a systematic review and meta-analysis. *Lancet* 2006;**367**:404–11.

29 Von Oppell UO, Masani N, O'Callaghan P *et al*. Mitral valve surgery plus concomitant atrial fibrillation ablation is superior to mitral valve surgery alone with an intensive rhythm control strategy. *Eur J Cardiothorac Surg* 2009;**35**:641–50.

30 Davies RR, Goldstein LJ, Coady MA *et al*. Yearly rupture or dissection rates for thoracic aortic aneurysms: simple prediction based on size. *Ann Thorac Surg* 2002;**73**:17–28.

31 LeMaire SA, Miller CC III,, Conklin LD *et al*. A new predictive model for adverse outcomes after elective thoracoabdominal aortic aneurysm repair. *Ann Thorac Surg* 2001;**71**:1233–8.

32 Demers P, Miller DC, Mitchell RS *et al*. Midterm results of endovascular repair of descending thoracic aortic aneurysms with first-generation stent grafts. *J Thorac Cardiovasc Surg* 2004;**127**:664–73.

33 Hosenpud JD, Bennett LE, Keck BM *et al*. The registry of the International Society for Heart and Lung Transplantation: eighteenth Official Report-2001. *J Heart Lung Transplant* 2001;**20**:805–15.

CHAPTER 10
Cardiac Rehabilitation

Niccolò Marchionni, Francesco Fattirolli, Francesco Orso, Marco Baccini, Lucio A. Rinaldi and Giulio Masotti
University of Florence and Azienda Ospedaliero – Universitaria Careggi, Florence, Italy

Cardiac diseases and rehabilitation services

Epidemiology

In 2001, cardiovascular diseases were still the first among the leading causes of death in men and women of all ages in the United States, with coronary heart disease (CHD) alone accounting for 54% of all cardiovascular deaths. The prevalence of cardiovascular diseases – including CHD, stroke and hypertension – increases with age up to more than 70% at age 75 years and older. A surveillance study performed by the National Heart, Blood and Lung Institute in 1987–2000 reported that the incidence of myocardial infarction also increases exponentially with age.[1]

Due to the remarkable advances in the management of acute CHD events, chronic heart failure (CHF) and cardiovascular risk factors, the specific mortality for heart disease has been declining continuously over the last two decades, especially among men. Furthermore, preventive medicine has shifted the age at which patients develop CHF but has not reduced, and indeed may have increased, its global epidemiological burden. As a consequence, growing numbers of cardiac patients currently survive longer, but with substantial functional limitations that are secondary to several manifestations of CHD, such as CHF, whose incidence has been increasing steadily, particularly in older populations, suggesting that we now face a real 'CHF epidemic'. The National Health and Nutrition Examination Survey (NHANES) epidemiological study reported that the prevalence of CHF is less than 5% among individuals aged 65 years or younger, but doubles among those older than 75 years,[2] and data from the World Health Organization (WHO) suggest that these figures differ little around the world, at least in more affluent countries.

As is discussed in this chapter, randomized clinical trials, and also meta-analyses and observational studies, have demonstrated that

Cardiovascular Disease and Health in the Older Patient: Expanded from 'Pathy's Principles and Practice of Geriatric Medicine, Fifth edition', First Edition. Edited by David J. Stott and Gordon D.O. Lowe.

integrated cardiac rehabilitation (CR) programmes are highly effective in accelerating functional recovery and in improving exercise tolerance, adherence with secondary prevention measures, health-related quality of life (HRQOL) and also long-term prognosis after acute cardiac events.[3–6] As a result, the most recent guidelines clearly define the core components and outcome measures of CR and secondary prevention programmes and indicate CR as an integral component of long-term care of patients with CHD and CHF.[7,8]

Utilization of cardiac rehabilitation services: An international perspective

Despite this considerable amount of evidence and the fact that CR programmes are recommended (class I) by the European Society of Cardiology (ESC),[9] American Heart Association (AHA) and American College of Cardiology (ACC)[10] in the management of CHD and CHF,[11] prescription of CR programmes and diffusion of CR services is still relatively limited.

The level of CR service coverage across the European Union can be estimated from a survey of 454 phase 2 (medium-term recovery after hospital discharge) and 383 phase 3 (long-term maintenance) centres in 13 countries. Fewer than 50% of eligible patients participate in CR rehabilitation programmes in most European countries, with services in particularly short supply in countries with the greatest burden of cardiovascular diseases.[12] According to another survey of the European Society of Cardiology, only 67% of patients are prescribed CR soon after coronary artery bypass surgery, and this proportion drops to 49%, 35% and 17% among those with recent myocardial infarction, coronary angioplasty or chronic myocardial ischaemia, respectively. Furthermore, utilization of CR services is widely variable cross-nationally, with an average participation after any type of CHD event ranging from 4% in Spain to 71% in Slovenia.[13] In the recently published results of the third EUROASPIRE Survey, the scenario is similar: less than 50% of CHD patients were advised to participate in a CR programme after hospitalization and about 75% of those advised attended at least half of the sessions; in summary, only about one third of the originally eligible population.[14] More importantly, the data are limited to patients younger than 70 years who, in that survey, were selected for obtaining information on CR service coverage. Given the almost systematic exclusion of older patients which has also been reported by the most recent meta-analyses of CR in patients with CHD[15] or CHF,[16] under-prescription is expected to be even more marked in the older subset of the clinical population of cardiac patients.

Under-prescription of CR is similar in the United States, where only about 20% of appropriate candidates of any age, and about 10–15% of those older than 70 years, are estimated to participate in CR programmes, despite this treatment being acknowledged and recommended as a key component of secondary prevention programmes also in subjects older than 75 years.[17]

Cardiac rehabilitation: Definition and aims

CR is defined as the 'sum of activities and interventions required to ensure the best possible physical, mental and social conditions so that patients with chronic or post-acute cardiovascular disease may, by their own efforts, preserve or resume their proper place in society and lead an active life'.[18]

In this perspective, CR and secondary prevention are aimed at (a) preventing the disability that may result from heart disease, particularly in older persons and in those with occupations implying physical exertion, and (b) preventing subsequent cardiovascular events. These goals can best be achieved through programmes combining the use of evidence-based prescription of drug therapy with exercise training and education, counselling, behavioural strategies and psychosocial interventions to help patients optimally control their coronary risk factors.[15] Therefore, CR is an integrated process of care, the aims of which are well beyond the simple functional assessment and prescription of exercise (Table 10.1), and which is currently indicated not only for cardiac patients already disabled or at increased risk of disability, but also for those with a diagnosis of CHD, intermittent claudication or with coronary risk factors. The benefits of CR programmes have been well documented in young and middle-aged CHD patients, whereas older patients rarely have been included in CR programmes and are poorly represented in clinical trials.[19,20] On the other hand, one randomized clinical trial did show that CR is at least as effective in older as in middle-aged patients.[21] Despite such evidence, older

Table 10.1 Aims and role of cardiac rehabilitation as an integrated secondary prevention tool.

- Clinical support to optimize pharmacological and non-pharmacological therapy
- Risk stratification, to define the probability of new events and deterioration of cardiac function, overall functional capacity and quality of life
- Assessment of physical exercise capacity, with exercise prescription in short-term training and long-term maintenance programmes
- Assessment of cardiovascular risk factors and implementation of counselling and education programmes to promote a healthy lifestyle
- Assessment of psychosocial and occupational profile, to design interventions aimed at promoting an active lifestyle
- Clinical and instrumental follow-up, to improve the efficacy of secondary prevention programmes

patients are still less likely to be referred to formal CR programmes and, when referred but not encouraged enough to participate, experience in general a poor compliance with programmes. At least in part, the scant referral of older patients to CR programmes could be related to their more compromised clinical and functional status, due to frailty and greater burden of comorbidity resulting in disability.

Although epidemiological data show that patients aged ≥75 years requiring cardiac care are increasing, only limited age-specific data are so far available from observational studies reporting CR in elderly individuals.[22] Most of these data refer to patients with an average age <75 years,[21,23,24] and from studies of post-infarction CR with small numbers >75 years of age.[21] Nevertheless, several studies have demonstrated that, compared with adults, older patients derive from exercise-based CR similar, and sometimes greater, relative improvements in exercise tolerance and self-reported physical function. Suaya *et al.* recently demonstrated in a large cohort of older US Medicare beneficiaries, who had been hospitalized for CHD events or myocardial revascularization, that CR users had a better 5-year survival.[25] After fully adjusting for a series of potential confounders, depending on the analytical procedure, mortality rates were from 21 to 34% lower in CR users than non-users: results similar to those observed in randomized controlled trials and meta-analyses in younger populations. Mortality reductions extended to all demographic and clinical subgroups, including patients with recent myocardial infarction, recent myocardial revascularization or CHF. Interestingly, the benefit was progressively greater with advancing age and reached the maximum at 85 years or more. Unfortunately, only 12% of the initial total population was prescribed CR. CR users with 25 or more sessions were 19% less likely to die over five years than matched CR users with 24 or fewer sessions ($p < 0.001$). The association of number of CR training sessions with outcome has recently been confirmed in another large cohort of older patients.[26]

The progressively shortened in-hospital stay after an acute myocardial infarction (from about 10 to only 4 days in the past 20 years)[27] reduces the risk of physical deconditioning, but also the time available to check physical activity and promote the lifestyle changes that are necessary to reduce cardiovascular risk; this reinforces the need for CR programmes that function as comprehensive, secondary prevention services and are based in-hospital, and also in the community or at home. Chow *et al.* recently have demonstrated that early lifestyle modifications (within 1 month after acute CHD events) strongly predict short-term prognosis, reducing the 6-month risk of myocardial infarction/stroke/death.[28] For this reason, behavioural modification should be given priority similar to other preventive medications immediately after acute coronary syndromes.

Owing to better clinical management of cardiac diseases leading to improved survival rates, and to increasing evidence on the beneficial effects of CR in a wide range of cardiac conditions, the delivery of CR has changed remarkably over the past 30 years. In the 1960s, patients recovering from uncomplicated myocardial infarction accounted for almost the totality of referrals for CR. Complicated post-infarction patients or patients recovering from myocardial revascularization have also been enrolled in CR programmes in later years. Patients once considered as too high risk to participate in CR programmes, such as those with persisting myocardial ischaemia, CHF or harmful arrhythmias, are currently enrolled in CR programmes based on more gradual, protracted and, most often, supervised exercise training.[6,29,30] Furthermore, as a result of the progressive ageing of the population, CR should now be provided to increasing numbers of older patients, characterized by more complicated coronary illness, comorbidities,[6,31] functional or cognitive impairment, emotional disorders or social isolation, which all may concur to reduce the enrolment rate in, and adherence to, standardized CR programmes. Paradoxically, although some of these factors represent specific indications to CR, female gender, older age, a low formal education and, most importantly, functional impairment, are all negative predictors of enrolment in CR. Therefore, CR centres have to become familiar with the aims and skills of multidimensional geriatric assessment, to implement strongly individualized programmes that may promote the extension of CR to frail, older individuals.

Studies have proved that CR is at least equally effective in younger and older cardiac patients,[31] even those as old as 86 years,[32] to improve their exercise tolerance and HRQOL. However, no one study has yet demonstrated the efficacy of CR with respect to outcomes that are most typically desirable in geriatric medicine, such as reverting or limiting the progression of functional dependence in frail, older individuals.

Secondary prevention strategies in integrated cardiac rehabilitation programmes

Guidelines indicate that secondary prevention should be based on non-pharmacological and pharmacological interventions that can reduce the risk of new events and disease progression and should be aimed at improving both the prognosis and HRQOL. Non-pharmacological interventions consist of education, counselling and psychosocial interventions targeted at smoking cessation, improving dietary habits, controlling body weight and increasing physical activity and long-term adherence to prescriptions.

Educational principles

A meta-analysis of 37 trials[33] found that CR programmes including psychological and/or educational interventions resulted in a significant reduction in incident cardiovascular events at 1–10 years, with studies with the greatest response to intervention showing the greatest impact. The desirable characteristics of the educational and counselling approach have been outlined after a meta-analysis demonstrating that the most important determinant of effectiveness is the quality of intervention,[34] defined as behaviourally oriented interventions adhering to the five principles of adult learning:

- relevance (tailored to patients' knowledge, beliefs, circumstances)
- individualization (tailored to personal needs)
- feedback (informed regarding progress with learning or change)
- reinforcement (rewarded for progress)
- facilitation (provided with means to take action and/or reduce barriers).

Behavioural techniques such as self-monitoring and personal communication, including written or audiovisual techniques, may further improve the outcome, with information provision alone found to be less effective.

Psychosocial interventions

Some anxiety and depression are found in at least 20–25% of patients with various forms of heart disease but, particularly when they persist, should not be accepted as an appropriate reaction to heart disease. Emotional disorders reduce exercise capacity,[35] HRQOL and adherence to secondary prevention measures and substantially increase the risk of new events. Depressive disorders are probably more common among older patients, who frequently suffer from isolation and financial constraints, which are negative prognostic factors after myocardial infarction. However, the long-term consequences of emotional disorders among older cardiac patients in CR programmes have been poorly addressed, and patients 75 years of age and older are at higher risk of under-recognition and under-treatment of depressive disorders.

Randomized trials proved that early psychological interventions improve the mood of middle-aged cardiac patients,[36] but information on efficacy at older ages is not available. However, particularly for most severe or disabling cases of persisting depression, psychological support therapies should be used in conjunction with antidepressants. Selective serotonin reuptake inhibitors, such as sertraline, which was proven to be safe and effective in a randomized trial enrolling patients depressed after an acute coronary syndrome, are probably the agents to be preferred.

Smoking cessation

A Cochrane review confirmed the beneficial effects of smoking cessation, which reduces the risk of new events by up to 40%,[37] comparable to what is seen with pharmacological correction of other cardiovascular risk factors. Smoking induces chronic dependence that makes relapses highly probable. Systematic encouragement of smoking cessation is based on the '5A-strategy' of Asking, Assessing, Advising, Assisting, Arranging. In this process, it is necessary to identify smokers, to evaluate the degree of their dependence and their willingness to quit, to support those who are trying to quit with behavioural counselling, prescription of nicotine substitutes and participation in educational meetings, with regular follow-up visits.

Healthy eating and diet

Dietary prescriptions, adapted to local habits and individualized as much as possible, should be aimed at controlling body weight and provision of all elements of proven efficacy in secondary prevention. Dietary habits should be assessed objectively, with the use of reproducible questionnaires and checking individual knowledge of nutrients and of possible substitutes. Education, rather than prescription, should be provided, limiting dietary restrictions to patients with defined metabolic abnormalities. Education and counselling should be provided by professional dieticians, who perform better than physicians in obtaining a long-term reduction in plasma cholesterol levels.

Increasing physical activity

Promoting a long-term increase in usual physical activity is a fundamental objective of integrated CR programmes finalized at secondary prevention. Regular physical exercise improves the lipid profile and delays the progression of CHD in middle-aged, male patients and reduces cardiovascular mortality in the general population. In the Harvard Alumni Health Study,[38] the relative (i.e. perceived) intensity of physical activity was a strong predictor of lower CHD rates, with a clear dose–effect relationship and an effect that was similar, if not superior, among subjects older compared with those younger than 70 years. Interestingly, the absolute intensity of physical activity did not perform as well as the relative intensity in distinguishing CHD risk groups, suggesting that physical activity recommendations need to be individually tailored. Standard recommendations of regular performance of activities at an intensity of at least 3 METs (Metabolic Equivalents, 1 MET corresponding to 3.5 ml of oxygen consumption per kilogram of body weight; see also below) may therefore be inappropriate, especially for older persons.[38]

Long-term adherence and follow-up

Once the process of short-term recovery is complete, the emphasis of CR shifts to long-term maintenance of physical activity, lifestyle changes and prophylactic drug therapy, in the perspective of 'comprehensive cardiac care' as the final goal, following evidence-based recommendations.

A systematic review of 12 randomized trials of secondary prevention programmes in CHD found that structured disease management programmes improve risk factor profiles and secondary preventive treatment, while reducing hospital readmissions and enhancing HRQOL.[39] The programmes included in the review differed considerably: all were multifaceted, with about half including medical and lifestyle treatments, and the rest were predominantly lifestyle and psychosocial interventions. Most were hospital based, but two conducted in UK primary care suggested that a structured approach benefits HRQOL and uptake of secondary prevention. Indeed, long-term adherence with recommendations and prescriptions made during CR is difficult to maintain, usually being reduced to 50–60% at 1 year and to 20–30% at 3 years. Therefore, to enhance long-term maintenance of the goals attained during CR, it is highly recommended that structured care and follow-up are provided in primary care and studies suggest that low-cost, physical training programmes carried out in the community are safe and help patients maintain the physical performance levels they had attained during hospital-based rehabilitation. The GOSPEL study, the results of which have recently been published, is the first trial to demonstrate that a multifactorial, continuously reinforced intervention up to three years after post-infarction CR is effective in decreasing the risk of several adverse outcomes, although statistical significance was reached for non-fatal reinfarction only.[7]

The structure of cardiac rehabilitation programmes

CR programmes usually consist of three phases, each representing a different step in the progression of individual patient care: in-hospital care, the early post-discharge and exercise training period and long-term follow-up. Common to each phase and irrespective of which model of CR is chosen, is the need for individually tailored interventions.

Phase I occurs during in-hospital stay, when a 'step change' (any acute coronary event, cardiac surgery or first diagnosis of heart failure) has occurred in a patient's cardiac condition. Medical evaluation and treatment, reassurance and information aimed at reducing emotional distress, risk factor assessment, mobilization and discharge planning are the key elements during this phase.

Phase II includes the early post-discharge period – when baseline assessment and initial counselling on self-management of heart conditions usually take place – and subsequent structured exercise programmes, which are carried out either in a hospital setting or in outpatient clinics or, at least for selected patients, at home.[32] Guidelines[29] suggest that, for greatest secondary prevention success, training must be associated with educational and psychological support and advice on risk factors, such as smoking cessation and weight management, vocational rehabilitation to assist return to work or retirement and referral to a psychologist, cardiologist or exercise physiologist. It has been demonstrated that phase II programmes of integrated, multicomponent CR can be undertaken safely and successfully also in the community.

Phase III involves the long-term maintenance of physical activity and lifestyle changes. Available evidence suggests that both must be sustained for benefits to continue. Membership of a local cardiac support group, which involves exercise in a community centre such as a gymnasium or leisure centre and structured care and follow-up in primary care, may help maintain physical activity and behavioural change.

Baseline assessment

Baseline evaluation is a process of crucial importance that has to be completed prior to enrolment in a cardiac rehabilitation programme. In this process, several clinical, functional and, particularly in older persons, emotional, cognitive and social elements must be taken into account, as these are used to assign the patient to the programme most appropriate for their clinical and functional conditions, to pursue reliable and clinically valuable outcomes, to reduce the probability of programme-related complications and to promote individual adherence to the programme. Exercise training programmes for older persons also need to take into account commonly associated comorbidities that can alter the modalities and intensities of the exercise that is required to produce a training effect. These include, but are not limited to, CHF, arthritis and osteoporosis, chronic lung disease, diabetes and peripheral or cerebrovascular disease.

Risk stratification

Risk stratification and assessment of exercise capacity are the two fundamental steps of baseline evaluation. These two steps are closely linked, as information gathered with assessment of exercise capacity is used not only for an appropriate exercise prescription for each individual patient, but also as one of the criteria for assigning each patient to one risk category. Risk stratification will serve, on the other hand, to optimize pharmacological therapy and possibly to indicate the need for invasive procedures (e.g. coronary angiography and myocardial revascularization; implantation of pacemakers or intracardiac defibrillators), but also as further information to be taken into account for exercise prescription.

In essence, risk stratification relies upon the evaluation of clinical stability, left ventricular function, presence of residual myocardial ischaemia or of sustained ventricular arrhythmias and exercise tolerance. Following the

Table 10.2 Criteria for baseline risk stratification of candidates to a cardiac rehabilitation programme.

Criterion[a]	Class of risk[a]		
	Low	Intermediate[b]	High[b]
Clinical course	Uncomplicated In-hospital course	Uncomplicated In-hospital course	• Severe complications (e.g. cardiac arrest; shock; cardiac/respiratory failure) during in-hospital course, OR • Persisting clinical instability (e.g. cardiac failure; renal failure)
LVEF (%)	≥50	31–49	≤30
Myocardial ischaemia	NO	YES • At intermediate (≥100 W) workload, OR • With ST-segment depression <2 mm, OR • Limited asynergies or perfusion defects on stress echocardiography or scintigraphy	YES • At low (<100 W) workload, OR • With ST-segment depression >2 mm, OR • Extensive asynergies or perfusion defects on stress echocardiography or scintigraphy
Ventricular arrhythmias	NO	NO	YES Sustained ventricular arrhythmias
Exercise capacity	≥6 METs	<6 METs	<4 METs

[a]LVEF, left ventricular ejection fraction; METs, metabolic equivalents.
[b]Presence of any condition listed causes patient assignment to that risk class.

criteria outlined in Table 10.2, patients are classified as at low, intermediate or high risk.

Assessment of exercise capacity

Baseline exercise capacity can be evaluated by several methods, among which the most commonly used are the ergometric stress test, the cardiopulmonary exercise test and the 6-minute walk test. Each of them is indicated in different conditions and provides different information.

The *ergometric stress test* is one of the most important diagnostic and prognostic instruments in cardiac patients, with the objectives of determining (a) the exercise capacity, which is used for defining baseline functional capacity, training prescription and evaluation of training results, and (b) the coronary reserve and the inotropic reserve. The cycle ergometer and the treadmill are the most common equipment for exercise stress testing, using protocols that may differ for the type of workload (constant versus increasing), the modality of delivering the workload (continuous versus at intervals), the rate of increase in workload (high versus low) and the type and level of endpoint (predetermined versus symptom-limited, sub-maximum versus maximum). The specificity of the test is reduced with increasing age and its sensitivity, which should theoretically increase with increased prevalence of CHD, may also be reduced. Indeed, it has been reported that a maximum, or symptom-limited, exercise stress test is possible in only about 50% of individuals >75 years of age, as a consequence of ageing-associated reduction in exercise capacity, detraining and increased prevalence of comorbidities which may limit exercise capacity. Furthermore, the current use of a predetermined (220 − age), maximum theoretical heart rate to assess the maximum intensity of physical exercise does not represent a robust reference method, particularly in older patients with intrinsic functional limitations. The type of equipment and the protocol should be chosen on an individual basis, in order to adapt to the expected, individual exercise tolerance. The test duration should not exceed 10–12 min and smaller increases in workload (e.g. 10 W per step) are recommended for patients with expectedly reduced functional capacity. The indications and contraindications and the diagnostic criteria for exercise stress testing are detailed in guidelines of the American College of Cardiology/American Heart Association.

The *cardiopulmonary exercise test* is an ergometric test with simultaneous measurement of oxygen consumption (VO_2), carbon dioxide production (VCO_2), respiratory quotient (VCO_2/VO_2) and pulmonary ventilation. This requires relatively expensive equipment, which needs frequent calibration. Most commonly, the workload is increased by 10 W every 1–2 minutes. The large variability in measurement of VO_2 – which is influenced by age, gender, level of fitness, severity of disease and comorbidity – is the main limitation to standardizing this test. Nonetheless, $VO_{2\,max}$ is the best available objective measure of aerobic capacity, although cardiac patients only rarely can exercise up to an intensity corresponding to their $VO_{2\,max}$. Therefore, the VO_2 at peak exercise indexed by body weight ($VO_{2\,peak}$, ml min^{-1} kg^{-1}) is a more frequently used measure of exercise tolerance. During exercise, the respiratory quotient increases progressively until it becomes >1, which corresponds to the anaerobic threshold (AT), a useful indicator of the workload that an individual can tolerate without overproducing lactic acid. Unfortunately, it cannot always be identified, particularly in patients with markedly reduced exercise tolerance ($VO_{2\,peak}$ <10 ml min^{-1} kg^{-1}). This test is particularly indicated to measure exercise tolerance and to define the prognosis of patients with CHF, and $VO_{2\,peak}$ or AT is also used to make the decision on patient inclusion in the waiting list for heart transplant.

With the *6-minute walk test*,[40] exercise tolerance is assessed by measuring the distance that a patient can walk at his/her fastest possible pace in 6 minutes. A stopwatch, a notepad and a measuring tape are the only materials required. The test has been standardized for application in a linear, enclosed, quiet and seldom travelled corridor, at least 30 m in length, which must be marked throughout its length, to determine the walked distance accurately. Two chairs positioned at the two extremities of the corridor further delimit the path and allow the patient to sit if they become so symptomatic during the test as to need some rest.[40] For safety purposes, the test is best carried out with continuous, telemetric control of heart rate and rhythm and peripheral oxygen saturation, and in association with use of scales aimed at quantifying the perception of fatigue; emergency equipment must be on hand. The main strengths of this test are that it is easy to carry out, does not require any special equipment and is based on a 'natural' activity of common daily life. For these characteristics, the test has been extensively used to evaluate exercise tolerance, especially in CHF and in older post-infarction or post-surgery patients, particularly when they are disabled to such an extent that they cannot perform reliably in a conventional ergometric stress test. The main limitation, on the other hand, is the low reproducibility, which is essentially due to variable motivation and self-assessment of fatigue and which is improved with the use of standardized encouragement by the test monitor.

The physical exercise training programme

Physical exercise training is the core component of CR programmes, essentially aimed at improving exercise tolerance and, through this goal, at reducing disability, improving quality of life and control of cardiovascular risk factors, thereby reducing long-term morbidity and mortality.

Efficacy and safety are the most important characteristics to be considered in prescribing the physical exercise training in a CR programme. Physical training is effective when it produces measurable benefits at the cardiocirculatory and skeletal muscle level and is safe when it is not associated with either short- or long-term harmful effects.

Baseline assessment data are used to design individually adapted, effective and safe training programmes. To this purpose, all factors that may limit the capability of exercising (e.g. presence and severity of angina or of concurrent diseases, such as disabling osteoarthritis) and the response to the baseline, symptom-limited exercise stress test to be used to calculate the individual training workload, are the elements to be taken into fundamental account. The energy expenditure during physical exercise is influenced by the type of exercise (e.g. isotonic versus isometric), the amount of skeletal muscles involved, aerobic capacity and also by the intensity, duration, frequency and modality of exercise sessions.

Intensity of exercise training sessions

Setting the intensity of exercise is a process of crucial importance, based on individual data and ideally leading to the prescribing of training at an intensity which is adequate for each patient. The intensity of exercise can be measured directly – as the amount of mechanical work produced (kg min^{-1}; W min^{-1}; J min^{-1}) – or indirectly – from measures of energy expenditure (such as kilocalories or METs) or from exercise-related changes in physiological variables (such as heart rate or VO_2). The method based on changes in heart rate is the simplest and the most commonly used in the clinical practice. Following this approach, a training exercise programme is prescribed at an intensity (i.e. load) that produces an increase in heart rate (defined as the 'target' heart rate) to 70–85% of the maximum heart rate that the patient has attained during a symptom-limited, baseline exercise stress test. The beneficial effects of training are maximized, exercise-related complications and lactic acid production in the peripheral organs are minimized and the onset of fatigue is delayed, by maintaining the heart rate within its target range. Alternatively, training is prescribed at an intensity that will produce an increase in VO_2 to 60–80% of the $VO_{2\,peak}$ that the patient has attained at baseline.

To reduce further the risk of complications, it is recommended that the intensity of exercise is increased gradually, allowing a few minutes of warm-up before reaching the training workload. Beyond a generic recommendation of starting a training programme at lower intensities with gradual increments during the following weeks, no conclusive data are available on how adapt the training intensity to an individual patient's clinical and functional profile. For practical purposes, however, it can be suggested that patients with CHD but without inducible myocardial ischaemia or left ventricular systolic dysfunction start their training at an intensity corresponding to 70–85% of maximum heart rate, those with inducible ischaemia exercise at an intensity almost corresponding to the ischaemic threshold, whereas those with systolic left ventricular dysfunction or overt CHF should exercise at lower intensities, that is at 70–80 and 60–70% of maximum heart rate, respectively.

In addition to aerobic exercise, strength exercise is also increasingly being recognized as a useful component of the training programme for selected patients and muscular strength and endurance improve with strength training of moderate intensity in low-risk patients, even at older ages. Information on safety and usefulness of strength training in high-risk patients is still limited, although it has been suggested that low-intensity weight training can be safely and effectively introduced in the circuit training programme for patients with CHD – even in the presence of inducible ischaemia or left ventricular systolic dysfunction – or for patients with CHF.

Duration of exercise training sessions

An individually prescribed duration of exercise sessions may range from 5 to 60 min, being indirectly proportional to the intensity of exercise. The duration of each session is usually shorter in the initial phase of training, to be increased gradually thereafter. An excessively prolonged duration may be associated with increased risk of lactoacidosis and orthopaedic complications. However, a reasonably prolonged exercise is necessary to activate the energy metabolism pathways: it is acknowledged that, for an intensity at about 80% of maximum heart rate, the optimum duration is between 20 and 30 min. A practical method for determining the most appropriate duration of sessions is to use the product of workload and duration of exercise to calculate the energy expenditure, which should be about 250–300 kcal per session or 1000–1500 kcal per week.

Frequency of exercise training sessions

In the initial phase of an exercise programme, when the exercise intensity is gradually increased, daily sessions, on at least 5 days per week, are to be preferred, also to check most accurately the cardiovascular response to exercise. This is particularly important because, during the initial phase of training, exercise-related changes in heart rate and arterial pressure may be substantially different from those observed during the baseline stress test. Following the initial phase, three sessions per week are usually adequate to maintain the training effect. It should be remembered that, if the training programme is interrupted, exercise capacity usually is reduced by 50% within 4–5 weeks.

Modality of exercise training sessions

A training programme can be set up following the continuous, the interval and the circuit training modalities. The continuous training modality, which is particularly effective in increasing cardiovascular and muscular endurance capacities, is carried out at moderate intensities, with a prolonged duration and without periods of recovery. In the interval training modality, periods of exercise at higher intensity are alternated with periods of recovery or of exercise at lower intensity. The circuit training programme is based on a series of different exercises (with or without equipment) carried out in a sequence. Circuit training is a programme of moderate intensity which improves not only the endurance capacity and muscular strength, but also neuromuscular coordination and agility. Despite these multiple positive effects, this training modality is still rarely used in CR.

Various equipment (e.g. cycle ergometer or treadmill) and various types of calisthenics have been used in training programmes mostly aimed at enhancing aerobic capacity.

The training is the main phase of the programme, aimed at improving the delivery of oxygen to the working muscles through both enhanced oxygen transportation capacity and extraction and at maximizing caloric expenditure. Continuous and rhythmic exercises involving large muscle groups, such as walking, stepping on a staircase and exercising on a cycle ergometer, are the most effective modalities of aerobic training. Calisthenics, particularly those involving large muscle masses, and also strength training and recreational activities, can also be usefully included.

A 5–10 minute cool-down phase at a lower workload should follow the training phase, for a gradual recovery of heart rate and arterial pressure to their baseline levels. A too brisk interruption of exercise can produce arterial hypotension and syncope, especially in older persons with blunted cardiovascular reflexes.

Progression and duration of training programmes

During the course of a training programme, the exercise intensity should be adapted to the patient's improved exercise capacity. Change in heart rate at sub-maximum exercise is the simplest method to be followed for this purpose. However, particularly in older patients and in those treated with beta-blocking agents, these may prove to be unreliable indicators of an improved aerobic capacity. Therefore, use of the Borg's scale, which assesses the rate of perceived exertion (RPE),[41] is a commonly recommended, simple method to confirm additionally that exercise tolerance has improved from baseline. With a maximum possible value of 20 on the scale, patients should exercise at an RPE of 13–15. A reduction in RPE can be the consequence of enhanced cardiovascular and muscular fitness, but also of improved emotional profile and of increased confidence with the schemes of exercises and use of equipment. In any case, when the RPE at sub-maximum workloads is reduced, the intensity of exercise can be safely increased, in order to obtain a further training effect. Assessment of RPE is of particular importance in frail, older patients with CHF or comorbidity or after prolonged bed rest for complicated cardiac surgery. In these subgroups, a standardized and reproducible assessment of perceived fatigue should guide the progression through strictly individualized rehabilitative programmes, initially setting the exercise intensity at an RPE of 9–11, which corresponds to about 60% of maximum heart rate and slowly progressing to an RPE of 12–13 over the following weeks.

The duration of training programmes is one of the most difficult characteristics to be exactly defined. Ideally, a training programme should be prolonged enough to induce positive changes in functional conditions.

However, this objective has to confront the organizational constraints of rehabilitation centres, which have to offer access to new patients following turnover programmes. Furthermore, exact information on the relationship between programme duration and attainable outcomes is still lacking, with the exception of documentation on variable increments in non-standardized measures of exercise tolerance reported by training programmes of variable duration. A period of 3–12 weeks is generally recommendable, with longer durations needed for patients at higher risk. At least three sessions per week at high workloads for 4 weeks are the minimum prescription to obtain a measurable and clinically valuable effect, and more sessions are necessary when – for safety reasons if faced with a markedly deteriorated functional profile or unstable clinical conditions – the workload has to be set initially at a low level. Following these general considerations, a programme duration of at least 3 weeks is sufficient for most low-risk patients after uncomplicated infarction or cardiac surgery, whereas for patients at higher risk or with CHF a duration of 4–6 and 8–10 weeks, respectively, is deemed to be more appropriate. The programme duration should be prolonged also for older patients, who are usually trained at lower initial intensities. It should be remembered that the duration of the training programme is also a function of many other clinical elements, such as the adaptive changes in heart rate and arterial pressure, the absence of symptoms, the RPE, the capacity of obtaining at least a 10–20% increase in exercise tolerance from baseline, the stability of the emotional profile and adherence to the structure of an overall preventive programme.

As already mentioned, long-term, community-based physical exercise maintenance programmes are effective in preserving the otherwise declining improvement in exercise tolerance attained with participation in hospital-based rehabilitation programmes.

Safety of training programmes

Patients are admitted to a training programme when in a stable clinical condition and in the absence of absolute contraindications to physical exercise (Table 10.3).

The safety of physical training in CHD patients has long been a source of considerable controversy. Studies in the 1970s and 1980s reported an incidence of non-fatal events ranging from 1 event per 34 000 h of exercise-patient to 28 events per 2 350 000 h of exercise-patient, with an incidence of fatal events ranging from 1 event per 116 000 to 1 event per 2 350 000 h of exercise-patient. Lower overall rates and absence of any fatality have been reported in two reviews[42,43] that were based on more recent studies. Whether continuous ECG monitoring may reduce the risk of complications is still unknown. Usually, high-risk patients are constantly monitored

Table 10.3 Contraindications to exercise training.

Absolute	• Acute myocardial infarction • Unstable angina • Uncontrolled ventricular cardiac arrhythmias • Severe aortic stenosis • Unstable heart failure • Pulmonary embolism or infarction • Myocarditis or pericarditis • Aortic dissection
Relative	• Uncontrolled arterial hypertension (SAP/DAP >180/110 mmHg) • Tachy- or bradyarrhythmias • High degree atrioventricular block • Electrolyte abnormalities • Hypertrophic cardiomyopathy • Mental or physical impairment leading to inability to exercise adequately

during the whole training programme, whereas low-risk patients are monitored only during the first few sessions. However, studies have suggested that the overall incidence of complications is low and similar across risk categories and that the few complications are represented mostly by 'minor' events such as angina, ST-segment depression or non-sustained cardiac arrhythmias. For the purpose of safety, multiple parameters must be taken under control during exercise training, in particular the linearity of the increase in heart rate and arterial blood pressure, ECG morphology and the RPE. Surveillance and monitoring must be especially close during the initial phase of the programme, when physical detraining or difficulties in learning how to carry out exercises may contribute to abnormal increases in heart rate or arterial pressure. Adapting exercise prescriptions to a limited functional capacity – particularly in older, disabled and comorbid individuals – further contributes to the feasibility and safety of exercise programmes. A skilled staff that includes several different professionals, such as physical therapists, nurses and technicians, and on-site devices and drugs that are necessary for immediate treatment of emergencies are the final elements that support programme safety.

Exercise training programmes in special cardiac conditions

Cardiac surgery

Exercise training after cardiac surgery can start when the clinical conditions have become stable and it is usually preceded by short programmes of respiratory physical therapy to recover respiratory dynamics and of low-intensity exercise to improve mobility and flexibility. Extensive neurological and cognitive evaluation is particularly recommended in older persons, in whom cerebral complications of prolonged anaesthesia and extracorporeal circulation are more likely to occur. In these patients, an early rehabilitation programme is aimed mainly at improving mobility and independence in activities of daily living. In the absence of specific contraindications that may occur after surgery (e.g. anaemia with Hb $<10\,g\,dl^{-1}$; pleural or pericardial effusion; delayed or complicated healing of surgical wounds), a 6-minute walk test is prescribed as soon as the patient is able to walk independently (on average, 10 days after surgery). A baseline, symptom-limited ergometric stress test is carried out 3–4 weeks after surgery, when the sternum has usually stabilized and thoracic pain has relieved. As previously described, data acquired during the stress test are used to select the appropriate intensity for exercise training, which low-risk patients can usually be taught to self-manage at home without risk. As for other categories of cardiac patients, assessment of cardiovascular risk factors, associated with education, counselling and behavioural strategies to help achieve the best optimal control of coronary risk factors, is an essential component of medium- and long-term rehabilitation programmes.

Chronic heart failure

CHF patients must be clinically stable while on optimized drug therapy for at least one month before their exercise capacity can be assessed for potential enrolment in a physical training programme. Particularly in the presence of permanent atrial fibrillation, the cardiopulmonary exercise test is the preferred method for assessment,[30] as it can evaluate aerobic capacity and, hence, exercise capacity also when the heart rate response to exercise is inappropriate or difficult to determine precisely. Endurance training with a cycle ergometer, with the intensity set at 50% of the maximum workload attained in a baseline cardiopulmonary exercise test, 15 min sessions of interval training (exercise for 30 s, followed by 60 s of recovery or very light work), is the most commonly adopted training modality for CHF patients, since it would induce the best possible training effect without excessively increased fatigue or undesirable metabolic effects. Alternative protocols include arm exercises, walking on treadmill, flexibility and respiratory exercises. More recently, studies have demonstrated some positive effects from association of endurance with strength training.[44] Since functional assessment of and exercise prescription for CHF patients require particularly high skills, these patients should participate only in programmes that are run by well-experienced rehabilitation centres. At least in the initial phase, the training programme should be carefully supervised. Studies have demonstrated the feasibility, safety and efficacy of home-based, low-intensity training programmes for CHF patients but, again, no specific data are yet available for older individuals.

The physiological effects of aerobic training

Effects of aerobic training in middle-aged and older adults with coronary heart disease

The beneficial physiological effects of physical training, namely improved exercise tolerance associated with less fatigue, less angina and increased sense of wellbeing, derive from both peripheral (vascular or skeletal muscle) and central (myocardial) adaptations.

Peripheral adaptations are mainly the consequence of improved skeletal muscle efficiency, leading to improved ability to extract oxygen from entering the blood supply and increased arteriovenous difference during physical exercise. This reduces the need for increasing cardiac output and hence the work that the heart has to do to bring an adequate amount of oxygen to the tissues at sub-maximum exercise. Central adaptations include increases in cardiac dimensions, stroke volume, cardiac output and indexes of left ventricular function,[45,46] which have been reported after training programmes of variable duration in middle-aged patients with CHD. The mechanisms of physiological adaptations to exercise training in older patients may be somewhat different from those seen in middle-aged patients. Probably because of the ageing-associated increase in myocardial and vascular stiffness, adaptability to central remodelling is reduced and exercise-induced adaptations in older coronary patients appear to be almost exclusively localized at the periphery. After three months of aerobic training, peak exercise cardiac output, peripheral vascular conductance and hyperaemic calf blood flow were unchanged in older, low-risk patients with CHD, despite the fact that their exercise tolerance, $VO_{2\,max}$ and arteriovenous oxygen difference had increased.[47] Histological analysis of skeletal muscle biopsies showed a marked increase in capillary density and in oxidative enzyme capacity that fully account for improved adaptation to exercise.[47]

Effects of aerobic training in patients with chronic heart failure

Reduced exercise tolerance with increased breathlessness and muscle fatigue are the symptomatic hallmarks in CHF patients, who limit their activity to avoid these symptoms. This may result in further detraining, possibly leading to a vicious circle of progressively reduced exercise tolerance.

The origin of these symptoms is multifactorial, involving central cardiac factors (left ventricular systolic and diastolic dysfunction with increased pulmonary capillary pressure), central pulmonary factors (impaired ventilatory mechanics and increased physiological dead space; altered ventilation/perfusion ratio; hypoxia of ventilatory muscles) and peripheral circulatory and muscular factors (impaired vasodilatation during physical exercise; metabolic and structural alterations of skeletal muscles). Peripheral pathophysiological changes appear to be the most important determinants of exercise capacity in CHF, as systemic and pulmonary haemodynamics correlate poorly with exercise capacity or exertional breathlessness and, while central haemodynamics improve rapidly with drug therapy, improvement in exercise capacity may be delayed for weeks or months.

Skeletal muscle hypoperfusion has been observed in CHF both at rest and during exercise. This is directly related to CHF severity, is the consequence – together with sympathetic overactivity and parasympathetic withdrawal – of increased activity of endothelial ACE and reduced endothelial production of nitric oxide, and is responsible for early occurrence of lactacidosis, which, in turn, produces muscular exhaustion and increases the ventilatory needs. It has also been demonstrated that unmyelinated and small myelinated afferents in muscle that are sensitive to metabolic changes related to work ('ergoreceptors') are responsible for the early circulatory response to exercise, including activation of the sympathetic vasoconstrictor drive, and that this reflex is exaggerated in CHF, probably because of sensitization by muscular acidosis during exercise. Limited physical activity, anorexia and increased circulating substances with known catabolic effect, all contribute to inducing a certain degree of muscular atrophy, which correlates with the reduction in strength and exercise tolerance. However, functional data suggest that muscular atrophy cannot fully account for the reduced exercise tolerance. When strength is measured per unit of muscular area, it correlates poorly with $VO_{2\,max}$ and exercise tolerance. This is consistent with qualitative alterations of muscular fibres, represented by a reduction in slow-reacting, type I fibres – responsible for muscular endurance, with prevalent oxidative metabolism – with a relative increase in fast-reacting type II fibres, whose metabolic pathways rely mainly on glycolysis.

Randomized trials have demonstrated that physical training determines a sustained improvement in functional class, maximum ventilation, exercise capacity[48] and quality of life in CHF patients, particularly when enrolled in long-term maintenance programmes. Although some improvement in left ventricular ejection fraction at rest and in maximum stroke volume during exercise has occasionally been described,[48] changes in central haemodynamics after training are generally modest. Thus, also in the case of

CHF, the major adaptations to training appear to be peripheral. Many of the peripheral vascular and muscular dysfunctions that concur to reduce exercise tolerance in CHF are fully reverted, or at least partially corrected, by training. In particular, the endothelial production of nitric oxide in response to exercise is remarkably enhanced and the exaggerated ergoreflex activity is attenuated, with both effects contributing to reducing the inappropriately increased peripheral vascular resistance. Exercise training also reduces the concentrations of circulating norepinephrine and atrial natriuretic peptide. Analysis of percutaneous muscular biopsies, coupled with measurement of $VO_{2\ max}$ during a symptom-limited cardiopulmonary exercise test, suggests that structural and functional changes in skeletal muscles are a further determinant of improvement in exercise tolerance observed with training in CHF. Indeed, ultrastructural morphometry demonstrated a training-associated increase in skeletal muscle cell mitochondria, suggesting that the improved functional capacity is linked to an increased oxidative capacity of skeletal muscles and a concomitant reshift to type I fibres.

Evidence-based results of cardiac rehabilitation in different cardiac conditions

Coronary heart disease

Most randomized trials of CR in CHD have included mixed populations of patients with recent myocardial infarction, myocardial revascularization or angina and are based on exercise-only or exercise in addition to psychological and educational interventions, which is usually termed comprehensive CR.

The most recent meta-analysis included 48 trials and 8940 patients.[15] Compared with usual care, CR was associated with a significant 20 and 26% reduction in all-cause and cardiac mortality, respectively, and with larger reductions in plasma lipids, systolic blood pressure and rates of persistent smoking cessation. Rates of non-fatal myocardial infarction and revascularization and changes in high- and low-density lipoprotein cholesterol levels, diastolic pressure or HRQOL were similar with CR and usual care. The effect of CR on total mortality was independent of CHD diagnosis, programme of exercise intervention, length of follow-up, trial quality and trial publication date. In contrast to previous reports of greater benefit from comprehensive rehabilitation than from exercise-only programmes, the benefits were independent of type of rehabilitation programme. The authors suggested[15] that this may be because the follow-up in most studies was too short to observe indirect effects, which may need a longer time to occur. However, there are two alternative explanations. One is that exercise-only CR is likely to include psychological and educational support, even though not offered in a structured manner. The other is that most of the exercise-only trials were conducted in the pre-thrombolytic era, whereas most of the comprehensive trials were more recent. This means that the benefits in the comprehensive rehabilitation trials are likely to be additional to the already great benefit of thrombolysis, prophylactic medication and/or coronary revascularization. Only one trial included in the meta-analysis deliberately enrolled significant numbers of patients older than 75 years of age. In particular, this was the first randomized controlled trial demonstrating the feasibility, safety and efficacy with respect to exercise tolerance and HRQOL of rehabilitation in post-myocardial infarction patients as old as 86 years of age.[32] The uniqueness of this trial is confirmed by the fact that the ages of patients enrolled in other trials ranged from 48 to 71 years and, accordingly, recommendations for further trials including subsets of older patients were made in Taylor *et al.*'s review.[15]

The precise mechanism(s) by which physical exercise training reduces mortality in CHD patients is still to be completely elucidated. Exercise training exerts direct beneficial effects on myocardial oxygen demand, development of coronary collateral vessels and coronary endothelial function, cardiocirculatory autonomic tone, coagulation and clotting factors and inflammatory markers. However, reduction in mortality may also be mediated via the indirect effects of exercise through improvements in the risk factors for atherosclerotic disease.

Cardiac surgery

Although almost two out of three enrollees in CR programmes in Europe are recovering from cardiac surgery, only a few studies have specifically addressed the efficacy of CR after surgery. Furthermore, most meta-analyses have not examined the results of post-surgery CR separately from those in other clinical subsets. These aggregated analyses have demonstrated that CR is associated with a significant reduction in long-term mortality.

Information on the efficacy of post-surgery rehabilitation in older patients is even more limited, despite the demonstration that older age, together with female gender and comorbidity, are independent risk factors for cognitive, neurological and functional complications, prolonged hospital stay, worse long-term prognosis and early hospital readmission after cardiac surgery, which are all elements that would recommend greater participation of older surgical patients in rehabilitation programmes. Nonetheless, a recent review[49] demonstrated that in addition to age, disability, lower formal education, cardiac dysfunction and poor quality of life are all predictors of non-participation in rehabilitation after coronary artery bypass operations, although patients with these conditions would benefit the most from integrated, multicomponent CR programmes.

Chronic heart failure

After the success with newer pharmacological agents such as ACE inhibitors, beta-blockers and anti-aldosteronic agents, a further 'therapeutic revolution' has occurred recently in the management of CHF, consisting of a profound change in recommendations about physical activity. From the previous orientation in favour of restrictions on physical activity, the newest guidelines recommend therapeutic exercise programmes for the current management of CHF.[11] This came after the demonstration that supervised exercise training improves the functional capacity and quality of life of CHF patients, without any risk of unfavourable clinical events or deteriorating cardiac function, but rather with an anti-remodelling effect.

A review pooled the results of 81 studies of exercise training in CHF,[16] which differed considerably in the intensity (from 40 to 90% of $VO_{2\,max}$), the frequency (from one to seven per week) and duration (from 15 to 120 min) of exercise training sessions and in the overall programme duration (from 2 to 104 weeks). Despite these differences and the different characteristics of patients enrolled, a relatively homogeneous and significant improvement in exercise tolerance was reported in all studies. Pooled analysis has also demonstrated the absence of relevant, exercise-related adverse events and significant, positive effects of training on combined endpoints (all-cause mortality plus new events). A meta-analysis[50] including nine randomized trials with 809 patients (395 exercise training versus 406 controls) determined the effect of exercise training programmes of at least 8 weeks with follow-up data for at least 3 months on survival in patients with CHF due to left ventricular systolic dysfunction. Exercise training significantly reduced all-cause mortality and the combined endpoint of hospital readmission by 35 and 28%, respectively, with no statistically significant subgroup treatment-specific effect. Age comparison was limited to patients younger and older than 60 years, since most of those enrolled in randomized trials were younger than 65 years. Moreover, most patients enrolled in randomized trials were highly selected individuals with little or no comorbidity, unlike older cardiac patients seen in everyday clinical practice, and the surrogate endpoints that have frequently been adopted in those trials (e.g. changes in $VO_{2\,max}$) do not provide evidence that such therapy affects outcomes that are especially valuable in older persons, such as functional capacity or quality of life. Several controversies still need to be addressed. Exercise training is recommended for NYHA functional class II or III patients, tailored to the individual's exercise tolerance, because it improves exercise capacity and quality of life. However, ExTraMATCH[50] and the HF-ACTION trial[51] have provided somewhat contradictory results about its effectiveness on morbidity and mortality in stable patients. Limited information about combined aerobic, strength, interval, resistance and respiratory exercise training is available. Although the safety of all of these exercise modalities is undisputed, the question of the most effective training mode remains to be answered.

Key points

- Cardiac rehabilitation is an integral component of secondary prevention and is indicated for patients with a wide variety of cardiac conditions, ranging from coronary artery disease to chronic heart failure.
- The best results are obtained with integrated, multicomponent cardiac rehabilitation programmes, which include exercise training together with counselling and psychosocial measures that may help patients maintain sustained changes towards a healthier lifestyle. Studies suggest also that long-term maintenance programmes carried out in the community after the in-hospital phase may achieve better long-term results.
- Robust evidence from randomized controlled trials and meta-analyses supports the efficacy of cardiac rehabilitation on clinically relevant outcomes such as reduced long-term morbidity and mortality, enhanced functional profile and improved control of cardiovascular risk factors. A limited number of economic analyses suggest that cardiac rehabilitation is also cost-effective.
- Most of this evidence derives from trials of middle-aged patients with only small numbers of patients older than 70–75 years of age.
- Future research programmes should therefore be aimed at specifically investigating the efficacy and effectiveness of cardiac rehabilitation in older, frail cardiac patients.

References

1 American Heart Association. (2004) *Heart Disease and Stroke Statistics – 2004 Update.* AHA, Dallas, TX, 2004, http://www.heart.org/ (last accessed 14 November 2011).

2 He J, Ogden LG, Bazzano LA *et al.* Risk factors for congestive heart failure in US men and women: NHANES I epidemiologic follow-up study. *Arch Intern Med* 2001;**161**:996–1002.

3 Jolliffe JA, Rees K, Taylor RS *et al.* (2001) Exercise-based rehabilitation for coronary heart disease. *Cochrane Database Syst Rev* **1** (Art. No.: CD001800).

4 Taylor RS, Brown A, Ebrahim S *et al.* Exercise-based rehabilitation for patients with coronary heart disease: systematic review and meta-analysis of randomized controlled trials. *Am J Med* 2004;**116**:682–92.

5 Witt BJ, Jacobsen SJ, Weston SA *et al.* Cardiac rehabilitation after myocardial infarction in the community. *J Am Coll Cardiol* 2004;**44**:988–96.

6 Ades PA. Cardiac rehabilitation and secondary prevention of coronary heart disease. *N Engl J Med* 2001;**345**:892–902.

7 Giannuzzi P, Temporelli PL, Marchioli R *et al.* Global secondary prevention strategies to limit event recurrence after myocardial infarction: results of the GOSPEL study, a multicenter, randomized controlled trial from the Italian Cardiac Rehabilitation Network. *Arch Intern Med* 2008;**168**:2194–204.

8 European Association of Cardiovascular Prevention and Rehabilitation Committee for Science Guidelines (EACPR); Corrà U, Piepoli MF, Carré F *et al.* Secondary prevention through cardiac rehabilitation: physical activity counselling and exercise training: key components of the position paper from the Cardiac Rehabilitation Section of the European Association of Cardiovascular Prevention and Rehabilitation. *Eur Heart J* 2010;**31**:1967–74.

9 Van de Werf F, Bax J, Betriu A *et al.* Management of acute myocardial infarction in patients presenting with persistent ST-segment elevation: the Task Force on the Management of ST-Segment Elevation Acute Myocardial Infarction of the European Society of Cardiology. *Eur Heart J* 2008;**29**:2909–45.

10 Anderson JL, Adams CD, Antman EM *et al.* ACC/AHA 2007 Guidelines for the Management of Patients with Unstable Angina/Non-ST-Elevation Myocardial Infarction. A Report of the American College of Cardiology/American Heart Association Task Force on Practice Guidelines (Writing Committee to Revise the 2002 Guidelines for the Management of Patients with Unstable Angina/Non-ST-Elevation Myocardial Infarction) developed in collaboration with the American College of Emergency Physicians, the Society for Cardiovascular Angiography and Interventions and the Society of Thoracic Surgeons endorsed by the American Association of Cardiovascular and Pulmonary Rehabilitation and the Society for Academic Emergency Medicine. *J Am Coll Cardiol* 2007;**50**:e1–157.

11 Dickstein K, Cohen-Solal A, Filippatos G *et al.* ESC Guidelines for the Diagnosis and Treatment of Acute and Chronic Heart Failure 2008: the Task Force for the Diagnosis and Treatment of Acute and Chronic Heart Failure 2008 of the European Society of Cardiology. Developed in collaboration with the Heart Failure Association of the ESC (HFA) and endorsed by the European Society of Intensive Care Medicine (ESICM). *Eur Heart J* 2008;**29**:2388–442.

12 Vanhees L, McGee HM, Dugmore LD *et al.* A representative study of cardiac rehabilitation activities in European Union Member States: the Carinex survey. *J Cardiopulm Rehabil* 2002;**22**:264–72.

13 EUROASPIRE II Study Group. Lifestyle and risk factor management and use of drug therapies in coronary patients from 15 countries; principal results from EUROASPIRE II Euro Heart Survey Programme. *Eur Heart J* 2001;**22**:554–72.

14 Kotseva K, Wood D, De BG *et al.* Cardiovascular prevention guidelines in daily practice: a comparison of EUROASPIRE I, II and III surveys in eight European countries. *Lancet* 2009;**373**:929–40.

15 Taylor RS, Brown A, Ebrahim S *et al.* Exercise-based rehabilitation for patients with coronary heart disease: systematic review and meta-analysis of randomized controlled trials. *Am J Med* 2004;**116**:682–92.

16 Smart N and Marwick TH. Exercise training for patients with heart failure: a systematic review of factors that improve mortality and morbidity. *Am J Med* 2004;**116**:693–706.

17 Williams MA, Fleg JL, Ades PA *et al.* Secondary prevention of coronary heart disease in the elderly (with emphasis on patients > or =75 years of age): an

American Heart Association scientific statement from the Council on Clinical Cardiology Subcommittee on Exercise, Cardiac Rehabilitation and Prevention. *Circulation* 2002;**105**:1735–43.

18 World Health Organization. Rehabilitation after cardiovascular diseases, with special emphasis on developing countries. Report of a WHO Expert Committee. *World Health Org Tech Rep Ser* 1993;**831**:1–122.

19 Ades PA, Waldmann ML, McCann WJ and Weaver SO. Predictors of cardiac rehabilitation participation in older coronary patients. *Arch Intern Med* 1992;**152**:1033–5.

20 Worcester MU, Murphy BM, Mee VK *et al.* Cardiac rehabilitation programmes: predictors of non-attendance and drop-out. *Eur J Cardiovasc Prev Rehabil* 2004;**11**:328–35.

21 Marchionni N, Fattirolli F, Valoti P *et al.* Improved exercise tolerance by cardiac rehabilitation after myocardial infarction in the elderly: results of a preliminary, controlled study. *Aging (Milano)* 1994;**6**:175–80.

22 Giallauria F, Vigorito C, Tramarin R *et al.* Cardiac rehabilitation in very old patients: data from the Italian Survey on Cardiac Rehabilitation-2008 (ISYDE-2008) – Official Report of the Italian Association for Cardiovascular Prevention, Rehabilitation, and Epidemiology. *J Gerontol A Biol Sci Med Sci* 2010;**65**:1353–61.

23 Frasure-Smith N, Lesperance F, Prince RH *et al.* Randomised trial of home-based psychosocial nursing intervention for patients recovering from myocardial infarction. *Lancet* 1997;**350**:473–9.

24 Stahle A, Mattsson E, Ryden L *et al.* Improved physical fitness and quality of life following training of elderly patients after acute coronary events. A 1 year follow-up randomized controlled study. *Eur Heart J* 1999;**20**:1475–84.

25 Suaya JA, Stason WB, Ades PA *et al.* Cardiac rehabilitation and survival in older coronary patients. *J Am Coll Cardiol* 2009;**54**:25–33.

26 Hammill BG, Curtis LH, Schulman KA and Whellan DJ. Relationship between cardiac rehabilitation and long-term risks of death and myocardial infarction among elderly Medicare beneficiaries. *Circulation* 2010;**121**:63–70.

27 Berger AK, Duval S, Jacobs DR Jr, *et al.* Relation of length of hospital stay in acute myocardial infarction to postdischarge mortality. *Am J Cardiol* 2008;**101**:428–34.

28 Chow CK, Jolly S, Rao-Melacini P *et al.* Association of diet, exercise and smoking modification with risk of early cardiovascular events after acute coronary syndromes. *Circulation* 2010;**121**:750–8.

29 Wenger NK, Froelicher ES, Smith LK *et al.* (1995) *Clinical Practice Guidelines 17. Cardiac Rehabilitation*, US Department of Health and Human Services, Public Health Service, Agency for Health Care Policy and Research and the National Heart, Lung and Blood Institute, Rockville, MD.

30 Giannuzzi P, Tavazzi L, Meyer K *et al.* Recommendations for exercise training in chronic heart failure patients. *Eur Heart J* 2001;**22**:125–35.

31 Pasquali SK, Alexander KP and Peterson ED. Cardiac rehabilitation in the elderly. *Am Heart J* 2001;**142**:748–55.

32 Marchionni N, Fattirolli F, Fumagalli S *et al.* Improved exercise tolerance and quality of life with cardiac rehabilitation of older patients after myocardial infarction: results of a randomized, controlled trial. *Circulation* 2003;**107**:2201–6.

33 Dusseldorp E, van Elderen T, Maes S *et al.* A meta-analysis of psychoeducational programs for coronary heart disease patients. *J Health Psychol* 1999;**18**:506–19.

34 Mullen PD, Simons-Morton DG, Ramirez G *et al.* A meta-analysis of trials evaluating patient education and counseling for three groups of preventive health behaviors. *Patient Educ Couns* 1997;**32**:157–73.

35 Marchionni N, Fattirolli F, Fumagalli S *et al.* Determinants of exercise tolerance after acute myocardial infarction in older persons. *J Am Geriatr Soc* 2000;**48**:146–53.

36 Mayou RA, Thompson DR, Clements A *et al.* Guideline-based early rehabilitation after myocardial infarction. A pragmatic randomised controlled trial. *J Psychosom Res* 2002;**52**:89–95.

37 Critchley J and Capewell S. (2004) Smoking cessation for the secondary prevention of coronary heart disease. *Cochrane Database Syst Rev* **1** (Art. No.: CD003041).

38 Lee IM, Sesso HD, Oguma Y and Paffenbarger RS Jr. Relative intensity of physical activity and risk of coronary heart disease. *Circulation* 2003;**107**:1110–6.

39 McAlister FA, Lawson FM, Teo KK and Armstrong PW. Randomised trials of secondary prevention programmes in coronary heart disease: systematic review. *BMJ* 2001;**323**:957–62.

40 Guyatt GH, Sullivan MJ, Thompson PJ *et al.* The 6-minute walk: a new measure of exercise capacity in patients with chronic heart failure. *Can Med Assoc J* 1985;**132**:919–23.

41 Borg GA. Psychophysical bases of perceived exertion. *Med Sci Sports Exerc* 1982;**14**:377–81.

42 Franklin BA, Bonzheim K, Gordon S and Timmis GC. Safety of medically supervised outpatient cardiac rehabilitation exercise therapy: a 16-year follow-up. *Chest* 1998;**114**:902–6.

43 Vongvanich P, Paul-Labrador MJ and Merz CN. Safety of medically supervised exercise in a cardiac rehabilitation center. *Am J Cardiol* 1996;**77**:1383–5.

44 Hülsmann M, Quittan M, Berger R *et al.* Muscle strength as a predictor of long-term survival in severe congestive heart failure. *Eur J Heart Fail* 2004;**6**:101–7.

45 Ehsani AA, Biello DR, Schultz J *et al.* Improvement of left ventricular contractile function by exercise training in patients with coronary artery disease. *Circulation* 1986;**74**:350–8.

46 Hagberg JM, Ehsani AA and Holloszy JO. Effect of 12 months of intense exercise training on stroke volume in patients with coronary artery disease. *Circulation* 1983;**67**:1194–9.

47 Ades PA, Waldmann ML, Meyer WL *et al.* Skeletal muscle and cardiovascular adaptations to exercise conditioning in older coronary patients. *Circulation* 1996;**94**:323–30.

48 Hambrecht R, Gielen S, Linke A *et al.* Effects of exercise training on left ventricular function and peripheral resistance in patients with chronic heart failure: a randomized trial. *JAMA* 2000;**283**:3095–101.

49 Pasquali SK, Alexander KP, Coombs LP *et al.* Effect of cardiac rehabilitation on functional outcomes after coronary revascularization. *Am Heart J* 2003;**145**:445–51.

50 Piepoli MF, Davos C, Francis DP and Coats AJ. Exercise training meta-analysis of trials in patients with chronic heart failure (ExTraMATCH). *BMJ* 2004;**328**:189.

51 O'Connor CM, Whellan DJ, Lee KL *et al.* Efficacy and safety of exercise training in patients with chronic heart failure: HF-ACTION randomized controlled trial. *JAMA* 2009;**301**:1439–50.

CHAPTER 11

Acute Stroke Care and Management of Carotid Artery Stenosis

David Doig and Martin M. Brown

Institute of Neurology, University College London, London, UK

Introduction

A stroke is defined as 'rapidly-developed clinical signs of focal or global disturbance of cerebral function, lasting more than 24 hours or until earlier death, with no apparent non-vascular cause' by the World Health Organization.[1] A stroke is therefore distinguished from a transient ischaemic attack (TIA), which is defined similarly, except that the focal neurological symptoms must recover fully within 24 hours. The term 'cerebrovascular accident' should be avoided because of its negative connotations. Stroke carries with it a significant personal, community and economic burden. It is estimated that, in the United States alone, around 795 000 patients suffer a stroke each year at a direct and indirect financial cost of over US$70 billion.[2] When considered separately from other cardiovascular diseases, stroke is the third leading cause of death in the Western world, and in the world as a whole it is the second most common cause of death. It is also the leading cause of disability in survivors. Stroke occurs at all ages from birth onwards, but becomes increasingly common with advancing age and is a major cause of suffering in the elderly population.

The management of acute stroke is evolving, and applied evidence from recent randomized controlled trials, along with better management of associated risk factors, has contributed to a relative reduction in age-adjusted morbidity and mortality from the condition in many countries. There exists now a good evidence base for hyperacute and acute interventions, as well as for pharmacotherapy with the aim of secondary prevention. Acute stroke

Cardiovascular Disease and Health in the Older Patient: Expanded from 'Pathy's Principles and Practice of Geriatric Medicine, Fifth edition', First Edition. Edited by David J. Stott and Gordon D.O. Lowe.

will, however, remain an important and common medical presentation as the proportion of the population aged over 65 years increases in many developed countries.

This review will address the aetiology of stroke, the immediate management of the patient presenting with an acute stroke, the initiation of secondary prevention measures, and the management of carotid artery stenosis. Intracerebral and subarachnoid haemorrhage are also discussed, as these conditions will also present with the rapid onset of a focal neurological deficit.

Stroke aetiology

It is important to recognize that the terms 'stroke' and 'TIA' describe the presentation of the patient and are not sufficient as a diagnosis on their own. This requires a description of the underlying pathology (haemorrhage or infarction), anatomy (vessel and territory involved) and aetiology (mechanism). Ischaemic stroke may occur as a result of a number of heterogeneous conditions. The major precipitant of cerebral ischaemia in the elderly population is atherosclerosis. Atheromatous plaque may occlude the artery at the site of build-up, but more commonly plaque rupture with superimposed thrombosis results in occlusion or embolization to a smaller, more distal, artery, precipitating cerebral ischaemia. Smaller 'lacunar' infarcts may be caused by microatheroma of the deep penetrating arteries of the brain or by hyaline degenerative disease of the arterioles, which together are known as small vessel disease. The pathogenesis of atherosclerosis is discussed in more detail later in this chapter. Alternatively, stroke may be caused by intracranial haemorrhage, cerebral venous thrombosis, or cardiac embolism.

Cardiac embolism may arise from thrombus formation in the left atrium promoted by arrhythmia (especially atrial fibrillation or flutter), valvular heart disease or valve prosthesis, or in myocardial infarction where mural thrombosis may develop on the injured myocardium. An inter-atrial or inter-ventricular septal defect (e.g. patent foramen ovale) may allow passage of an embolus from the venous circulation to the left side of the heart, with the potential for subsequent paradoxical embolization to the cerebral vessels.

A number of other conditions may either cause ischaemic stroke or mimic its signs and symptoms, and should be considered in the differential diagnosis. Information from history, examination and investigation pointing to an alternative cause should be pursued vigorously, as the appropriate

Table 11.1 Classification of causes of stroke.

Cerebral infarction

Extracranial arterial embolism (internal carotid artery, aorta or vertebral artery)
- Atherosclerosis, arterial dissection, fibromuscular dysplasia, vasculitis, arterial trauma

Cardiac embolism
- Mural thrombus following myocardial infarction, rheumatic heart disease, calcific or prosthetic mitral or aortic valves, endocarditis, atrial fibrillation, atrial myxoma

Paradoxical embolism
- Deep vein thrombosis with atrial septal defect

Trauma
- Fat embolism

Iatrogenic embolism
- Cardiac surgery, cardiac catheterization, cerebral angiography

Intracranial arterial thrombosis
- Large-vessel occlusion – atherosclerosis, vasculitis, dissection, hypercoagulable states, sickle cell disease, Moyamoya disease
- Small-vessel occlusion – hypertensive arteriosclerosis, diabetes, CADASIL, vasculitis

Vasospasm
- Subarachnoid haemorrhage

Haemodynamic ischaemia
- Internal carotid artery occlusion, tandem stenoses, bilateral vertebral arterial occlusion, systemic hypotension (e.g. cardiac arrest), severe stenoses with poor collateral supply

Cerebral venous thrombosis
- Hypercoagulable states, puerperium, intracranial sepsis, malignancy

Intracranial haemorrhage

Subarachnoid haemorrhage
- Aneurysm, arteriovenous malformation, bleeding disorders, vascular malignancies, vasculitis, illegal drug use

Intracerebral haemorrhage
- Cerebral amyloid angiopathy, cavernous angioma, hypertensive small-vessel disease, cerebral venous thrombosis, venous anomalies and other causes as for subarachnoid haemorrhage

and timely management of the underlying pathology may alter the chance of recurrent disease (Table 11.1).

Stroke mimics

Conditions that may mimic stroke but which are not of vascular origin include space-occupying lesions (e.g. subdural haematoma, tumour or

Table 11.2 Differential diagnosis – stroke 'mimics'.

Traumatic
- Subdural haematoma
- Head injury

Metabolic
- Metabolic encephalopathy
- Toxic encephalopathy
- Hypertensive encephalopathy
- Hypoglycaemia

Structural
- Cerebral tumour
- Arteriovenous malformation

Infective
- Focal encephalitis
- Cerebral abscess

Functional

Genetic disorders
- Familial periodic paralyses
- Mitochondrial encephalopathy
- Porphyria

Disorders of neural and neuromuscular function
- Epileptic seizure and post-ictal neurological deficit
- Multiple sclerosis
- Central pontine myelinolysis
- Acute polyneuropathy
- Myasthenia gravis
- Motor neurone disease

abscess), hypoglycaemia, functional disorders and epilepsy, especially post-ictal paresis (Table 11.2).

Prognosis of stroke

The mortality following first ischaemic stroke may be as high as 41% after 5 years,[3] with vascular causes of death (stroke and myocardial infarction) most common during the first few weeks following the event.[3] The risk of recurrent stroke is highest in this acute period. When patients are divided into groups depending on the aetiology of their stroke, those with significant large artery (carotid) atherosclerosis are at highest risk of recurrence within the first month. Recurrence is least likely in those with small-vessel disease as a cause of their stroke.

Clinical evaluation and stroke syndromes

Evaluation of the patient should begin with a detailed history. In the case of the aphasic, obtunded or confused patient, a witness history should be obtained from the ambulance staff, relative, friend or carer. It is important to establish the exact time of onset of symptoms, the progression or regression of a deficit over time, and any associated features such as headache, loss of consciousness or possible seizure. Important details from past medical history will be the presence of other cardiovascular, neurological or haematological disease, medications taken, family history, and ascertainment of risk factors. It is important to establish the patient's baseline social function with respect to activities of daily living to plan future treatment, including resuscitation status, as well as rehabilitation.

Examination should focus on establishing the nature and severity of the neurological deficit to aid in confirming the clinical diagnosis of stroke and establishing the likely site and size of cerebral lesion. Examination of other systems, especially the heart, may give clues to an underlying cause, or prompt further investigation.

The severity of neurological deficit should be assessed using a formal tool such as the National Institute for Health Stroke Severity (NIHSS) Score.[4,5] This examination should be performed at the time of presentation, and grades the patient response in a number of domains which comprise level of consciousness, gaze and vision, motor power, ataxia, language and speech, and extinction and inattention, using specific validated techniques of examination. Higher scores are associated with more profound deficit and worse outcome, although the prominence of language domains in the score may underestimate the severity of the impact of right hemispheric syndromes. The NIHSS score is used to select patients for thrombolysis (see below) and monitor the patients' early progress. Other scales, including the Barthel Index[6] and modified Rankin Scale[7] (Tables 11.3 and 11.4), grade disability and handicap and are used to guide rehabilitation and measure the progress or outcome of treatment.

Identifying the likely size and location of the arterial territory involved from the symptoms and signs is an important aid to determining the mechanism and prognosis of stroke. The commonest arterial syndromes are described in the next section. Occlusion and rupture of vessels (i.e. infarction or haemorrhage) result in similar syndromes, which are indistinguishable clinically. However, in the next section, the description concentrates on ischaemic stroke for simplicity.

Total middle cerebral artery (MCA) syndromes

Occlusion of the trunk of the middle cerebral artery (MCA), carries the most grave prognosis and may cause infarction of a large area of brain

Table 11.3 The Barthel Index.[6]

	Bowels
0	Incontinent (or needs to be given enemata)
1	Occasional accident (once per week)
2	Continent
	Bladder
0	Incontinent or catheterized and unable to manage
1	Occasional accident (maximum once per 24 h)
2	Continent (for over 7 days)
	Grooming
0	Needs help with personal care
1	Independent face/hair/teeth/shaving (implements provided)
	Toilet use
0	Dependent
1	Needs some help, but can do something alone
2	Independent (on and off, dressing, wiping)
	Feeding
0	Unable
1	Needs help cutting, spreading butter, etc.
2	Independent (food provided within reach)
	Transfer
0	Unable – no sitting balance
1	Major help (one or two people, physical), can sit
2	Minor help (verbal or physical)
3	Independent
	Mobility
0	Immobile
1	Wheel chair independent including corners, etc.
2	Walks with help of one person (verbal or physical)
3	Independent (but may use any aid, e.g. stick)
	Dressing
0	Dependent
1	Needs help, but can do about half unaided
2	Independent (including buttons, zips, laces, etc.)
	Stairs
0	Unable
1	Needs help (verbal, physical, carrying aid)
2	Independent up and down
	Bathing
0	Dependent
1	Independent (or in shower)
Total	(0–20)

Table 11.4 The Modified Rankin Scale.[7]

Grade[a]	Description
0	No symptoms at all
1	No significant disability despite symptoms: able to carry out all usual duties and activities
2	Slight disability: unable to carry out all previous activities but able to look after own affairs without assistance
3	Moderate disability: requiring some help, but able to walk without assistance
4	Moderately severe disability: unable to walk without assistance and unable to attend to own bodily needs without assistance
5	Severe disability: bedridden, incontinent and requiring constant nursing care and attention

[a]In clinical trials, a grade of 6 is often added to record patients who have died.

tissue supplied by its superficial cortical branches and the deep lenticular branches supplying basal ganglia and internal capsular white matter. There is cortical dysfunction (such as a speech or spatial disorder depending on the hemisphere involved), motor and/or sensory deficit of the face and arm or arm and leg, and homonymous visual field defect. There may also be a decreased level of consciousness secondary to oedema and brainstem compression, which usually develops over the course of the first 24 to 48 hours after onset. Total MCA territory infarction is frequently fatal, with a 1-year mortality of up to 40%, depending partly on the care provided.[4]

Partial MCA syndromes

Branch occlusions of the MCA are heterogenous in their presentation. If the upper division of the MCA is affected then typically there is no visual field defect. If the lower division of the MCA is affected then typically there is a reduced motor or sensory component to symptoms and signs. Branch occlusion is more commonly caused by embolism than local thrombus. Prognosis is variable, with a 1-year mortality of up to 16%, but 55% of patients are independent at 1 year.[4]

Lacunar syndromes

Occlusion of small perforating arterioles supplying the basal ganglia, external or internal capsule and the pons results in small infarcts known as lacunes. These have been defined on brain imaging as deep subcortical infarcts less than 15 mm in maximum diameter. They are caused by occlusion of the smaller perforating arteries either secondary to microatheroma at the vessel origin or secondary to more distal lipohyalinosis in which degenerative pathological changes occur in the tunica media and adventitia of the vessels. These two pathologies are difficult to distinguish clinically or radiologically and together are often known as *small vessel disease*. This term is also frequently used by radiologists to describe the appearances of patchy or confluent low attenuation on CT, or high signal on T_2 and FLAIR MRI, in the periventricular deep white matter. These changes are also known as leukoaraiosis and are thought to be another manifestation of lipohyalinosis, as are microhaemorrhages seen on gradient echo (T_2*) MRI. Leukoaraiosis, lacunes and microhaemorrhages are independently associated with cognitive impairment. Hypertension is a major risk factor for lacunar infarction, leukoaraiosis and microhaemorrhage. The latter are also associated with cerebral amyloid angiopathy.

Four common presentations of lacunar infarction, known as lacunar syndromes, are described. Pure motor stroke presents with unilateral face, arm and leg weakness. The weakness may not involve all three sites, but should involve at least two contiguous sites, that is face and arm, or arm and leg. Pure sensory stroke gives rise to hemisensory loss on the contralateral side. A larger infarct may give rise to a mixed motor/sensory stroke, but the characteristic feature of lacunar infarction remains, which is that there is no disturbance of higher (cortical) function and no visual field deficit. The fourth common type of lacunar stroke, ataxic hemiparesis, describes limb ataxia in combination with a hemiparesis and/or dysarthria. These syndromes arise from lacunar infarction (or occasionally small haemorrhages) in either the internal capsule or the pons, and imaging is required to distinguish these sites. Numerous rarer lacunar syndromes are described, including unilateral chorea and hemiballismus – from lacunes in the basal ganglia.

Lacunar stroke carries a good prognosis for survival, with a 1-year mortality of about 10%, but 50% of survivors remain dependent.[4]

Posterior circulation syndromes

Vertebrobasilar (or posterior) circulation syndromes result from ischaemia of the brainstem, cerebellum, and/or occipital lobes and therefore the symptoms experienced are varied depending on the vessels and territories affected. Brainstem infarction from basilar artery or perforating vessel occlusion can result in cranial nerve dysfunction, eye movement disorders and/or nystagmus, with or without bilateral motor and/or sensory deficit. Pontine infarction secondary to basilar artery thrombosis may cause the 'locked-in' syndrome. This produces quadriplegia, but with preservation of eye movements and blinking which may facilitate communication. Occlusion of one of the posterior cerebral arteries results in hemianopia, while occlusion of both posterior cerebral arteries results in cortical blindness. In some patients, the posterior cerebral artery supplies the median temporal lobe, in which case the visual field defect may be accompanied by mild or, if bilateral, severe memory impairment (amnesia). In about 5% of individuals, the posterior cerebral artery is supplied by the ipsilateral internal carotid artery via a dominant posterior communicating artery. In such cases, occipital infarction and hemianopia may result from carotid disease.

Cerebellar infarction may result in gait ataxia, but not necessarily any other cerebellar signs. Occlusion of the posterior inferior cerebellar artery (PICA) may produce the characteristic lateral medullary (Wallenberg) syndrome. This comprises vestibular dysfunction, ataxia, ipsilateral loss of pain and temperature sensation from the face, ipsilateral Horner syndrome, and contralateral loss of pain and temperature sensation in the arm and leg. Dysarthria and dysphagia are not specific for brainstem lesions and can occur with any motor syndrome.

In contrast to anterior circulation syndromes, thrombosis of the basilar artery may be responsible for a higher proportion of strokes than embolism from a distant site. The 1-year mortality for posterior circulation infarction is 19% with 62% of patients independent at 1 year.[4]

Thalamic syndromes

The blood supply of the thalamus is carried by branches of the vertebrobasilar system as well as the tuberothalamic artery that arises from the posterior communicating artery. Thalamic nuclei participate in sensory and motor function, language, cognitive function, alertness, memory, mood and motivation.[8] Thus the clinical syndrome that results from thalamic infarction depends on the specific nuclei involved. Unilateral infarction may cause memory loss or confusion, language disturbance when the dominant hemisphere is affected and spatial deficit when the non-dominant hemisphere is affected. The *thalamic syndrome* describes the combination of contralateral sensory loss and hemiparesis associated with the development of distressing post-stroke pain in the affected limbs. Bilateral infarction of the thalamus may result in coma with subsequent severe amnesia.[8]

Prehospital care

In many countries where hyperacute stroke treatments such as thrombolysis are available, the spotlight of public health has fallen on the early recognition of stroke by both the general public and allied health professionals.

Validated clinical tools such as the FAST ('Face, Arm, Speech Test') screening test[9] allows paramedics and the public to identify symptoms of stroke and can allow triage to the correct facility with early warning of the patient's arrival. FAST instructs the user to evaluate facial movement, upper limb power and speech to identify a neurological deficit, and paramedic findings on examination correlate well with subsequent examination findings by a trained physician. It may, however, be less sensitive for the detection of posterior circulation events,[9] which has led to the development of the ROSIER ('Recognition of Stroke in the Emergency Room') Scale, which incorporates a measure of hemianopia and may be more suitable for use by physicians in the emergency department. Prospective validation of this scale in 173 patients referred with suspicion of stroke showed sensitivity of 93% (95% CI, 89–97%) and specificity of 83% (95% CI, 77–89%) for the diagnosis of stroke.[10]

A number of other, similar, screening tools in Melbourne (MASS), Cincinatti (CPSS) and Los Angeles (LAPSS) have also been described in the literature.

Initial investigations and imaging

The investigation of stroke and TIA are similar and are designed to establish the pathology, anatomy and mechanisms of symptoms, and plan treatment. All patients should have urea, electrolytes, creatinine, full blood count, clotting screen, serum glucose and erythrocyte sedimentation rate carried out when they are first seen. A fasting glucose and fasting cholesterol should be done as soon as possible to exclude hypercholesterolaemia and diabetes. Electrocardiography will confirm the clinical assessment of heart rhythm or document evidence of ischaemia or acute myocardial infarction. If symptoms or clinical signs suggest respiratory involvement, such as heart failure or aspiration pneumonia, a chest X-ray should be added to these investigations. Further biochemical investigation of rarer causes of ischaemic stroke or stroke mimics will be directed by the clinical picture.

The immediate concern in acute stroke is the rapid differentiation of ischaemic from haemorrhagic stroke, which is most quickly and reliably demonstrated by non-contrast CT imaging. CT is sensitive and specific for haemorrhage within the first 8 days after stroke,[11] after which time reliability of detection decreases. MRI as an alternative is discussed below. All patients admitted with suspected stroke should undergo cranial imaging as soon as possible after admission, and definitely within 24 hours.[11,12] An immediate emergency scan is required for patients being considered for thrombolytic therapy, or for those at risk of intracerebral haemorrhage by virtue of their presentation, including reduced conscious level, sudden onset of severe headache, a history of trauma, known coagulopathy or therapeutic anticoagulation.

Early signs of ischaemic stroke on CT include hyperdensity of a cerebral artery (showing thrombus in situ), slight hypodensity of the brain parenchyma leading to loss of the clear definition of the insular ribbon and lentiform nucleus, sulcal effacement reflecting tissue swelling, and mass effect from more pronounced oedema (Figure 11.1).[13] A large hypodense

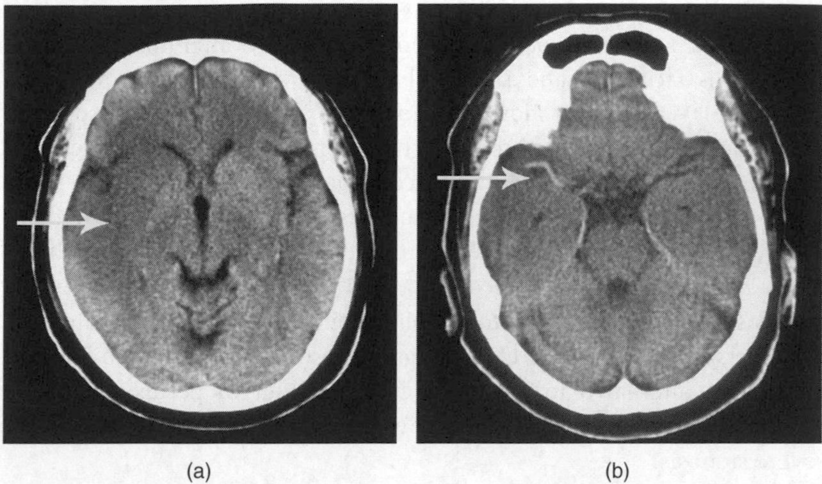

Figure 11.1 (a) Early changes of right MCA territory infarction on CT scan. (b) MCA hyperdensity in the same patient.

area seen on CT reflects a poor prognosis, and is sometimes used as a contraindication to thrombolysis because the risk of subsequent haemorrhage may be increased. This is because hypodensity reflects increased water content of the tissue and suggests both established infarction and the breakdown of the blood–brain barrier in this region. If the hypodensity is clearly delineated, this indicates that the infarction is well established and not hyperacute.

CT angiography (CTA) may be carried out in the same session as non-contrast CT to visualize acute intracranial vessel occlusion, as well as extravascular and intravascular stenosis or dissection. Acute CT perfusion imaging may also have a role in the future, allowing assessment of the extent of hypoperfusion in an arterial territory.

CT has the limitation that it is normal within the first few hours after onset in 30–40% of patients.[13] MRI is much better at detecting early changes of infarction and small infarcts, especially in the posterior fossa. MRI is also the technique of choice to identify haemorrhage if the scan is done more than 8 days after onset. Several MRI sequences can be combined in one examination, termed 'multi-modal MRI', to produce a variety of clinically useful images. T2 sequences provide good anatomical definition and show established infarction well, but are not very sensitive to early changes. Diffusion-weighted imaging (DWI) is much more sensitive than CT to the early and chronic changes of infarction. DWI becomes abnormal within a few minutes of onset of infarction, and shows areas of restricted extracellular movement of water molecules, secondary to ischaemic membrane pump failure and cell swelling from excessive intracellular water, as bright areas. When the infarction is complete and cell lysis has occurred, usually between 7 and 14 days after onset, diffusion of water is facilitated and DWI will then show infarcts as dark areas. However, DWI may also show older infarcts as bright areas because of the phenomenon of 'T2 shine through'. The same MR sequences are therefore used to generate apparent diffusion coefficient (ADC) maps which show acute infarction as dark, and older infarcts as brighter areas.[14] Gradient echo imaging (GRE or T2*) is very sensitive to new and old haemorrhage. Fluid-attenuated inversion recovery (FLAIR) imaging is highly sensitive to areas of gliosis secondary to established infarction and periventricular small vessel disease (Figure 11.2). Magnetic resonance angiography (MRA) provides an alternative to CTA for vascular imaging. MR perfusion imaging can show areas of impaired blood flow secondary to arterial occlusion or severe stenosis.

Thus MRI has considerable advantages over CT, as well as avoiding ionizing radiation. If available in the emergency situation, MRI with DWI can replace CT or may be used as an additional investigation. It should be considered a routine investigation in stroke patients in whom CT has failed to establish the diagnosis and is the investigation of choice after TIA. Limitations of MRI include patient tolerability, increased cost compared to CT, and the requirement to exclude patients with metallic foreign bodies or implants.

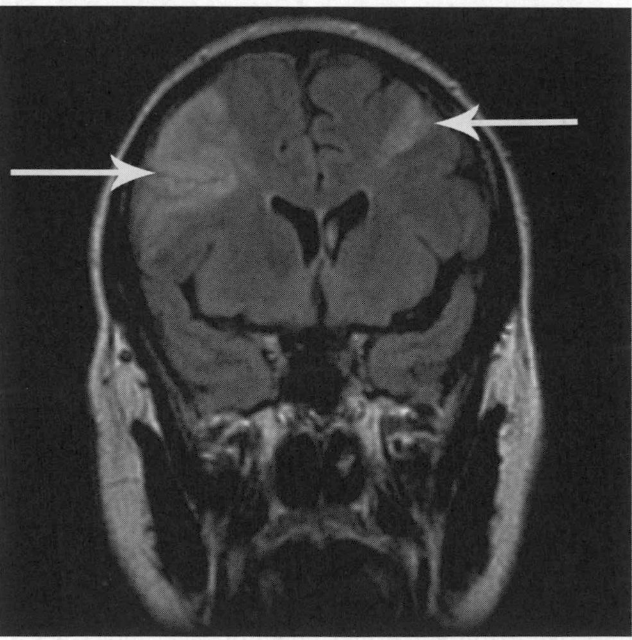

Figure 11.2 Multiple areas of cerebral infarction on FLAIR MR imaging.

In-hospital care

As with any acutely unwell patient presenting to hospital, the standard initial assessment and resuscitation of a patient with suspected stroke begins with attention to the airway, breathing and circulation.

Airway

The airway in a stroke patient may be obstructed secondary to a reduced level of consciousness, or a build-up of secretions that cannot be effectively swallowed. Simple airway manoeuvres – for example chin lift or jaw thrust – may be enough to clear the airway, or the use of an airway adjunct may be required. Patients with ongoing airway problems may warrant consideration of the involvement of an anaesthetist as an airway specialist.

Breathing

Effective breathing, and therefore effective oxygenation of the blood and brain, may be compromised by a number of mechanisms. A stroke affecting the respiratory centres of the brainstem may cause apnoea or bradypnoea. Problems with swallowing may precipitate aspiration pneumonia. In addition, hypoxaemia may arise through an associated condition such as heart failure, or pulmonary embolism. Initial management is directed at treatment of the underlying cause, although guidelines recommend the application of inhaled oxygen only where a new desaturation below 92–95% exists on pulse oximetry.[12]

Circulation

In ascertaining the heart rhythm and blood pressure, some of the risk factors for stroke are being assessed. A finding of an elevated blood pressure is almost universal in patients within 48 hours of stroke onset. This may occur either secondary to the stroke itself, or reflect pre-existing hypertension. The management of high blood pressure in acute stroke is discussed later in this chapter.

Less common is the finding of hypotension. This may reflect severe dehydration, blood loss or cardiac failure, and should lead to a search for the underlying cause, as well as immediate treatment aimed at restoring the mean arterial blood pressure. The aim is to minimize secondary damage to the ischaemic penumbra in the brain, as in the presence of a fixed intracranial pressure the cerebral perfusion pressure is dependent on the mean arterial blood pressure.

Blood sugar

Hypoglycaemia should be excluded – and treated if present – in all patients with neurological deficit, as it is an easily reversible cause of symptoms that mimic stroke. Hyperglycaemia following ischaemic infarction is associated with increase in infarct size and poor outcome. Raised blood glucose is a common finding at the time of presentation, and severe hyperglycaemia is a contraindication to rt-PA administration. However, the benefit of early correction of blood glucose in stroke patients at the time of presentation remains uncertain. Preliminary investigation of the effects of 'tight' control of blood sugar levels in a stroke patient population has highlighted the high incidence of unintended hypoglycaemia as a consequence,[15] a factor which may offset any potential benefit of the treatment. Control may be achieved by the administration of an insulin infusion or by the administration of subcutaneous insulin, but close monitoring of blood glucose is mandated. It has been suggested that non-diabetic patients receive less intensive correction of blood glucose levels, since hyperglycaemia at the time of presentation may not reflect underlying insulin deficiency or resistance and may be a transient state with a return to baseline levels.[15]

Environment

Fever, defined as a core temperature of greater than 37.5 °C, should prompt a search for a source, as fever carries increased mortality and worse neurological outcome, and may indicate an underlying aetiology for the stroke, such as endocarditis. Lower respiratory tract infection and urinary tract infection are common complications of stroke. Antibiotic prescription should be considered, but the effect on clinical outcome of active lowering of the temperature with antipyretics is not clear.

Early attention should also be paid to nutrition and hydration. For those patients in whom a swallowing disorder is suspected it is appropriate to provide nutrition via a nasogastric tube, and request a formal specialist assessment of swallowing. Regardless of the mode of administration of nutrition, normal hydration should be maintained.[12]

Thrombolysis and recanalization

The introduction of intravenous alteplase (recombinant tissue plasminogen, rt-PA) as treatment for acute ischaemic stroke has transformed stroke care. However, its benefits in acute stroke are tempered by the risk of precipitating intracranial haemorrhage and the strict licensing conditions that govern its safe use. The NINDS (National Institute of Neurological Disorders and Stroke) rt-PA Stroke Study[16] included patients under the age of 80 years old with a carotid arterial, or vertebrobasilar arterial distribution stroke, not in coma, who could start treatment within a 3-hour time window and randomized patients to receive either intravenous thrombolysis with alteplase or placebo. Impairment was measured using the NIH (National Institutes of Health) Stroke Score. Intracranial haemorrhage occurred in 6.4% of thrombolysed patients within the first 36 h, compared to 0.6% of those randomized to placebo. However, patients treated with t-PA were around 30% more likely to have minimal or no disability at 3 months.[16] Pooled analysis of the NINDS trial with several other trials of thrombolytic therapy confirmed that, when given within 3 h, intravenous thrombolysis significantly reduces the risk of death or dependency with a linear relationship time from stroke onset to treatment and degree of benefit, perhaps extending out beyond 3 h.[17] The ECASS-3 trial has subsequently confirmed that intravenous alteplase can be given safely to patients under the age of 80 between 3 and 4.5 h after onset with a small overall benefit.[18]

Contraindications to thrombolysis include the presence of intracranial haemorrhage, seizure at the time of onset of neurological deficit, recent major surgery or major trauma, severe hypoglycaemia or hyperglycaemia, pancreatitis or pericarditis, recent gastrointestinal or urinary tract bleeding, concurrent anticoagulation with raised INR, severe thrombocytopenia, and recent myocardial infarction (Table 11.5). Very severe, mild deficit or rapidly resolving symptoms may also be contraindications. Hypertension, with blood pressure >180/110 mmHg, should be treated cautiously before

Table 11.5 Contraindications to thrombolysis with tPA.

1	Symptoms only minor or rapidly improving
2	Haemorrhage on pretreatment CT (or MRI)
3	Visible changes on pretreatment CT (or MRI) of infarction >one-third of MCA territory
4	Suspected subarachnoid haemorrhage
5	Active bleeding from any site
6	Recent gastrointestinal or urinary tract haemorrhage within 21 days
7	Platelet count less than $100 \times 10^9\,l^{-1}$
8	Recent treatment with heparin and APTT above normal
9	Recent treatment with warfarin and INR elevated
10	Recent major surgery or trauma within the previous 14 days
11	Recent post-myocardial infarction pericarditis
12	Neurosurgery, serious head trauma or previous stroke within 3 months
13	History of intracranial haemorrhage (ever)
14	Known arteriovenous malformation or aneurysm
15	Recent arterial puncture at non-compressible site
16	Recent lumbar puncture
17	Blood pressure consistently above 185 mmHg systolic or 110 mmHg diastolic
18	Abnormal blood glucose (<3 or >20 mmol l^{-1})
19	Suspected or known pregnancy
20	Active pancreatitis
21	Epileptic seizure at stroke onset

Source: Adapted from the NINDS protocol.[16]

the administration of thrombolytics. Aspirin is contraindicated within the first 24 h after alteplace administration because of an increased risk of death.[19] If intracranial haemorrhage should result, management guidelines vary, but the discontinuation of ongoing infusion of thrombolytic agent is mandatory. Blood samples should be analysed to provide an up-to-date clotting profile, and consideration should be given to the administration of reversal agents (for example cryoprecipitate). In the event of a severe haemorrhage neurosurgical consultation may be necessary.

The Third International Stroke Trial (IST-3) sought to determine whether thrombolysis provides benefit up to 6 h from the onset of symptoms, and the effectiveness of this therapy in patients over the age of 80, who were not included in previous trials. Despite early hazards of intracranial haemorrhage and increased risk of death, thrombolysis within 6 h improved long-term functional outcome. This benefit did not seem to be diminished in elderly patients.[20]

Providing access to thrombolysis for stroke requires the provision of hyperacute stroke units (HASUs) and well-developed pathways organized to deliver urgent access to brain imaging and stroke expertise, with the aim of achieving door-to-needle time from arrival of the patient to the start of alteplase infusion of less than 30 min, with facilities to monitor patients appropriately following administration of alteplase.

Newer modalities of treatment such as endovascular mechanical extraction of thrombus, intra-arterial thrombolysis and acute stenting to recanalize an occluded vessel continue to undergo evaluation and are not yet part of the routine treatment of acute stroke. These treatments require the involvement of an interventional neuroradiology service.

Neuroprotective drugs

The ischaemic penumbra, an under-perfused area of brain surrounding an area of infarcted tissue which is potentially salvageable, offers a target for therapeutic intervention.[21] In general, it is thought that the higher the residual perfusion of an area, the longer ischaemia may be tolerated before leading to cessation of neuronal electrical activity, failure of ion homeostasis and cell death. In addition to thrombolysis to restore perfusion of this area, a number of 'neuroprotective' agents have been trialled with disappointing results. Biochemically or physiologically logical treatments, for example using calcium channel inhibitors to reduce vasogenic oedema, have not translated into a clinical improvement. Included in the definition of neuroprotection is therapeutic hypothermia, which remains an experimental procedure. However, tight control of physiological parameters as described above, for example prevention of hypoxia, is likely to have an important role in limiting secondary damage after ischaemia.

Neurosurgery for ischaemic stroke

Neurosurgical intervention in ischaemic stroke is generally considered in two circumstances. In large middle cerebral artery territory infarction, cerebral oedema develops over the immediate days following the event as brain cells swell and lyse, and may result in midline shift and increased intracranial pressure, sometimes referred to as *'malignant MCA infarction'*. Should cerebral oedema be severe, transtentorial herniation may result in death from brainstem compression. Neurosurgery in patients at imminent risk of brain herniation consists of a duraplasty and the formation of a large bone flap to allow room for swelling of the cranial contents.

A pooled analysis of three randomized controlled trials of craniectomy for malignant MCA infarction (DECIMAL, DESTINY and HAMLET)[22] showed a significantly improved outcome, as measured by the modified Rankin Scale (mRS) which records disability and death on a scale of 0–6 (where 0 is no symptoms and 6 is death), in the surgical groups versus standard medical treatment. Neuroimaging criteria used in the trials differed, but all aimed to quantify the volume of brain tissue involved as either an absolute volume (greater than 145 cm^3) or a relative volume (more than two-thirds of the MCA territory). These are patients with a poor prognosis, and mortality in this group is high. The primary endpoint of the analysis was death or disability. The absolute risk reduction of a bad outcome (mRS $\leq$4) in the surgical group versus the control group was 51% (95% CI, 34–69%) and more patients survived in the surgical group (78% vs 29%).[22] The authors concluded that this represented a number-needed-to-treat (NNT) of two for both mRS $\leq$4 and to prevent one death. Only patients younger than 60 benefited from decompression, with patients over the age of 50 years old suffering a higher rate of death or severe disability after surgery compared to those under 50.

Posterior fossa infarction may also warrant consideration of neurosurgery. The volume of the posterior fossa is small compared to that of the rest of the cranium, and oedema secondary to a large cerebellar infarct is tolerated poorly, with the potential for brainstem compression and obstruction of the fourth ventricle and resultant hydrocephalus.

Palliative care

Unfortunately, there are patients who suffer a stroke so extensive that they will not recover. In these circumstances, treatment is directed at the relief of pain or other distressing symptoms such as restlessness, mood disturbance or confusion. For those that survive the first few days, spasticity, pressure areas and incontinence, amongst other neurological consequences, may need specific attention. An open discussion with family members about prognosis and continuing communication is essential. Good communication with ward staff and clear documentation in the notes may prevent unnecessary investigation or intervention. Involvement of local inpatient palliative care services may be beneficial, but there is relatively little published research or guidance in this area.

Stroke units

Care of the patient with stroke has been revolutionized with the introduction of specialized stroke units, which seek to standardize management and co-ordinate a multidisciplinary team of experts. Features of stroke unit care include early mobilization, medical, nursing and allied professional staff specialized in stroke care, and specific investigation such as assessment of swallowing.[23] In an acute stroke unit, there should also be regular monitoring of physiological variables such as oxygen saturation, blood pressure and temperature. It is unknown exactly which of these interventions is most responsible for an improvement in outcome, and there are additional unmeasurable factors, such as the professional dedication and continuing education of ward staff, that may also contribute. There is also specific attention given to the modification of risk factors for recurrent stroke, such as blood pressure management and antithrombotic therapy. However, it is clear that the majority of benefit relates to early intervention and therefore current NICE guidelines in the United Kingdom recommend that all stroke patients should be admitted without delay directly to an acute stroke unit.[12]

Systematic review of smaller stroke unit studies in 1997 suggested an overall benefit for stroke unit care, and paved the way for the widespread implementation of stroke units. At the conclusion of follow-up, the combined odds ratio of death in a stroke unit versus conventional care was 0.82 (95% CI, 0.69–0.98). The odds ratio of death or dependency was 0.71 (95% CI, 0.61–0.84).[23] There was no statistically significant difference in the calculated length of stay of patients in either group, and subgroup analysis did not reveal a difference in groups of different sex, age or stroke severity, leading to the conclusion that stroke unit care is effective and that it should be offered to all stroke patients regardless of individual characteristics (Figure 11.3). Subsequent updated reviews have found similar results.

Secondary prevention

Patients who present with minor stroke or TIA have a high risk of early recurrence. As many as 10% of patients may experience a further event

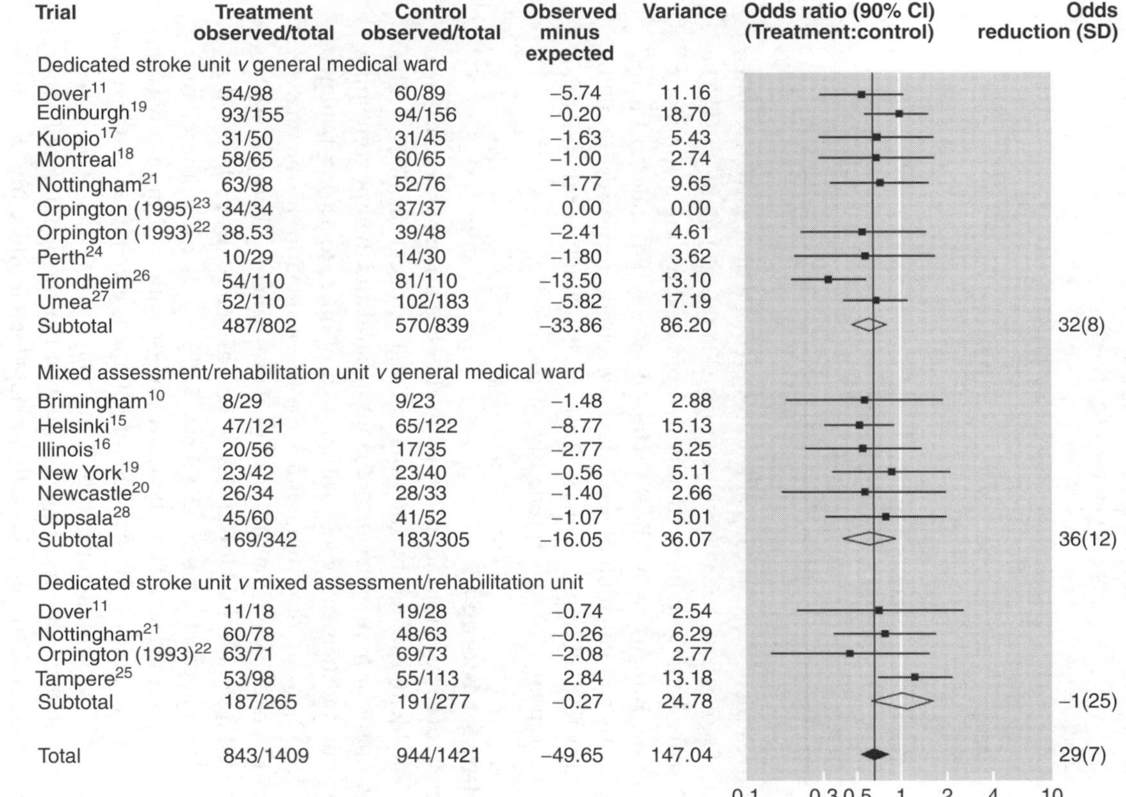

Trial
Treatment observed/total
Control observed/total
Observed minus expected
Variance
Odds ratio (90% CI) (Treatment:control)
Odds reduction (SD)
Dedicated stroke unit v general medical ward
Dover[11] 54/98 60/89 –5.74 11.16
Edinburgh[19] 93/155 94/156 –0.20 18.70
Kuopio[17] 31/50 31/45 –1.63 5.43
Montreal[18] 58/65 60/65 –1.00 2.74
Nottingham[21] 63/98 52/76 –1.77 9.65
Orpington (1995)[23] 34/34 37/37 0.00 0.00
Orpington (1993)[22] 38.53 39/48 –2.41 4.61
Perth[24] 10/29 14/30 –1.80 3.62
Trondheim[26] 54/110 81/110 –13.50 13.10
Umea[27] 52/110 102/183 –5.82 17.19
Subtotal 487/802 570/839 –33.86 86.20 32(8)
Mixed assessment/rehabilitation unit v general medical ward
Brimingham[10] 8/29 9/23 –1.48 2.88
Helsinki[15] 47/121 65/122 –8.77 15.13
Illinois[16] 20/56 17/35 –2.77 5.25
New York[19] 23/42 23/40 –0.56 5.11
Newcastle[20] 26/34 28/33 –1.40 2.66
Uppsala[28] 45/60 41/52 –1.07 5.01
Subtotal 169/342 183/305 –16.05 36.07 36(12)
Dedicated stroke unit v mixed assessment/rehabilitation unit
Dover[11] 11/18 19/28 –0.74 2.54
Nottingham[21] 60/78 48/63 –0.26 6.29
Orpington (1993)[22] 63/71 69/73 –2.08 2.77
Tampere[25] 53/98 55/113 2.84 13.18
Subtotal 187/265 191/277 –0.27 24.78 –1(25)
Total 843/1409 944/1421 –49.65 147.04 29(7)
0.1 0.3 0.5 1 2 4 10

Figure 11.3 Systematic review of the randomized trials of organized inpatient care after stroke: odds ratio (95% confidence interval) of death or requiring institutional care at the end of scheduled follow-up in patients receiving stroke unit compared with conventional care. Reproduced from The Stroke Unit Trialists' Collaboration (1997),[23] with permission from BMJ Publishing Group Ltd.

Table 11.6 The ABCD2 score.[24]

Feature		ABCD2 score
Age	≥60 years	1
	<60 years	0
Blood pressure	SBP >140 or DBP >90 mmHg	1
	SBP <140 and DBP <90 mmHg	0
Clinical features	Unilateral weakness	2
	Speech disturbed without weakness	1
	Others	0
Duration	≥60 min	2
	10–59 min	1
	<10 min	0
Diabetes	Diabetic	1
	Not known to be diabetic	0
Total		Range 0–7

without treatment. Certain clinical features predict a high early risk and a number of scores have been developed to predict those at highest risk. The ABCD2 score is the one most commonly used in the United Kingdom[24] (Table 11.6). Patients with ABCD2 score of ≥4 should undergo further investigations and initiation of secondary prevention measures should be organized within 24 hours of onset. Rapid access clinics are therefore an essential component of a comprehensive stroke service.

Antiplatelet therapy

The benefit of early aspirin administration, after exclusion of haemorrhagic stroke, was demonstrated by the International Stroke Trial (IST).[25] This study compared aspirin with subcutaneous heparin and therapy combining both aspirin and heparin, given within 48 h of onset in 19 435 patients, with a control group receiving neither aspirin or heparin. In the analysis of aspirin versus 'avoid aspirin' groups, those patients allocated aspirin experienced a significantly lower risk of recurrent stroke at 14 days than patients not allocated aspirin (2.8% vs 3.9%).[25] There is therefore a small but significant benefit to early treatment with aspirin, a low-cost intervention. Typically an initial dose of 300 mg is given, followed by the initiation of long-term therapy with 75 mg daily.

Subsequent work has aimed to identify whether the addition of further therapy, in the form of dipyridamole or clopidogrel, offers any increased benefit in longer term secondary prevention after ischaemic stroke or TIA. Aspirin combined with modified release dipyridamole in the ESPRIT study produced an absolute risk reduction of 1% (95% CI, 0.1–1.8%) compared to aspirin alone for the primary outcome of death from stroke, myocardial infarction or other vascular conditions, without an increase in the risk of haemorrhage.[26] The risk ratio for the primary outcome was similar when the trial results were compared with previous studies in a meta-analysis. At higher doses given acutely, dipyridamole exhibits vasodilatory properties, and thus caution is advised in patients who are known to have coronary arterial disease. The principal side effect limiting the tolerability of dipyridamole is headache.

Clopidogrel has also been investigated as an alternative to the combination of aspirin and dipyridamole. The PRoFESS study[27] reported a similar rate of recurrent stroke in patients randomized to treatment with clopidogrel or treatment with aspirin and extended-release dipyridamole, with similar rates of major haemorrhage. A previous study (MATCH) had demonstrated an increased risk of bleeding with the combination of clopidogrel and aspirin in long-term use compared to clopidogrel alone, hence the use of clopidogrel monotherapy in the PRoFESS study.[28] Therefore, clopidogrel as monotherapy provides an alternative to the combination of aspirin and dipyridamole for secondary prevention of stroke and is the antiplatelet of choice because of its better side effect profile.

Secondary prevention after stroke requires appropriate management of vascular risk factors and treatment focused on identification of the likely cause of the TIA or stroke. Thorough investigation of patients presenting as stroke or TIA is an important component of secondary prevention measures (Table 11.7).

Blood pressure management

There is good evidence that lowering blood pressure reduces the risk of recurrent stroke, whatever the initial level of blood pressure. Secondary prevention with an antihypertensive drug is typically initiated 7–14 days

Table 11.7 NICE guidelines for early management and investigation of TIA.[12]

- Start daily aspirin (300 mg) immediately
- Introduce measures for secondary prevention as soon as the diagnosis is confirmed, including discussion of individual risk factors
- Specialist assessment within 24 h of onset, including decision on brain imaging, for patients at high risk of stroke (ABCD2 score of ≥4 crescendo TIA)
- Specialist assessment within 1 week of symptom onset, including decision on brain imaging, for patients at lower risk of stroke (ABCD2 score of ≤3 or presenting more than 1 week after symptoms have resolved)
- Use diffusion-weighted MRI for brain imaging, except where contraindicated. For these people, use CT scanning
- If the person is identified as a candidate for carotid endarterectomy on specialist assessment, perform carotid imaging within 1 week of symptom onset
- Make sure that carotid imaging reports state clearly which criteria (ECST or NASCET) were used when measuring the extent of carotid stenosis

after stroke onset, when any acute, transient, blood pressure elevation will have settled. The benefits and risks of acute blood pressure lowering in the hypertensive patient presenting acutely with stroke are less certain. Lowering of blood pressure levels initially within the normal range, as well as good control of hypertension, with the combination of a diuretic and an angiotensin-converting enzyme (ACE) inhibitor drug, reduced the long-term risk of recurrent stroke by 40% in the PROGRESS trial.[29] An ACE inhibitor alone is not nearly as effective, probably because the benefit depends on how much blood pressure is lowered.

Physiological changes in the cerebral circulation occur at the time of stroke, and cerebral autoregulation may be impaired. In an acute stroke, lowering mean arterial blood pressure may reduce cerebral perfusion pressure and, in areas with critically reduced blood flow (the ischaemic penumbra), this may lead to infarction. However, in patients with evidence of cardiac dysfunction or acute myocardial infarction the balance of risks may be altered to favour hypotensive therapy. Severe hypertension (systolic blood pressure >180 mmHg or diastolic blood pressure >105 mmHg) is a contraindication to thrombolytic therapy. If blood pressure is therapeutically lowered in acute stroke, reductions in blood pressure should be closely monitored and rapid falls avoided.

Cholesterol management

The finding of an elevated serum cholesterol level should prompt involvement of a dietician or nutritionist. There is good evidence that lowering serum cholesterol levels of >3.5 mmol l^{-1} with, for example, simvastatin 40 mg at night results in a substantial reduction in the long-term risk of recurrent stroke and myocardial infarction of about one third.[30,31]

Diabetes management

Management of prolonged fasting hyperglycaemia is in accordance with guidelines for the standard management of diabetes. The evidence suggests that tight control of blood sugar levels over the long term in diabetes has more of an effect on reducing rates of myocardial infarction than stroke rates, whereas the opposite is the case for hypertension. The blood pressure readings in diabetic patients during follow-up after stroke should therefore be maintained at or below the target of 130/80 mmHg.

Anticoagulation

In acute stroke, unfractionated heparin, given subcutaneously, reduces the rate of recurrent stroke and pulmonary embolism, but at the expense of an increase in cerebral haemorrhage of similar magnitude that offsets potential benefit. There is also a significant increase in extracranial bleeding. Low molecular weight heparin (LMWH) has similarly failed to demonstrate a therapeutic benefit at treatment dose. The balance of evidence, therefore, does not favour heparin use in acute stroke. Anticoagulation is therefore reserved for the patient with atrial fibrillation (AF) at risk of stroke, or for those in whom another indication exists (e.g. prosthetic heart valve, deep vein thrombosis or pulmonary embolism).

The only situation where anticoagulation with warfarin has been found to be more effective than antiplatelet therapy is in the prevention of stroke recurrence after TIA or ischaemic stroke associated with AF. Randomized trials have shown that any benefit in the first 2 weeks after onset of stroke is offset by an increase in cerebral haemorrhage. Initiation of warfarin should therefore be delayed until after 2 weeks, except after TIA and minor stroke, when it is logical to start immediately. Warfarin reduces the risk of recurrent stroke in suitable patients with AF by about 70%.[32] Aspirin and other antiplatelet agents are much less effective in preventing recurrent stroke in patients with AF, but provide an alternative for those who cannot or will not take warfarin. There is an assumption that has not been tested in randomized trials that other causes of cardioembolic stroke will also benefit from anticoagulation, including patients with recent myocardial infarction, congestive valvular heart disease and cardiomyopathies. Safe anticoagulation will require patient participation, monitoring and adjustment of therapy, and an acceptably low risk of falls.

Carotid artery stenosis

Carotid artery stenosis is responsible for 20–30% of cases of anterior circulation ischaemic stroke and TIA, and between 5 and 10% will need endarterectomy (or stenting) to prevent recurrence. The arterial narrowing is usually caused by atherosclerosis, which becomes more prevalent with age and is accelerated by risk factors. Dissection is an important cause in younger patients.

Atherosclerosis

Atherosclerosis is the commonest arterial disorder in developed countries and, when complicated by thrombosis and embolism, may result in ischaemic stroke, myocardial infarction or peripheral arterial disease. The process of atheroma formation occurs over many years, beginning with low-density lipoprotein (LDL) cholesterol moving into the subendothelium, often at sites of endothelial injury or haemodynamic stress. In the cerebral circulation this occurs at sites of arterial branching, especially the bifurcation of the common carotid artery into the internal carotid artery (ICA) and external carotid artery (ECA). The LDL is oxidized by macrophages and smooth muscle cells. Production of growth factors and cytokines attracting more immune cells, foam cell accumulation and smooth muscle proliferation all result in the growth of an atherosclerotic plaque.[33] Risk factors that accelerate the formation of atherosclerosis include cigarette smoking, diabetes mellitus, age, dyslipidaemia and hypertension. Genetic predisposition may also be a factor.

Plaques with a fatty core and a fibrous cap then spread along and around the arterial wall, encroaching on the media and ultimately leading to narrowing of the vessel lumen and stiffening of the arterial wall. A defect in the fibrous cap, due to rupture or erosion, predisposes to thrombosis at that site. Platelets adhere to the vessel wall and are activated, initiating blood coagulation. This is the site of action for antiplatelet agents used in the secondary prevention of stroke. Thrombosis may initially be incorporated into the plaque, but as the plaque grows, the lumen of the vessel may become obstructed, causing a narrowing or stenosis. The atherothrombotic plaque may completely occlude the artery, or embolization from the plaque may cause either transient or permanent obstruction of a smaller distal artery, resulting in cerebral or ocular symptoms. Most strokes and TIAs secondary to carotid stenosis occur as a result of thromboembolism. Hypoperfusion of arterial territories is a relatively rare cause of symptoms compared to other sites, because of collateral supply via the circle of Willis.

Arterial dissection

A rare cause of carotid artery stenosis in the elderly population, dissection may be spontaneous, traumatic or associated with underlying connective tissue disease (such as Marfan syndrome or Ehlers-Danlos syndrome). Most commonly, dissection occurs following minor neck or head trauma associated with sudden rotation of the neck. The ICA is torn against the second cervical vertebra and a haematoma forms in the arterial wall, which can narrow the vessel lumen, leading to thrombosis. Alternatively, an intimal free flap may promote thromboembolism. There may be a delay of up to several days, between the event and symptoms in the territory of the anterior cerebral circulation. Diagnostic clues suggesting dissection include a Horner syndrome resulting from compression or ischaemia of the sympathetic chain which surrounds the carotid artery in the neck. Cross-sectional MRI with fat-suppressed sequences is the investigation of choice, revealing a characteristic crescent-shaped haematoma in the carotid arterial wall (Figure 11.4).

Subsequent management is controversial, with most centres anticoagulating patients with heparin and subsequently warfarin, but there is no good evidence of benefit in preventing recurrent stroke compared with aspirin. Stenting may be an option for some patients resistant to medical treatment.

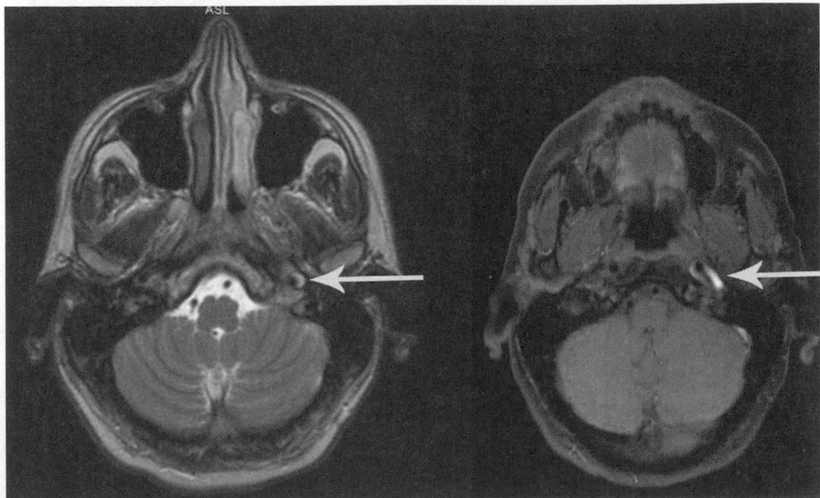

Figure 11.4 Carotid artery dissection on MR imaging – there is left carotid dissection from the high cervical to at least the laceral segment.

Investigations

Carotid artery atheroma may be found after investigating a neurological event, be sought on imaging after clinical examination reveals a carotid bruit, or may be an incidental finding during preoperative work-up for procedures such as cardiac bypass surgery. Auscultation for carotid bruit, however, is not a reliable screening test for significant carotid stenosis. A localized bruit is indeed usually caused by a narrowing of the artery, but the extent and significance of the stenosis cannot be predicted by the presence of a bruit. A very tight stenosis, for example, may not cause a bruit, or an ECA stenosis of little clinical significance may cause a loud bruit.

The level where the carotid artery divides into ICA and ECA branches varies, but in most patients it is possible to examine the common carotid artery, bifurcation and proximal portions of the ICA and ECA with ultrasound. B-mode Duplex ultrasound with Doppler measurement of flow velocities in these arteries is therefore commonly used to screen for ICA stenosis. Although the artery itself may be visualized using plain ultrasound, estimation of the degree of stenosis with accuracy is difficult. Indirect evidence is therefore gathered through measurement of the velocity of flow in the longitudinal direction.[34] As the systolic pulse passes a stenosis, the velocity of blood will tend to increase, and it is the absolute velocity of flow both distal to the stenosis and prior to the stenosis that are assessed (Table 11.8). Grading of stenosis for a given examination varies according to the method used. It is important to note which method is being applied.

It is also possible to derive measurement of the intimal-medial thickness of the carotid artery from B-mode ultrasound, which can be used to

Table 11.8 Derived figures for Doppler ultrasound criteria for grading ICA diameter reduction.[34]

Diameter reduction (%)	Peak systolic velocity ($cm\,s^{-1}$)	End diastolic velocity ($cm\,s^{-1}$)	PSV_{ICA}/PSV_{CCA}[a]
0–29	<100	<40	<3.2
30–49	110–130	<40	<3.2
50–59	>130	<40	<3.2
60–69	>130	40–110	3.2–4.0
70–79	>230	110–140	>4.0
80–95	>230	>140	>4.0
96–99		'String flow'	
100		'No flow'	

[a]ICA = internal carotid artery; CCA = common carotid artery, PSV_{ICA}/PSV_{CCA} = ratio of the velocities.

measure plaque thickness or progress, and to visualize portions of the vertebral arteries in some subjects, but the clinical utility of the latter is limited by the superiority of other contrast methods.[34]

Ultrasound is a safe, non-invasive and relatively inexpensive technique, but its utility remains limited by the requirement of a high degree of operator skill. Results are subject to inter-observer variation, and technical limitations of the procedure include acoustic shadowing caused by calcified plaque and difficulty in studying a tortuous vessel where flow velocities may appear increased.[34]

Because of these limitations, most units confirm abnormal findings on ultrasound with a second non-invasive imaging modality before considering surgery or stenting for carotid stenosis. Catheter angiography may be required if the non-invasive investigations are discordant or difficult to interpret.

Magnetic resonance angiography (MRA), with or without intravenous contrast, was the first alternative non-invasive technique used for the investigation of arterial pathology in the neck and head to confirm the presence of carotid artery stenosis (Figure 11.5) in patients who have undergone preliminary ultrasound investigation, but MRA may also be used as a screening investigation. The limitations of MRA include patient tolerability, and safety with metallic implants. Technical limitations include misinterpretation of swallowing artifact or turbulent flow as stenosis. MRA and/or Duplex ultrasound are increasingly being replaced by CT angiography (CTA) with intravenous contrast because it is often combined with CT in the initial evaluation of stroke.

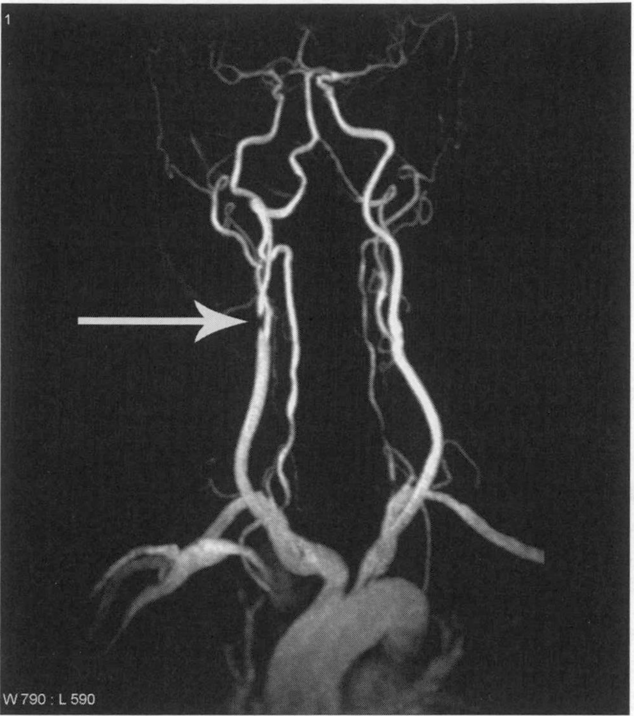

Figure 11.5 Carotid artery stenosis.

The limitations of CTA include contrast toxicity (including renal impairment), contrast allergy and poor visualization of stenosis if there is heavy plaque calcification.

Catheter angiography is the 'gold standard' investigation for carotid artery stenosis, but this procedure carries with it a significant risk of stroke or TIA of between 0.5% and 2%, depending on indications. The catheter may dislodge atheromatous plaque, dissect the arterial wall or thrombus may form on the catheter. The intravenous contrast administered carries the same risks as for other indications, namely, headache, nausea, bradycardia and renal failure. For these reasons angiography is normally preceded by non-invasive investigation, and should only be performed in experienced neurovascular units.

Carotid endarterectomy

The case for intervention

To warrant intervention, the risk of stroke that accompanies carotid endarterectomy (CEA) must be less than the natural risk of stroke in the patient receiving best medical management, and the benefit of surgery must be sufficient to justify the costs to healthcare providers and risks to the patient.

Symptomatic patients

Large randomized clinical trials have demonstrated a benefit of CEA for severe symptomatic carotid artery stenosis compared to medical treatment alone. In the European Carotid Surgery Trial (ECST),[35] over 3000 patients with any degree of carotid stenosis who had a TIA or minor stroke in the 6 months prior to randomization were randomized to receive CEA or best medical management alone. Concurrently, the North American Symptomatic Carotid Endarterectomy Trial (NASCET)[36] randomized over 2800 patients with >30% carotid stenosis who had symptoms within 3 months of randomization to CEA or best medical management. A meta-analysis of these trials indicates a clear advantage of CEA over medical management for the patients with more severe stenosis, so long as the peri-operative risk of stroke or death is no more than 5%.[37] NICE guidelines for the management of carotid stenosis are given in Table 11.9.

ECST and NASCET used different denominators to measure the severity of stenosis, but the NASCET method in which the diameter of the stenosis is compared to the diameter of the distal ICA has become the standard method. The absolute risk reduction of ipsilateral ischaemic stroke or death

Table 11.9 NICE guidelines for the management of carotid stenosis.[12]

- All people with suspected non-disabling stroke or TIA who after specialist assessment are considered as candidates for carotid endarterectomy should have carotid imaging within 1 week of onset of symptoms
- People who present more than 1 week after their last symptom of TIA has resolved should be managed using the lower risk pathway
- People with stable neurological symptoms from acute non-disabling stroke or TIA who have symptomatic carotid stenosis of 50–99% according to the NASCET (North American Symptomatic Carotid Endarterectomy Trial) criteria or 70–99% according to the ECST (European Carotid Surgery Trialists' Collaborative Group) criteria should:
  - be assessed and referred for carotid endarterectomy within 1 week of onset of stroke or TIA symptoms
  - undergo surgery within a maximum of 2 weeks of onset of stroke or TIA symptoms
  - receive best medical treatment (control of blood pressure, antiplatelet agents, cholesterol lowering through diet and drugs, lifestyle advice)
- People with stable neurological symptoms from acute non-disabling stroke or TIA who have symptomatic carotid stenosis of <50% according to the NASCET criteria or <70% according to the ECST criteria should:
  - not undergo surgery
  - receive best medical treatment (control of blood pressure, antiplatelet agents, cholesterol lowering through diet and drugs, lifestyle advice)
- Carotid imaging reports should clearly state which criteria (ECST or NASCET) were used when measuring the extent of carotid stenosis

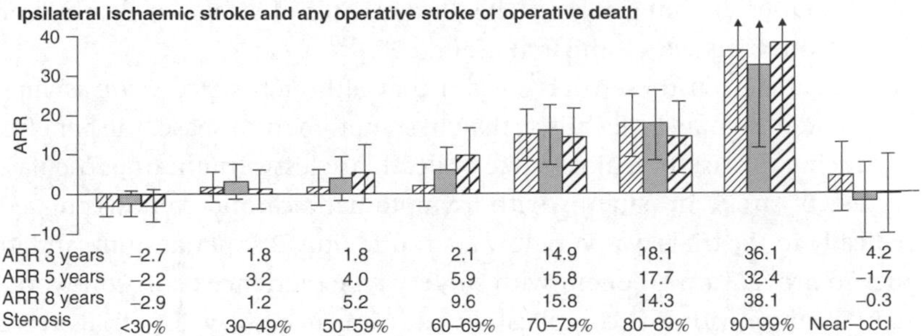

ARR 3 years	−2.7	1.8	1.8	2.1	14.9	18.1	36.1	4.2
ARR 5 years	−2.2	3.2	4.0	5.9	15.8	17.7	32.4	−1.7
ARR 8 years	−2.9	1.2	5.2	9.6	15.8	14.3	38.1	−0.3
Stenosis	<30%	30–49%	50–59%	60–69%	70–79%	80–89%	90–99%	Near–occl

Figure 11.6 Effect of surgery on absolute risk of main trial outcomes at 3, 5 and 8 years' follow-up by degree of symptomatic carotid stenosis, in analysis of pooled data from ECST and NASCET. Reprinted from Rothwell *et al.* (2003)[37], Copyright 2003, with permission from Elsevier.

in those patients with NASCET 70–99% stenosis undergoing CEA was 16% ($p < 0.001$)[37] (Figure 11.6). Patients with 50–69% NASCET stenosis also achieved a risk reduction, but the margin of benefit was slimmer. Below this stenosis threshold, there was evidence of overall harm. In subgroup analyses, male gender, advancing age and recent symptoms were identified as factors conferring additional benefit to the procedure.

Asymptomatic patients

The benefits of surgery for asymptomatic carotid stenosis, and symptomatic stenosis with more than 6 months since last symptoms, are less clear-cut than for symptomatic stenosis. Two large randomized controlled trials have addressed this issue.[38,39]

In the Asymptomatic Carotid Atherosclerosis Study (ACAS), over 1600 patients with asymptomatic carotid stenosis of 60% or more were randomized to receive CEA or best medical treatment. The results showed that surgery significantly reduced the overall 5-year risk of ipsilateral stroke or any peri-operative stroke or death from 11% to 5.1% ($p = 0.004$), but not the risk of major stroke. The complication rate in the surgical arm approached 3% at 30 days when preoperative angiography was included in the analysis.[38]

The Asymptomatic Carotid Surgery Trial (ASCT) randomized over 3000 patients to a policy of immediate or deferred carotid endarterectomy (until surgery seemed to be more clearly indicated, for example in the presence of related symptoms), for asymptomatic 60–99% stenosis. The results showed a benefit to immediate surgery in terms of reducing the 5-year risk of all strokes and peri-operative death from 11.8% to 6.4% ($p < 0.0001$). However, subgroup analysis showed no evidence of benefit in patients older than 75 years, or in women after taking into account the risks of surgery. There was a less marked benefit in terms of reducing the risk of fatal or disabling stroke. The 30-day rates of stroke or death after CEA in both trials were similar at around 3%.[39]

The results from these trials suggest that although surgery for asymptomatic stenosis may be less risky than in symptomatic disease, the benefits of reducing the risk of major stroke or death are less certain. In particular, the rate of stroke in patients with asymptomatic carotid stenosis treated medically in the trials was very low at around only 2% per annum, and in order to provide a net benefit with surgery an experienced surgeon working in a centre with low complication rates was necessary. The trials were conducted several years ago at a time when statins were not in widespread use, blood pressure was less well controlled and dual antiplatelet therapy was not used routinely. It is therefore likely that with better medical management, the rates of ipsilateral stroke associated with asymptomatic carotid stenosis will be even lower than recorded in the trials, which could negate any potential benefit of surgery.

These results together suggest that patients with asymptomatic stenosis aged over 75 or those with less than 60% stenosis should not be offered surgery. Those who otherwise meet inclusion criteria may be offered surgery, but in the knowledge that their risk of stroke with best medical treatment is low. If patients, and their neurologists and surgeons, opt for medical management then they should be educated about the symptoms of TIA and stroke and urged to present to a doctor should these occur.

Carotid artery stenting

Carotid artery stenting has developed as an alternative to the more established procedure of CEA. In theory there are several potential benefits to the patient of this approach. This procedure is normally carried out under local anaesthesia, avoiding the risks of a general anaesthetic. Patients may recover faster from a procedure performed under local anaesthesia, thereby reducing the length of hospital stay. The other major advantage of an endovascular approach is that there is no need for an incision in the neck and the incidence of haematoma, infection and cutaneous or cranial nerve injury are reduced. Complications at the site of endovascular access in the groin are rare.

However, there are few interventionists with extensive experience of angioplasty and stenting in the carotid artery, although experience with endovascular surgery elsewhere in the body is increasing. Endovascular treatment of carotid stenosis may lead to distal embolization of thrombus to the brain during the passage of the catheter through a tight stenosis, and simple balloon angioplasty has been replaced with stenting and the use of cerebral protection devices (either filters or occlusion devices) to try and mitigate this problem. Stents are thought to cause less arterial dissection than balloon angioplasty, but transcranial Doppler studies have shown that embolization frequently occurs during deployment of the stent and during post-stent dilation. The utility of cerebral protection devices is debated, and research in this area has not always shown an improved outcome with the use of a protection device.

Although the recovery time following successful endovascular intervention is short, the cost benefits of a reduced length of inpatient stay may be overshadowed by the higher costs of the stent and protection device equipment. Another problem with endovascular treatment is the greater potential for restenosis of the treated artery compared to surgery, although the clinical significance of this is not clear.

The carotid stenting versus carotid endarterectomy trials have consistently shown an excess rate of stroke after stenting for recently symptomatic stenosis compared with endarterectomy. In a pooled analysis of the European based trials, the overall risk of stroke or death within 30 days of stenting was 7.7% compared with 4.4% after endarterectomy (risk ratio 1.74; 95% CI, 1.32–2.30).[40] However, there is a small excess of myocardial infarction after endarterectomy (risk <1%) and cranial nerve injury.

However, in symptomatic patients, the risks of stroke or death associated with the procedure were identical after stenting and endarterectomy in patients younger than 70 years, while all the excess risk of stroke appeared to be associated with older age. A more recent North American trial, CREST, showed very similar results. Thus, stenting may be an option for younger patients. However, although the long-term effectiveness of stenting at preventing stroke recurrence appears similar to endarterectomy, there is an increased risk of restenosis after stenting and more long-term data are required to determine how often this leads to symptoms. Trials are examining the role of stenting for asymptomatic carotid stenosis. Stenting is also an option for treatment of symptomatic carotid stenosis in patients not suitable for endarterectomy, for example stenosis secondary to radiotherapy, fibromuscular dysplasia, dissection and high cervical lesions not amenable to surgery.

Vertebral and intracranial arterial stenting

Surgical access to the vertebral artery origin is difficult and procedures carry high morbidity. Stenting therefore provides a preferable option for the treatment of symptomatic extracranial vertebral arterial stenosis, which most commonly occurs at the vertebral artery origin.[41] Stenting of intracranial arteries, for example basilar or middle cerebral artery, carries a risk of vessel dissection or rupture in addition to the risk of embolization of fragments of plaque. Stenting of these vessels is therefore usually reserved for patients with recurrent symptoms despite medical therapy. However, the benefits are uncertain and randomized trials are needed to establish the benefit of endovascular intervention for vertebral and intracranial stenosis.

Intracranial and subarachnoid haemorrhage

Spontaneous intracerebral haemorrhage

A typical history is given of sudden onset of severe headache, with the subsequent rapid development of focal neurological deficit. However, headache may be absent and in some cases the deficit progresses more slowly, sometimes over several days, especially when the haemorrhage is associated with anticoagulation or a coagulopathy. Intracerebral haemorrhage may also present as collapse. No one clinical feature reliably differentiates haemorrhage from infarction, and imaging is essential to distinguish between the two.

Spontaneous intracerebral hemorrhage (ICH) may be divided into those occurring in the absence (primary) or presence (secondary) of an identified underlying structural abnormality. ICH is also associated with oral anticoagulant therapy. In this situation, tissue damage is limited by rapid identification of the condition and reversal of anticoagulation, although treatment dilemmas arise when the patient is anticoagulated for a high-risk condition such as acute pulmonary embolism, or prosthetic heart valve. Consideration may have to be given to the eventual reintroduction of anticoagulation despite haemorrhagic risk, or alternative strategies such as the placement of an inferior vena caval filter for DVT.

The initial management of cerebral haemorrhage is broadly similar to that of ischaemic stroke, apart from antiplatelet and anticoagulant therapy, which are clearly contraindicated. However, further investigation, including some form of angiography, should be undertaken in selected patients to exclude an underlying vascular abnormality which may require surgical or neuroradiological intervention to reduce the chances of a recurrent bleed. An intracranial aneurysm or arteriovenous malformation (AVM) should be particularly suspected in the younger patient with cerebral haemorrhage. Risk factors such as hypertension promote bleeding from aneurysms and AVMs and therefore should not necessarily influence the decisions about further investigation. The latter should be made after discussion with a neurovascular team at the local neuroscience centre.

Poor prognosis is conferred by a large volume of blood, intraventricular extension or reduced level of consciousness at the time of presentation. However, patients are often referred to neurosurgical colleagues for consideration of intervention, and evidence has been sought in randomized controlled trials for this aggressive approach. The STICH trial recruited 1033 patients from neurosurgical centres with supratentorial intracerebral haematoma over 2 cm in diameter, occurring within the previous 72 hours, and randomized to early surgery or initial conservative (medical) management.[42] 26% of the surgical group had a favourable outcome (good recovery or moderate disability on the Glasgow Outcomes Scale) compared to 24% of the conservative treatment group. This small difference between the groups did not reach statistical significance. However, there was a suggestion that patients with haematomas 1 cm or less from the cortical surface were likely to have a favourable outcome and these patients are being included in the second STICH trial.[42]

Cerebellar haemorrhage may present with occipital headache, truncal ataxia and conjugate gaze palsy, followed after an interval by impairment of consciousness and subsequent neurological deterioration as an expanding haematoma compromises the ventricular system causing hydrocephalus and brain herniation. Surgical evacuation of a cerebellar haematoma is a life-saving measure.

Subarachnoid haemorrhage

The incidence of subarachnoid haemorrhage (SAH) is ~6 per 100 000 per year.[43] Bleeding into the subarachnoid space is often the result of rupture of an intracranial aneurysm. There may be a familial component to aneurysm development, but hypertension and smoking are the predominant risk factors for aneurysmal rupture. As in intracerebral haemorrhage, presentation is typically with sudden onset of severe headache, which may be accompanied by nausea and vomiting, neck stiffness, visual disturbance, altered conscious level and collapse. Subarachnoid bleeding may also be the result of trauma, dural fistula, arteriovenous malformations (AVMs), cerebral venous thrombosis, or there may be no clear cause found.

SAH is frequently fatal, with mortality rates in many series around 35–65%.[43] A significant portion of the survivors remain dependent, and complications such as delayed cerebral ischaemia secondary to vasospasm, rebleeding of the affected vessel, and the development of hydrocephalus may lead to a poorer outcome. At the time of presentation, outcome appears to be predicted by Glasgow Coma Scale score, age and the volume of intracranial blood. However, non-aneurysmal perimesencephalic haemorrhage, in which the bleeding is confined to the basal cisterns around the midbrain, and there is no extension of the haemorrhage to the lateral Sylvian fissures or to the anterior part of the interhemispheric fissure, is associated with a good outcome. The cause is uncertain.

CT of the head is the preferred initial investigation, and the pattern of bleeding may suggest a site of origin. CT angiogram may be added to this to localize the site of bleeding and identify a target for acute intervention.

In the well patient, if clinical suspicion for SAH remains despite the lack of evidence on brain imaging then lumbar puncture should be undertaken to look for xanthochromia. Lysis of the red blood cells in the cerebrospinal fluid (CSF) produces oxyhaemoglobin and bilirubin giving a yellow colour to the CSF after centrifugation between 12 hours and 14 days after SAH. MRI imaging with gradient echo T2 sequences or FLAIR (fluid attenuated inversion recovery) technique can also demonstrate SAH accurately. MRI is most useful in the setting of delayed presentation, with negative CT but positive lumbar puncture where a site of bleeding is sought.[43]

Management of SAH should be discussed with the neurovascular team at the local neuroscience centre and consists of treatment to secure the aneurysm, or other source of bleeding, and the prevention of secondary cerebral damage. Neurosurgery may be considered for those patients with an intracerebral haematoma secondary to SAH, or surgical ventricular drainage for those who develop hydrocephalus. Surgical solutions to prevent rebleeding include operative clipping of the aneurysm, but there is increasing use of endovascular exclusion of the aneurysm using platinum coils. The ISAT study demonstrated lower morbidity and mortality after endovascular coiling compared to neurosurgical clipping for aneurysms suitable for both treatments.[44] The only agent shown in a randomized trial to prevent cerebral ischaemia after SAH is nimodipine, a calcium channel antagonist, continued for 3 weeks.[45] The oral or nasosgastric enteral route is preferred over intravenous administration to avoid precipitating hypotension. Its effect in reducing cerebral vasospasm may be the mechanism for the reduction in risk of a poor outcome.

Conclusion

Acute stroke can be a devastating disease, and the safe and effective evidence-based management of this condition and its consequences is fundamental. Stroke is a medical emergency, and early presentation of symptoms with prompt recognition by healthcare providers will allow the patient to be considered for treatments that limit disability or improve outcome, such as intravenous thrombolysis. Subsequent multidisciplinary care in a stroke unit will allow access to the best medical management of risk factors, reducing the risk of recurrent stroke, allowing timely further investigation, and permitting better access to rehabilitation therapies. Rare causes of stroke, such as cerebral venous thrombosis, should always be kept in mind because they may need different management.

If, during investigation, a tight carotid artery stenosis is discovered, there is good evidence to guide the patient's further management. Selected

Table 11.10 NICE stroke guidelines – key priorities for implementation.[10]

- In people with sudden onset of neurological symptoms, a validated tool, such as FAST (Face, Arm, Speech Test), should be used outside hospital to screen for a diagnosis of stroke or TIA
- All people with suspected stroke should be admitted directly to a specialist acute stroke unit following initial assessment, either from the community or from the A&E department
- Brain imaging should be performed immediately for people with acute stroke if any of the following apply:
  - indications for thrombolysis or early anticoagulation treatment
  - on anticoagulant treatment
  - a known bleeding tendency
  - a depressed level of consciousness (Glasgow Coma Score <13)
  - unexplained progressive or fluctuating symptoms
  - papilloedema, neck stiffness or fever
  - severe headache at onset of stroke symptoms
- On admission, people with acute stroke should have their swallowing screened by an appropriately trained healthcare professional before being given any oral food, fluid or medication

symptomatic patients benefit from carotid endarterectomy. Carotid artery stenting provides an alternative for patients considered at high peri-procedural risk of stroke from endarterectomy. All patients with TIA or stroke who might be suitable for surgical or endovascular treatment should therefore be investigated for carotid stenosis, initially with non-invasive methods.

Intracranial haemorrhage, including subarachnoid and cerebral haemorrhage, is likewise a threat to life. Those patients who survive an intracranial haemorrhage without major disability may need further investigation to determine the presence of a treatable aneurysm or AVM.

NICE stroke guidelines with key priorities for implementation are given in Table 11.10.

Key points

- Acute stroke is a major cause of death and disability in the older population.
- Selected patients benefit from thrombolysis after early brain imaging to distinguish between infarct and haemorrhage.
- Multidisciplinary care on a stroke unit improves outcome.
- Early treatment of severe carotid artery stenosis may prevent recurrent stroke.
- Patients with stroke and TIA should be managed as emergencies by a specialized stroke service to prevent early brain damage and recurrent stroke.

References

1 WHO MONICA Project Principal Investigators. The World Health Organization MONICA Project (Monitoring Trends and Determinants in Cardiovascular Disease): a major international collaboration. *J Clin Epidemiol* 1988;**41**(2):105–14.

2 Lloyd-Jones D, Adams RJ, Brown TM *et al.* Heart Disease and Stroke Statistics – 2010 Update. A report from the American Heart Association. *Circulation* 2010;**121**:e1–e170.

3 Dhamoon MS, Sciacca RR, Rundek T *et al.* Recurrent stroke and cardiac risks after first ischemic stroke: The Northern Manhattan Study. *Neurology* 2006;**66**:641–6.

4 Bamford J, Sandercock P, Dennis M *et al.* Classification and natural history of clinically identifiable subtypes of cerebral infarction. *Lancet* 1991;**337**:1521–6.

5 National Institutes for Health (NIH) *Stroke Scale.* Available at: http://www.ninds.nih.gov/doctors/NIH_Stroke_Scale_Booklet.pdf (accessed June 2012).

6 Mahoney F and Barthel D. Functional evaluation: the Barthel Index. *Md State Med J* 1965;**14**:56–61.

7 van Swieten JC, Koudstaal PJ, Visser MC *et al.* Interobserver agreement for the assessment of handicap in stroke patients. *Stroke* 1988;**19**:604–7.

8 Schmahmann JD. Vascular syndromes of the thalamus. *Stroke* 2003;**34**:2264–78.

9 Nor AM, McAllister C, Louw SJ *et al.* Agreement between ambulance paramedic- and physician-recorded neurological signs with face arm speech test (FAST) in acute stroke patients. *Stroke* 2004;**35**:1355–9.

10 Nor AM, Davis J, Sen B *et al.* The recognition of stroke in the emergency room (ROSIER) scale: development and validation of a stroke recognition instrument. *Lancet Neurol* 2005;**4**:727–34.

11 Wardlaw JM, Keir SL, Seymour J *et al.* What is the best imaging strategy for acute stroke? *Health Technol Assess* 2004;**8**(1).

12 National Institute for Health and Clinical Excellence (NICE). (2008) *Stroke: Diagnosis and initial management of acute stroke and transient ischaemic attack (TIA),* NICE Clinical Guideline 68, NICE, London.

13 Lövblad K-O and Baird AE. Computed tomography in acute ischaemic stroke. *Neuroradiology* 2010;**52**:175–87.

14 Kloska S, Wintermark M, Engelhorn T and Fiebach J. Acute stroke magnetic resonance imaging: current status and future perspective. *Neuroradiology* 2010;**52**:189–201.

15 Johnston K, Hall C, Kissela B *et al.* Glucose Regulation in Acute Stroke Patients (GRASP) trial: a randomized pilot trial. *Stroke* 2009;**40**:3804–9.

16 Kwiatkowski TG, Libman RB, Frankel M *et al.* for the National Institute of Neurological Disorders and Stroke Recombinant Tissue Plasminogen Activator Stroke Study Group. Effects of tissue plasminogen activator for acute ischemic stroke at one year. *New Engl J Med* 1999;**340**:1781–7.

17 The ATLANTIS, ECASS, and NINDS rt-PA Study Group Investigators. Association of outcome with early stroke treatment: pooled analysis of ATLANTIS, ECASS, and NINDS rt-PA stroke trials. *Lancet* 2004;**363**:768–74.

18 Hacke W, Kaste M, Bluhmki E *et al.* Thrombolysis with alteplase 3 to 4.5 hours after acute ischemic stroke. *New Engl J Med* 2008;**359**(13):1317–29.

19 Wardlaw J, del Zoppo G, Yamaguchi T and Berge E. Thrombolysis for acute ischaemic stroke. *Stroke* 2004;**35**:2914–15.

20 The IST-3 Collaborative Group. The benefits and harms of intravenous thrombolysis with recombinant tissue plasminogen activator within 6 h of acute ischaemic stroke

(the Third International Stroke Trial [IST-3]): a randomised controlled trial. *Lancet* 2012;**379**(9834):2352–63.

21 Astrup J, Siesjö BK and Symon L. Thresholds in cerebral ischemia – the ischemic penumbra. *Stroke* 1981;**12**:723–5.

22 Vahedi K, Hofmeijer J, Juettler E *et al.* Early decompressive surgery in malignant infarction of the middle cerebral artery: a pooled analysis of three randomised controlled trials. *Lancet Neurol* 2007;**6**:215–22.

23 The Stroke Unit Trialists' Collaboration. Collaborative systematic review of the randomised trials of organised inpatient (stroke unit) care after stroke. *BMJ* 1997;**314**:1151–9.

24 Giles M and Rothwell P. Using the ABCD system to evaluate transient ischaemic attack. *Nat Rev Neurol* 2009;**5**:470–1.

25 International Stroke Trial Collaborative Group. The International Stroke Trial; a randomised trial of aspirin, subcutaneous heparin, both, or neither among 19 435 patients with acute ischaemic stroke. *Lancet* 1997;**349**(9056):1569–81.

26 ESPRIT Study Group. Aspirin plus dipyridamole versus aspirin alone after cerebral ischaemia of arterial origin (ESPRIT): randomised controlled trial. *Lancet* 2006;**367**:1665–73.

27 Sacco RL, Diener H-C, Yusuf S *et al.* for the ProFESS Study Group. Aspirin and extended-release dipyridamole versus clopidogrel for recurrent stroke. *New Engl J Med* 2008;**359**:1238–51.

28 Diener H-C, Bogousslavsky J, Brass LM *et al.* Aspirin and clopidogrel compared with clopidogrel alone after recent ischaemic stroke or transient ischaemic attack in high-risk patients (MATCH): randomised, double-blind, placebo-controlled trial. *Lancet* 2004;**364**:331–7.

29 PROGRESS Collaborative Group. Randomised trial of a perindopril-based blood pressure-lowering regimen among 6105 individuals with previous stroke or transient ischaemic attack. *Lancet* 2001;**358**:1033–41.

30 The Stroke Prevention by Aggressive Reduction in Cholesterol Levels (SPARCL) Investigators. High-dose atorvastatin after stroke or transient ischaemic attack. *New Engl J Med* 2006;**355**:549–59.

31 Heart Protection Study Collaborative Group. Effects of cholesterol-lowering with simvastatin on stroke and other major vascular events in 20 536 people with cerebrovascular disease or other high-risk conditions. *Lancet* 2004;**363**:757–67.

32 EAFT (European Atrial Fibrillation Trial) Study Group. Secondary prevention in non-rheumatic atrial fibrillation after transient ischaemic attack or minor stroke. *Lancet* 1993:**342**(8882):1255–62.

33 Faxon D, Fuster V, Libby P *et al.* Atherosclerotic Vascular Disease Conference: Writing Group III: Pathophysiology. *Circulation* 2004;**109**:2617–25.

34 Sidhu P. Ultrasound of the carotid and vertebral arteries. *Br Med Bull* 2000;**56**(2):346–66.

35 European Carotid Surgery Trialists' Collaborative Group. Randomised trial of endarterectomy for recently symptomatic carotid stenosis: final results of the MRC European Carotid Surgery Trial (ECST). *Lancet* 1998;**351**(9113):1379–87.

36 Barnett HJM, Taylor DW, Eliasziw MA *et al.* Benefit of carotid endarterectomy in patients with symptomatic moderate or severe stenosis. *New Engl J Med* 1991;**339**(20):1415–25.

37 Rothwell PM, Eliasziw W, Gutnikov SA *et al.* Analysis of pooled data from the randomised controlled trials of endarterectomy for symptomatic carotid stenosis. *Lancet* 2003;**361**(9352):107–16.

38 Executive Committee for the Asymptomatic Carotid Atherosclerosis Study. Endarterectomy for asymptomatic carotid artery stenosis. *JAMA* 1995;**273**(18): 1421–8.

39 MRC Asymptomatic Carotid Surgery Trial (ACST) Collaborative Group. Prevention of disabling and fatal strokes by successful carotid endarterectomy in patients without recent neurological symptoms: randomised controlled trial. *Lancet* 2004;**363**(9420):1491–502.

40 Bonati LH, Dobson J, Algra A *et al.* Short-term outcome after stenting versus endarterectomy for symptomatic carotid stenosis: a preplanned meta-analysis of individual patient data. *Lancet* 2010;**376**:1062–73.

41 Jenkins J, Patel S, White CJ *et al.* Endovascular stenting for vertebral artery stenosis. *J Am Coll Cardiol* 2010;**55**(6):538–42.

42 Mendelow AD, Gregson BA, Fernandes HM *et al.* Early surgery versus initial conservative treatment in patients with spontaneous supratentorial intracerebral haematomas in the International Surgical Trial in Intracerebral Haemorrhage (STICH): a randomised trial. *Lancet* 2005;**365**:387–97.

43 van Gijn J and Rinkel GJE. Subarachnoid haemorrhage: diagnosis, causes and management. *Brain* 2001;**124**:249–78.

44 Molyneux AJ, Kerr RSC, Yu L-M *et al.* International subarachnoid aneurysm trial (ISAT) of neurosurgical clipping versus endovascular coiling in 2143 patients with ruptured intracranial aneurysms: a randomized comparison of effects on survival, dependency, seizures, rebleeding, subgroups and aneurysm occlusion. *Lancet* 2005;**366**(9488):809–17.

45 Pickard JD, Murray GD, Illingworth R *et al.* Effect of oral nimodipine on cerebral infarction and outcome after subarachnoid haemorrhage: British aneurysm nimodipine trial. *BMJ* 1989;**298**:636–42.

CHAPTER 12
Stroke Rehabilitation

Lalit Kalra
King's College, London, UK

Introduction

Stroke is the leading cause of severe disability in most of the developed world. The World Health Organization (WHO) estimated that in 2002, 15.3 million people had a stroke worldwide, with more than one third, 5.5 million, resulting in death.[1] Population projections for Europe suggest that the proportion of the population aged 65 and over will increase from 20% to 35% by 2050 and this demographic shift will increase the number of acute stroke episodes from 1.1 to more than 1.5 million per year by 2025.[2] In addition to a high mortality, stroke is also associated with significant disability amongst survivors. Nearly 40% of stroke survivors had severe and 20% had moderate disability, which consumed nearly a third of all healthcare resources in a large community study in patients >80 years of age.[3] Stroke is also an expensive disease. The estimated average cost of a stroke varies between countries and the average cost of a stroke ranged from US$468 to $146 149 in a review of 120 studies across the world.[4] The average cost of stroke varied between $2822 in Eastern Europe and $12 883 in Japan to $22 377 in the United Kingdom, $24 548 in Sweden and $28 253 in the United States.[5] These costs do not take informal costs of care into account; when such costs are included, the total cost of stroke nearly doubles.[6] An estimation of total costs of stroke using a long-running community-based South London Stroke Register estimated that stroke costs in the United Kingdom totalled £9 billion per year with productivity losses due to morbidity and mortality accounting for £1.3 billion.[7]

Recent years have seen several developments to improve the management of stroke patients and reduce mortality, disability and costs associated with this disease. These range from advances in imaging techniques which improve diagnostic capabilities[8] and acute interventions aimed at reducing the size of brain injury[9], to improved acute care[10] and organized rehabilitation aimed at reducing residual dependence.[11] Despite the proven

Cardiovascular Disease and Health in the Older Patient: Expanded from 'Pathy's Principles and Practice of Geriatric Medicine, Fifth edition', First Edition. Edited by David J. Stott and Gordon D.O. Lowe.

efficacy of thrombolysis and optimism about physiological manipulations in the acute phase of stroke, these interventions will have only a modest impact on eventual outcome in the vast majority of stroke patients because of the limitations on their use.[12] On the other hand, over 300 randomized controlled trials provide a sound foundation for evidence-based practice in stroke rehabilitation, supplementing and often confirming decades of clinical experience.[13] Hence, early and planned multidisciplinary rehabilitation remains the cornerstone of stroke management in the foreseeable future because it is applicable to most stroke survivors and has a strong evidence base for effectiveness in all patients, regardless of stroke severity.

The neurological basis of recovery

The principle that underlies all rehabilitation is that the brain has an inherent capacity to recover lost function after stroke.[14] This is based on observations that most survivors regain some or many of the functions lost as a result of the stroke. Recovery is of two types: intrinsic, which involves neuronal regeneration and setting up of new axonal connections; and adaptive, in which alternative strategies, usually behavioural changes, are used to overcome disability.[15] The majority of patients show both intrinsic and adaptive recovery, the proportion of each being dependent upon factors such as age, the severity of stroke, cognitive abilities and rehabilitation input after stroke. Intrinsic mechanisms consists of restitution, which includes repair of partially damaged pathways and strengthening of existing pathways, mediated by local changes in blood flow, neurogenesis and cell migration, growth factor release, metabolism or neurotransmitter concentrations. Diaschisis or substitution is the development of new, but functionally related, pathways in the unaffected areas of brain to take over the lost function. Studies in experimental models have shown a number of cellular and histological changes, such as axonal sprouting and formation of new dendritic connections, in the unaffected hemisphere of chronic stroke models, which probably are responsible for long-term recovery in these animals.[16] The degree of recovery due to intrinsic mechanisms is variable and may be incomplete in a significant number of patients. In these circumstances, re-education in compensatory techniques, either by changed use of the affected side or retraining of the unaffected side, becomes an important behavioural adaptation to improve function and reduce the level of disability posed by the impairment.[17]

The development of advanced neuroimaging techniques, such as PET and functional MRI, has helped to demonstrate the processes of reorganization of neural activity after stroke in human subjects.[18] These studies have shown that unilateral motor tasks are associated with activation

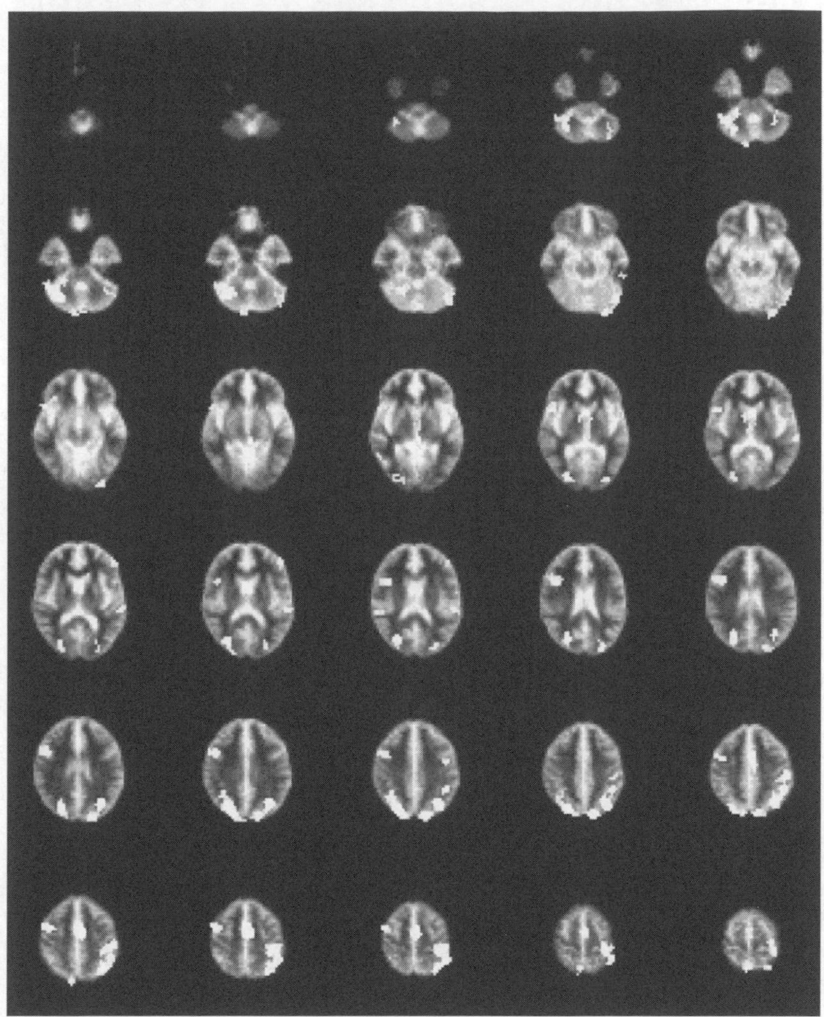

Group brain activation map in 5 subjects showing activation of the cerebellum, superior temporal gyrus, prefrontal cortex, SMA, PMC, lateral premotor cortex and somatosensory cortex on performance of the CRT

Figure 12.1 Activation on functional MRI during a choice reaction task (CRT) in a normal subject.

(increased metabolic activity) primarily in the contralateral sensorimotor cortex and the ipsilateral cerebellum in healthy subjects (Figure 12.1). The contralateral premotor cortex, ipsilateral somatosensory cortex and bilateral supplementary motor areas also participate in hand and finger motor tasks, particularly when the task increases in complexity. In recovered stroke patients, activation on these tasks is seen in the peri-infarct cortex and supplementary areas of the affected side (Figure 12.2) and also

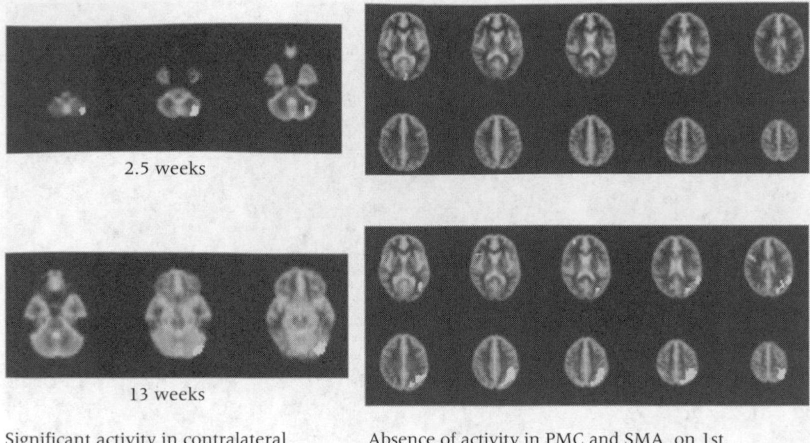
2.5 weeks
13 weeks
Significant activity in contralateral cerebellum persistent at 13 weeks
Absence of activity in PMC and SMA on 1st examination, remarkable increase Left PMC and PMA

Figure 12.2 FMRI on CRT using affected hand in a patient with small lacunar infarct in the left internal capsule.

in additional regions including the ipsilateral sensorimotor and premotor cortex (Figure 12.3). The cerebellum, thalamus and prefrontal areas play an important part in restoration of function. The process of reorganization is dynamic, there is an evolution of changes with time and several different patterns have been described. These include activation, and later extinction, of bilateral cerebellar and prefrontal areas, an initial increase followed by a decrease in activation of motor areas and progression from early contralesion activity to late ipsilateral activity.[19–22] All these changes appear to be associated with recovery, although their exact significance and relevance to recovery remains a subject of debate. It is now clear that there are multiple motor circuits in the brain that serve similar functions. Conventional pathways dominate in healthy subjects and inhibit the activity of alternate pathways in other areas of the brain. Disruption of traditional pathways in cerebral ischaemia reduces or eliminates the inhibition normally exerted by these pathways and allows activation of alternate pathways in the pre-motor areas of the affected side and primary motor areas on the unaffected side. Hence, the paradigm for function has shifted from strict cerebral localization to that of interactive functioning of diverse cortical areas activated by the constantly changing balance of inhibitory and excitatory impulses.

New evidence suggests that neurogenesis represents a key factor in plasticity of the normal brain in response to environmental stimuli, and that newly generated nerve cells form synaptic contacts which become fully integrated into existing neuronal circuitry.[15,23] Stroke-induced neurogenesis takes place in the subventricular zone and ischaemic boundary of adult human brains and has been demonstrated even in elderly patients

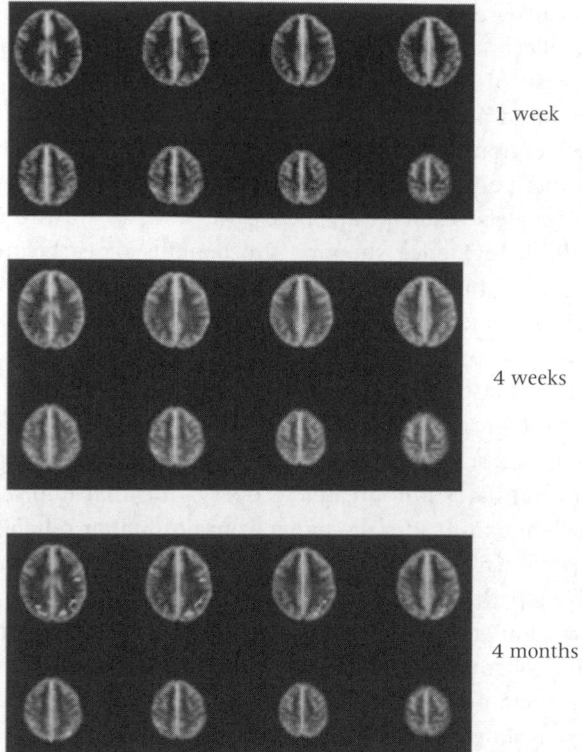

No activity in primary motor cortex or SMA associated with poor performance at 4 weeks but increased activity in ipsilateral parietal and occipital areas associated with clinical improvement at 4 months

Figure 12.3 FMRI on CRT using affected hand in a patient with cortical infarct in the right hemisphere.

up to 90 years of age.[24] Ischaemic injury to the brain sets up orchestrated waves of cellular and molecular events characterized by a reduction in growth-inhibitory molecules and activation of growth-promoting genes by neurons. Angiogenesis appears to be the first step in regeneration closely followed by the production and migration of neural progenitors.[25] Neural progenitors interact with other cells such as the astrocytes and oligodendrocytes and other growth factors, creating a microenvironment that promotes neurite outgrowth which repairs damaged connections or establishes new signalling pathways.[25]

An important concept in rehabilitation is that of 'brain plasticity', which implies that it is possible to modulate or facilitate reorganization of cerebral processes by external inputs.[23,26] This concept is supported by studies which show that activation can be facilitated by sensory stimulation, repetitive movement of the affected limbs or the use of drugs which modify neurotransmitter release.[27–29] Absence of adequate external inputs may have a negative effect – primate studies have shown that lack of afferent stimulation because of loss of voluntary activity impedes recovery in function after induced ischaemic injury to the brain.[30,31] The timing and intensity of intervention may also be important. Although some studies have suggested that very early attempts at intensive movement training in experimental models result in an increase in the size of the cortical lesion,[32] the bulk of evidence supports the benefits of early initiation of rehabilitation in animal models.[33] This emerging picture fits in well with theoretical concepts about motor learning, which emphasizes the importance of repetition, attention and goal-directed activity.

The observations made in animal experiments provide increasing support for some of the basic underpinnings of stroke rehabilitation; that is, the earlier rehabilitation is started the better the recovery, that greater intensity of treatment translates into greater recovery, and that improvement can continue for some time after discharge from hospital or rehabilitation centre.[34] Feys *et al.*, using a randomized controlled design, showed that adding an early, repetitive and targeted stimulation to the arm during the acute phase after a stroke resulted in a clinically meaningful and long-lasting effect on motor function in patients, even after 5 years of observation.[35] A meta-analysis of the effects of augmented exercise therapy after stroke has shown that such treatment has a small but favourable effect on activities of daily living (ADL) within the first 6 months after stroke.[36] Intensive language training has been shown to significantly improve language functioning and this correlated with cortical perilesional reorganization or plasticity.[37] In an observational study, Bode *et al.*[38], investigated the importance of therapy content and intensity after controlling for stroke severity and found that content and amount of therapy are important predictors of greater-than-expected gains in self-care and cognition. A small functional MRI study has demonstrated that drugs can modify reactivation and recovery; a single dose of fluoxetine resulted in significantly greater activation in the ipsilesional primary motor cortex and significantly improved motor skills on the affected side in patients with pure motor hemiparesis.[39]

To summarize, advances in basic sciences and clinical research are beginning to merge and show that the human brain is capable of significant recovery after stroke, provided that the appropriate treatments and stimuli are applied in adequate amounts and at the right time. There is also evidence to suggest that advances in pharmacotherapeutics and robotic assistive technology can further enhance and hasten the process of recovery, and will change the focus of rehabilitation from the intuitive methods employed at present to new strategies firmly rooted in the neuroscience of recovery.

Patterns of recovery

Recovery is fastest in the first few weeks after stroke, with a further 5–10% occurring between 6 months and 1 year. About 30% of survivors are independent within 3 weeks, and by 6 months this proportion rises to 50%.[40] Late neurophysiological recovery can continue for several years but is at a much slower rate and seldom results in dramatic changes in overall functional ability.[41] Completeness of recovery depends largely on the severity of the initial deficit. The more severe the initial deficit, the less likely it is that complete recovery will occur. The pattern of recovery is not uniform and shows considerable variation between individuals and also between different deficits in the same individual. There is currently no validated method for predicting the precise mode or degree of recovery for a given individual. In addition, there can be considerable variation in day-to-day progress of individual patients, which may mask overall recovery or at times give rise to false optimism. This problem can be overcome by monitoring patients over time, as overall trends are more important than 'one-off' assessments. Recovery may be affected adversely by the development of stroke-related complications. Comorbidity in elderly patients is another variable that affects overall recovery and rehabilitation.

The rate of recovery varies for different impairments and disabilities. Some problems such as homonymous hemianopia, dysphagia and sitting balance resolve very quickly in stroke survivors, whereas arm paralysis and language impairment recover more slowly and less completely. Perceptual problems may persist or take a very long time to recover. If all stroke survivors are considered, 62% are independent in self-care at 3 months and 66% at the end of 1 year, despite persistence of neurological deficit in some patients.[42]

Objectives of rehabilitation

Rehabilitation in stroke is not simply a matter of being treated by a therapist or a group of therapists but involves a whole range of approaches to managing disability, provided by a coordinated multidisciplinary team and tailored to restore patients to their fullest possible physical, mental and social capability.[43] The goals of rehabilitation are to:

- maximize patients' role fulfillment and independence in their environment within the limitations imposed by underlying impairment and availability of resources;
- make the best possible physical, psychological and social adaptation to any difference between the roles desired and the roles achieved following stroke;

- ensure the long-term well-being and quality of life of stroke survivors and their families by providing the necessary knowledge, skills and support using a range of health, social and voluntary services resources.

An important objective of the rehabilitation process is to monitor the relevance, quality and effectiveness of the services provided in order to ensure that they meet the expectations of patients and their families and obtain the best possible value for the money and effort being expended.

The revised World Health Organization International Classification of Impairments, Disabilities, and Handicaps (ICIDH) provides a conceptual model for stroke rehabilitation.[44] In this model, the terms disability and handicap have been replaced by limitations in activities and restriction in participation. The focus of attention shifts from pathology to handicap and from patient to environment during the course of rehabilitation.[45] The key areas that rehabilitation impacts upon are limitation of activity (disability) and restriction of participation (handicap). Disability is the lack of ability to perform an activity in the manner or within the range that the person was able to accomplish prior to the stroke and relates to function. In this context, the ability to undertake basic activities of self-care is fundamental to any physical rehabilitation programme. Handicap is the social consequence of disability and constitutes the limitations faced by stroke patients in fulfilling their normal role in society. It is not always possible to differentiate handicap from disability, and most pragmatic approaches tend to combine these two dimensions, referring to them as social disability.

Rehabilitation in stroke is essentially a multidisciplinary activity which has been described as a problem-solving educational process focusing on disability and intended to reduce handicap.[46] The basic principles that should be applied throughout rehabilitation of stroke patients are:

- documentation of impairments, disabilities and handicaps and, where possible, measuring them using simple, valid scales;
- maximization of independence and minimization of learned dependency;
- adopting a holistic approach to patients which takes into account their physical and psychosocial background, support mechanisms, as well as their environment;
- supporting caregivers and helping them to develop physical and psychological skills to provide long-term, sustainable support to stroke patients.

Process of rehabilitation

Rehabilitation has four important components: assessment, planning, intervention and evaluation.

Assessment

Assessment is fundamental to ascertain the precise nature and severity of deficits and define treatment goals prior to commencement of a rehabilitation programme because it provides a logical basis for treatment and management of stroke patients. The major reasons for undertaking assessments in stroke patients are to:

- define the type of patient, the extent of disability and the potential for recovery and/or responding to intervention (prognostication);
- identify main areas of difficulty and their underlying causes as well as the expectations of the patient and the family;
- monitor the process of rehabilitation (evaluation) and assess the degree of recovery or residual disability at the end of the rehabilitation process (outcome).

A large number of neurological, physical and functional assessments are currently available and can be divided into global assessments (which determine the overall impact of stroke) and specific assessments (which deal with a single level or domain of impairment or disability). Composite scores for global disease severity are unreliable because of the dominance of speech and language function over other indexes and because, when quite different disabilities are combined into one score, much specific information is lost.[47] Most scores also mix a variety of impairments and disabilities without considering their interactions.

The importance of knowing what information is wanted and why, that is, the purpose of a measure, is central to choosing any measure in rehabilitation. It is also important to decide on the least amount of information needed to achieve this purpose. The necessary characteristics of suitable measures are validity, reliability, sensitivity, simplicity and communicability. It is best to use existing measures wherever possible provided that they are valid for the purpose in mind, reliable in the circumstances proposed and relevant to the objectives of intervention. Moreover, the use of established measures makes communication and interpretation of data easier.

Predicting when a stroke patient has reached their full potential for recovery and may not benefit from further therapy inputs is an imprecise science. Estimation of the functional capacity for recovery is particularly important for chronic stroke patients (more than 1 year after stroke), especially as these are the patients most likely to be denied further rehabilitation inputs. Unfortunately imaging and electrophysiological techniques to aid such predictions have generally proven to be expensive and unhelpful in clinical practice. However, it may be possible to combine these modalities to develop algorithms for patient selection for both research and clinical programmes. A recent example of this was the combined use of transcranial magnetic stimulation (TMS) and MRI to determine the integrity of corticospinal tracts and predict functional recovery potential.[48] The study showed that motor evoked potentials to TMS in the affected limb in the presence of little or no asymmetry in the fractional anisotropy map of the internal capsule on MRI (indicative of minimal long tract damage) was associated with a potential for improvement up to 3 years after stroke.

Planning

Planning is the process of goal setting based on identification of aims, objectives and targets.[49] Goals can be set at different levels; most patients will have immediate goals which relate to basic personal activities of daily living such as achievement of sitting balance, independent transfers and independence in toiletting activities. As patients continue to improve goals need to be set for higher levels of function which incorporate not only independence in household activities but also the ability to undertake social, leisure and occupational pursuits. The ultimate goal of the rehabilitation programme is to improve overall well-being and participation but many rehabilitation programmes often stop once patients have achieved independence in personal activities of daily living. It is important that planning takes into account not only the immediate needs of the patients but also their potential needs when they return to their own environment. This often involves adapting rehabilitation to the home setting and addressing the needs of caregivers, many of whom will play an important role in providing ongoing support and management of disability at home.[50] The areas of practical importance in goal setting are:

- *Accommodation*: Where will the patient live and what physical adaptations will be needed?
- *Personal support*: What is the level of support available for existing caregivers and what extra help will be essential for the patient?
- *Life satisfaction*: What roles will the patient be fulfilling within his or her social setting and how will they be occupying their time?

Many difficulties arise in stroke rehabilitation because the goals of intervention are not set in advance or because these goals have not been discussed and agreed on by all relevant parties. Goals of rehabilitation vary according to the expectations of those involved. The goal of hospitals may be to discharge patients as soon as possible, whereas the goal of patients may be to return to their previous functional status even if this is unattainable. The goal of caregivers may be to minimize the level of input they need to provide even at the cost of institutionalization. Many of the difficulties ultimately faced in managing patients and in evaluating the effectiveness of interventions can be traced back to conflicts between the goals and objectives of different parties. An essential function of the whole rehabilitation team is to identify and modify unrealistically high (and sometimes unjustifiably low) expectations of patients and their families by making them more aware of the nature of residual deficit and expected prognosis as soon as these are reasonably clear. The two major problems that arise in goal setting include failure to use a common language in communication between various professionals or between professionals and patients and, second, failure to agree on a time frame within which the rehabilitation process must be accomplished.

Intervention

The minimum requirement of any stroke intervention is to provide care necessary to maintain *status quo* and prevent deterioration of the patient's condition or functional ability due to poor management or complications. Further intervention should be aimed at facilitating recovery and improving outcome by minimizing disability and preventing handicap. Although a large amount of time and resources are devoted to various therapy interventions after stroke, evidence suggests that these resources are not used optimally in many settings and many of the potential gains of therapy input are not realized because of organization and systems limitations.[51,52] There is also limited evidence on individual interventions because despite the large number of studies available, most studies have small and heterogeneous samples, small amounts of formal therapy have been given in any trial and the interventions most often become a comparison between different intensities of treatment. In addition, there is considerable diversity of outcome measures used in these studies and limited comparability of study designs.[53]

At present, there are many rehabilitation techniques available, some with more robust evidence than others in trial conditions but none that have been shown to be superior to any other in the major areas of physical therapy or in speech and language function in clinical practice. A summary list of current approaches has been given in Table 12.1 and some of the more commonly used approaches have been summarized.

Early mobilization

Early mobilization is a key rehabilitation strategy associated with good functional outcomes in several observational and controlled studies.[55] Despite this, mobilization protocols remain poorly defined and vary across units and across patients. A review which combined data from observational studies and meta-analyses was not able to find any positive, unequivocal benefit associated with early mobilization, independent of other aspects of stroke care[56] but concluded that early mobilization after

Table 12.1 A summary of rehabilitation techniques in stroke.[54]

- **Early mobilization**
  - Key strategy associated with good functional outcomes
  - Meta-analyses over 55 years: no positive independent benefit
  - Not harmful for most stroke patients
- **Restoration of motor function**
  - Balance and motor therapy ± sensory feedback effective for function and mobility
  - CIMT clinically relevant improvements in arm motor function
  - Robotic devices
- **Neuromuscular stimulation**
  - rTMS is associated with functional recovery in motor deficit, visuospatial neglect or aphasia
- **Motor imagery**
  - Positive effect arm function, promise for leg function
  - Virtual environments and tasks
  - Effects greater when combined with conventional therapy
- **Spatial Neglect**
  - Spatial techniques have limited success (prism adaptation)
  - Generalized attention enhancing techniques may be better

stroke was not harmful for most stroke patients and may contribute as part of routine stroke unit care in achieving good long-term outcome in stroke patients.

Restoration of motor function

Restoration of motor function is a primary objective of stroke rehabilitation and there are several pooled data analyses of studies on various strategies for improving motor performance in stroke patients.[57] A prospective meta-analysis of the effectiveness of bilateral movement training in post-stroke motor rehabilitation showed that bilateral movements alone or in combination with auxiliary sensory feedback were effective in improving functional and mobility outcomes in stroke patients.[58]

Treadmill training has been shown to improve gait and walking speeds significantly in hemiparetic patients when used as an adjunct to conventional treatment. There are many approaches to gait training but the most effective combination of training parameters, for example amount and timing of body support during the gait cycle, belt speed and acceleration, remains unknown.[59] The applicability of treadmill training in clinical practice is limited by the availability of specialist equipment and the technique may be suitable only for a small proportion of young stroke patients with relatively modest impairments.

Constraint induced movement therapy (CIMT) has been one of the most important and well-researched therapeutic approaches to restoring motor function. CIMT is based on the assumption that immobilization of the unaffected side to prevent learned 'non-use' and promote use of the affected limb results in faster (and more complete) recovery. The most convincing evidence for CIMT comes from the Extremity Constraint-Induced Therapy Evaluation (EXCITE) Trial.[60] The study showed that CIMT intervention in stroke patients was associated with statistically significant and clinically relevant improvements in arm motor function that persisted for at least one year. Despite this successful demonstration in a clinical trial, there continue to be doubts about the extent to which individualized CIMT is practical or cost-effective.[61] A meta-analysis has also suggested that recovery with CIMT is proportional to the amount of exercise given to the affected limb and it may be possible to achieve comparable benefits by less hazardous and less frustrating conventional therapy methods.[62]

Neuromuscular stimulation

Peripheral neuromuscular electrostimulation techniques appear to improve aspects of functional motor ability, motor impairment and normality of movement in recovering stroke patients.[63] A review of the use of repetitive transcranial magnetic stimulation (rTMS) in patients with post-stroke motor deficit, visuospatial neglect, or aphasia showed that low frequency rTMS to restore inhibition applied over the unaffected hemisphere or high-frequency rTMS to reactivate hypoactive regions applied over the affected hemisphere were associated with functional recovery.[64] There was great variation regarding the number of rTMS sessions required for a sustained effect and the timing of rTMS application after stroke.

Motor imagery

Recent years have seen several small clinical studies exploring the concept of motor imagery in stroke rehabilitation.[65] Most tasks involved mentally rehearsing movements of the arm and intervention periods varied from 2–6 weeks. The meta-analysis of these studies shows that mental practice has a positive effect on recovery of arm function and may have promise for improving leg function after stroke. The effects of motor imagery training appear even greater when combined with a conventional stroke rehabilitation programme in subacute stroke patients.[66]

Spatial neglect

A major advance in neglect rehabilitation is the shift of the conceptual paradigm from a spatial lack of awareness to a more generalized reduction in attentional abilities.[67] Non-spatial attention training has been shown to be associated with improvements in neglect, underpinned by changes in cortical activation patterns areas known to be associated with attention.[68] The clinical implications are that it may be possible to overcome spatial neglect in stroke patients by interventions that improve generalized or sustained attention. The expectation is that these techniques may prove to be more effective and have a sustained effect compared with conventional spatially oriented methods which did not result in sustained improvements in neglect that could be transferred to functional tasks.

Organized (stroke unit) care

Evidence suggests that organiszd care, such as that provided on stroke units, both facilitates neurological recovery and expedites discharges.[69] The conceptual rationale for organized stroke care is the awareness that stroke affects several domains of human performance and results in multiple impairments, many of which have significant interactions in determining the level of disability.[46] It is also clear that no single discipline has all the skills, resources and expertise required to manage all aspects of recovery from stroke. Facilitation of recovery is further compounded by the different speeds at which impairments recover as discussed previously, demanding a staged approach to interventions and therapy inputs. Rehabilitation goals are also shaped by the personal needs of stroke patients, the environment they will return to and the personal support available after discharge. Hence, the complex interdisciplinary process of stroke rehabilitation requires a multidisciplinary approach and collaborative policy of coordinated delivery of treatments based on comprehensive assessments and delivered by staff trained in stroke management in consultation with patients and their caregivers. This level of coordination of care is another argument to support the development of organized stroke services.[70]

The last two decades have seen a number of randomized controlled trials which suggested that organized care offered advantages to patients with stroke. However, many of these studies were too small to demonstrate a robust statistical benefit. Hence the Stroke Unit Trialists' Collaboration (SUTC) was set up to pool data from these and other ongoing studies from Australia, North America and Europe.[71] Despite the variation in methods of organized care and patient selection criteria, the meta-analysis of pooled data from 29 trials which included 6536 patients shows odds reductions in mortality of 0.86 (95% CI, 0.71–0.94), death or dependence of 0.78 (95% CI, 0.68–0.89) and death or institution of 0.80 (95% CI, 0.71–0.90) at 1 year associated with organized care, which are independent of age and gender.[72] More importantly and in contrast with thrombolysis for acute stroke, these benefits are seen for all stroke patients regardless of stroke aetiology or the duration between stroke onset and intervention. This expectation of the translation of trial efficacy into clinical effectiveness in mainstream practice has been further demonstrated in longitudinal studies.[73,74]

One of the difficulties faced in the interpretation of the evidence is that organized stroke care, especially stroke units, may mean different things to different people.[71] Definitions vary from 'a team of specialists who are knowledgeable about the care of stroke patients and who consult throughout a hospital or the community wherever a patient may be' to 'a geographic location within the hospital designated for stroke and stroke-like patients who are in need of medical and rehabilitation services and the skilled professional care that such an unit can provide'. There is also considerable controversy over the number and diversity of disciplines that need to be involved in stroke care, and differences in staff composition between different settings have limited the generalization of findings in individual settings.

There are also difficulties in assessing the independent benefits of different types of organization of stroke care, mainly because the comparators for organized care in different studies range from general medical wards to different types of organized care. This heterogeneity of comparisons makes it difficult to determine if one type of stroke care organization is superior to other methods of organizing stroke care, as there is no common yardstick against which the benefits of different strategies of stroke care can be measured. Langhorne *et al.* have shown that there is a definite benefit associated with comprehensive and rehabilitation stroke units and mixed rehabilitation units, all of which show an odds ratio of 0.85 to 0.89 in favour of organized care.[75] There may also be a possible benefit with acute (semi-intensive) units, although this just failed to achieve statistical significance (OR 0.88; 95% CI, 0.76–1.01). Mobile stroke teams were associated with no benefit in this analysis (OR 0.98; 95% CI, 0.95–1.05). There are no trials of acute intensive care, so this strategy of organizing stroke care remains untested. However, review of data suggests that emphasis on acute intensive care alone may not be adequate to change overall outcomes and that continuity of care is needed to realize the full potential of organized stroke unit care.

The amount of formal therapy received by stroke patients is small even in specialist stroke units. An important paper reported that patients spend more than 50% of their time in bed, 28% sitting out of bed, 13% in therapeutic activities and are alone for 60% of the time during the therapeutic day, even in a stroke unit.[76] The impact of a rehabilitation culture on therapy input was elegantly illustrated in the CERISE study, a comparison of stroke rehabilitation units across four settings in Europe.[77,78] The study showed that motor recovery outcomes after stroke varied significantly across Europe, and were not proportional to the therapy resources allocated to stroke but determined by the actual amount of treatment provided to stroke patients. For example, although the greatest amount of therapy resources being committed to stroke rehabilitation is in the United Kingdom compared with other centres (70 hours/week), stroke patients received the least amount of therapy input (1 hour/day) compared with others. Stroke patients in the United Kingdom spent nearly 65% of the therapeutic day sitting, lying or sleeping and had greater contact with visitors compared with therapists. In contrast, therapy input in Germany was structured and strictly timed resulting in significantly more time being spent with patients and with the best outcomes in Europe.

To summarize, there is consensus that well-organized and well-planned rehabilitation guided by well-defined goals based on adequate assessment and sensitive negotiation with patients and caregivers and provided in a specialist unit reduces disability and long-term institutionalization. There is, however, little evidence supporting any specific treatment technique for stroke patients. A pragmatic functional approach individualized for each patient's needs is recommended, and strict adherence to theories with little scientific basis or clinical evidence of effectiveness should be discouraged. There is evidence suggesting that early, intensive intervention by therapists may speed recovery and hasten discharge from the hospital without increasing the total amount of therapeutic input. However, observational studies suggest that therapy time may not always be optimally deployed and rehabilitation can be made more effective and efficient by addressing issues around the process of rehabilitation.

Evaluation

Evaluation is the process of monitoring a patient's progress (or lack of it) and assessing the effectiveness of the rehabilitation process itself. Objective assessment of effectiveness of stroke rehabilitation has proven difficult for several reasons. These include the confounding effect of spontaneous recovery from stroke, difficulty in defining the extent of need, and perceptions of good outcome, which may vary with the perspective of different observers. The wide variety of impairments and disabilities associated with stroke, as well as the large number of instruments available to measure each impairment and disability, have also contributed significantly to the lack of a common assessment for outcome in stroke rehabilitation. A sensible approach is to use simple assessments more frequently during the rehabilitation process to monitor and adjust the treatment programme. A review of studies on stroke rehabilitation has shown the predominance of activities of daily living (ADL) scales in monitoring rehabilitation.[79] This may be because the level of independence in ADL is not only the basis for more complete recovery but is also important in determining the care needs of, and resource use by, patients who continue to be dependent. Widespread use of ADL scales is further supported by the general agreement on the core ADL components (bladder and bowel function, feeding, cleanliness, dressing and mobility), high inter-rater reliability in clinical settings which is not influenced by the method of data collection, and communicability within multidisciplinary teams. On the other hand, ADL scales blur the distinction between impairment and disability, have a low ceiling effect and cannot identify the reasons why patients fail to achieve goals.

There is little consensus on the most relevant outcome, the method of measurement, or the most appropriate timing of such assessment in stroke patients.[45] The perception of a favourable outcome may vary depending upon professional, patient or carer perspectives and how long after stroke it is assessed. Although it has been recommended that outcomes should be measured at different levels within the ICIDH framework, patients will value their ability to undertake desired activities or to participate in social roles more than improvements in specific areas of performance. Even within the ICIDH framework, the rate and extent of change may vary between the different levels and continue over months. Consequently, it is important to consider the timing of any assessments and the influence of factors known to affect the chosen outcome measures. Measures at the level of activities (disability) are widely used for outcome and have the advantage of objectivity, reliability and sensitivity besides being simple and relevant to the patient. Measurement of participation and quality of life, however, may be more relevant and appropriate over the longer term. Appropriate timing of assessments is important and the natural history of recovery from stroke must be considered when selecting the time of assessment. Spontaneous recovery, especially in patients with greater severity of stroke, may not plateau until 6 months after the event. Most experts agree that 6 months is the most appropriate time point at which to measure neurological and functional outcome. Wider interactions with environment and society become important after this stage and measurement of participation, life satisfaction and emotionality should preferably take place at a time when the patient's social condition has stabilized.

Common problems in stroke rehabilitation

Stroke-related disorders that are important during rehabilitation include visual problems (hemianopia or inattention), dysphagia with the risk of aspiration and infection, communication problems, venous thromboembolism, urinary and bowel problems, spasticity and contractures, pressure sores, shoulder pain, associated reactions, cold hemiplegic arm and oedema of the limbs.[80] The main neurological complications include depression, seizures, behavioural changes and central pain. Stroke patients are also at a higher risk of falls which, in association with osteoporotic bone changes in the hemiplegic limb, often result in fractures on that side. Various studies have shown that complications occur in about 60% of stroke patients undergoing rehabilitation and are more frequent in patients with severe disability.[81]

Dysphagia

Dysphagia is a common complication of stroke; recent reviews show that its incidence ranges from 21–55% on clinical tests and 44–78% on videofluoroscopy (VF).[82] Although aspiration and dysphagia are not synonymous, many of the problems associated with dysphagia in stroke patients are because of aspiration and their close relationship means that there is considerable overlap between the assessment and management of these two conditions. In addition, a substantial number of patients have silent aspiration (aspiration without cough or any outward sign of difficulty) and are at an increased risk of developing complications because clinical swallowing assessments underdiagnose the problem and appropriate preventive strategies are not applied.[83] Dysphagia is associated with significantly higher mortality and morbidity in stroke patients, longer hospital stays, increased demands on feeding resources and higher admissions to nursing homes.[84] Evidence indicates that detection of aspiration and institution of appropriate management strategies reduces pneumonia, mortality, length of hospital stay and overall healthcare expenditure.[82] Dysphagia is also associated with malnutrition, poor participation in rehabilitation and worse functional outcome in survivors.[85,86] Although acute dysphagia improves in 80% of survivors, data from a 5-year follow-up of 1288 stroke patients in the South London Stroke Register showed that dysphagia at stroke onset was associated with a three- to fivefold increase in institutionalization at 5 years.[87] The prolonged duration of hospital stay, higher institutionalization and increased need for statutory support after discharge associated with dysphagia are estimated to cost the UK NHS £200 million per year.[88]

VF is the gold standard for assessment of dysphagia[89] but is not a feasible screening option in clinical settings.[83] The water swallowing test is routinely used in clinical practice but its diagnostic accuracy has been questioned.[83] However, it is likely to remain the mainstay of bedside screening because it is safe, relatively straightforward and easily repeated.[90] Decreases in blood oxygenation during swallowing and reduced ability to clear airways of aspirate have been observed in dysphagic patients, suggesting that oximetry may help in the diagnosis of aspiration.[91] Direct flexible endoscopy of the vocal cords and aspiration is another technique avialable to clinicians but requires expertise and validation in larger clinical studies.[92]

Current management options for dysphagia are limited.[2,14] Compensatory techniques and dietary modifications under the supervision of speech and language therapists and dieticians remain the mainstay of treatment of dysphagia in stroke patients. Patients with persistent dysphagia require alternative means of nutrition (e.g. nasogastric or percutaneous endoscopi garbrotomy (PEG) tubes). Other measures to alleviate swallowing problems include stimulation of the pharynx by mechanical or thermal means, cortical stimulation with magnetic fields to stimulate the swallowing reflex and insertion of artificial electrical pacemakers to trigger laryngeal elevation.

Dysphasia

Dysphasia is a defect in language function manifesting as impairment in speech production, comprehension, reading or writing in the absence of motor disturbances of voice production or writing, visual or auditory deficits, and intellectual or cognitive impairment. Impaired ability to understand speech is common in dysphasic patients. The difficulty in comprehension increases with increasing linguistic complexity of the speech presented and length of sentences used. The extent to which a dysphasic patient can understand what is being said is frequently overestimated, which can result in misunderstandings between patients and their families or professionals involved in patient care. It is important that communication problems are identified early in stroke patients because many therapy interventions are dependent on this function.

The more severe forms of dysphasia are often easy to diagnose on clinical examination in most stroke patients. The diagnosis of mild dysphasia may be more difficult, especially if the patient has a high-level language deficit. It is also important to differentiate dysphasia from confusion secondary to cognitive impairment. Enquiries about the patient's language background (native language, profession, social and educational status), previous speech problems and hand dominance should be part of the examination. Problems in comprehension are particularly difficult to assess. A bedside measure can be obtained by assessing the patient's ability to respond to commands of increasing complexity, either in content or in linguistic structure. It should be remembered that in some patients errors may occur because of dyspraxia or memory problems. All patients suspected of having dysphasia should be assessed by speech and language therapists regardless of the severity of the impairment. Appropriate treatment of dysphasic patients consists of individualized therapy programmes supervised by speech and language therapists, development of simple communication strategies to enable multidisciplinary rehabilitation, and educating caregivers in communication techniques appropriate to the patient's level of impairment.

Urinary Dysfunction in stroke

Urinary dysfunction is a common problem in stroke rehabilitation and occurs in approximately 37%–79% stroke patients. Common problems include incontinence, frequency, retention and infections. Many stroke patients regain continence in the first 2 weeks after stroke but as many as 15–20% patients may still be incontinent at 6 months. Urinary dysfunction, especially incontinence is associated with greater morbidity and poor functional outcomes at 3 months. Risk factors for urinary dysfunction include older age, increasing stroke severity, pre-morbid functional impairment, pre-existing urinary problems, diabetes mellitus, use of beta-blockers or antidepressants and post-void bladder residue of greater than 150 ml.

Several stroke and non-stroke related mechanisms contribute to urinary dysfunction during rehabilitation. Stroke related mechanisms include an "uninhibited bladder" due to lack of cortical control, hyperreflexia from disrupted neuromicturition pathways or stroke-related motor, cognitive, and language deficits. Non stroke related factors are bladder hyporeflexia caused by neuropathy due to age, diabetes or medication, depression, apathy or confusion, dependence on caregivers for transfers and mobility, difficulty to void in a socially appropriate manner and medications such as diuretics, anticolinergics or beta blockers.

There are very few randomised controlled trials on the efficacy of different interventions to improve bladder function after stroke. A stepwise approach is recommended starting with behavioural interventions followed by medication and even surgical interventions if required. The most common interventions include bladder training, continence nurse practitioner care, sensory-motor biofeedback techniques and various pharmacological treatments. There is some evidence to support the use of many of these techniques but no single treatment has been shown to be superior to others.

Caution needs to be exercised in the use of indwelling catheters in stroke patients undergoing rehabilitation. Early use of indwelling catheters inhibits regaining continence, increases risk of infections and causes inflammatory changes to the bladder wall that increase the risk of incontinence and infections. Routine use of indwelling catheters in stroke rehabilitation is not recommended and should be limited to patients who cannot be treated with other means. This includes patients with urinary outlet obstruction, those with skin breakdown in whom frequent bed or clothing changes would be difficult or painful and in patients were incontinence interferes with monitoring of fluid and electrolyte balance.

Perception

Perception is an important but neglected aspect of stroke management. The outcome of rehabilitation frequently depends on effective management of perceptual problems rather than on motor recovery alone. Despite this, perceptual problems are poorly understood and difficult to assess objectively because of the paucity of valid assessment instruments. Their management is equally difficult and a subject of great controversy. Perceptual problems after stroke can be divided into (1) neglect, which is the disregard of, and failure to attend to, one half of external space; (2) agnosias, which comprise problems with interpreting sensory data from the environment or the body (visual, tactile, autotopagnosia); and (3) apraxias, the collection of problems involving formulating, initiating or sequencing motor activity. Visuospatial dysfunction can be particularly disabling in stroke patients, as it affects their ability to judge distances and relationships between objects or between self and objects in a three-dimensional setting, causing severe restrictions in daily living activities. Patients with anosognosia are also difficult to rehabilitate because of the lack of awareness of any problems.

It is not known whether these deficits respond to general stimulation or to specific remedial measures. Recent research suggests that neglect may be amenable to therapeutic interventions such as prism correction, electrical stimulation and increasing attentional activities but further studies are required to confirm these findings. Although visuospatial problems delay or compromise functional recovery in most patients, some individuals eventually make full functional recovery despite residual impairments. There is no effective treatment for apraxia. Management currently focuses on increasing the patient's awareness of the condition and its effects. This requires early recognition of the problem and teaching of adaptive skills and coping strategies to patients and their relatives.

Tone and spasticity

The management of muscle tone is an integral part of therapy input in stroke patients. Muscle tone is a dynamic, complex process that is part of an overall pattern of posture and movement which plays a vital role in recovery from stroke. Appropriate management of tone is one of the fundamental principles of the Bobath method of facilitative physiotherapy, which gives priority to normalization of tone and improving symmetry even at the cost of postponing standing or walking. However, this pre-occupation with normalization of tone is not supported by evidence and there are several other approaches that combine early mobilization with active muscle tone management during rehabilitation.[93]

The management of abnormal tone and spasticity is difficult, as it depends on achieving the right balance between hypo- and hypertonia between different muscle groups. The problem is compounded by the fact that spasticity varies between different groups of muscles, times of day, emotional state of the patient, activity being undertaken and posture of the limb. Inappropriate exercise can result in inappropriate tone patterns to the ultimate detriment of the patient. If not managed correctly, spasticity leads to bad gait patterns, contractures and loss of function. Management of spasticity should be undertaken jointly by doctors and physiotherapists. Spasticity should be considered in relation to other impairments and in the context of therapy goals because interventions directed solely at reduction of spasticity are unlikely to result in significant functional gains.

Treatment of abnormal tone is initiated by physiotherapists, who can offer a range of interventions including physical therapy, attention to posture and seating and conventional orthoses. Drug therapy can be used in conjunction with physical manœuvres and adjusted to achieve optimal effects. Its main drawback is its lack of selectivity; since all muscle groups are affected equally, there may be undesirable hypotonia in some muscle groups (e.g. drugs for reducing spasticity in arm muscles may affect walking). In general, improvements in localized treatment of spasticity which can be administered selectively to specific muscle groups without major adverse effects have resulted in options like baclofen and dantrolene being replaced by botulinum therapy.[94]

The focal injection of botulinum toxin inhibits the release of acetylcholine into the synaptic cleft, resulting in a reversible paresis of the muscles relevant for the spastic deformity. It has has proven effective and well tolerated in several placebo-controlled trials for the treatment of focal upper and lower limb spasticity, although it has not been shown to improve motor function.[94] In a systematic review of 11 double-blind randomized placebo-controlled trials that included 782 patients, botulinum toxin reduced upper limb spasticity in patients post-stroke, but the improvement in functional ability was not established.[95] There were insufficient data to establish botulinum efficacy on lower limb spasticity.

Electrical stimulation techniques are a useful adjunct to other treatments, particularly for treating spastic equinus deformities. In some cases phenol nerve blocks can produce good results especially when standard treatments fail or botulinum toxin produces beneficial short-term effects. In patients refractory to medical treatments surgical interventions such as abalation of peripheral nerves, tenotomies or reconstruction of tendons and joints may be required.

The hemiplegic shoulder

Shoulder pain, restriction of movement and subluxation of the shoulder joint are common problems in stroke patients. In hypotonic patients, the loss of muscle strength around the shoulder joint and the weight of the paralysed arm may result in malalignment of the humeral head in the shallow glenoid cavity, predisposing to inferior subluxation of the shoulder. There is considerable variation in the reported incidence of subluxation in stroke patients, but it is estimated that one in every five patients is affected. Shoulder pain is more common and inconsistently related to subluxation. It is encountered in rehabilitation settings with disconcerting frequency and may be a result of spasticity in the shoulder muscles, glenohumeral subluxation, reflex sympathetic dystrophy (the shoulder-hand syndrome), or orthopaedic causes such as rotator cuff injury, arthritis or adhesive capsulitis made worse by immobility. Contributory factors include careless handling of patients and incorrect position of the hemiplegic arm. Management should be undertaken in collaboration with physiotherapists and includes measures such as proper positioning of the arm during periods of inactivity, avoidance of abnormal arm movements which cause excessive strain on the shoulder joint or inappropriate pulling of the hemiplegic arm during transfers and early passive exercise to prevent joint stiffness and contractures. Treatment with analgesics, strapping, non-steroidal anti-infammatory drugs and steroid injections may help in some patients.

Depression

Estimates of depression in stroke vary widely and it is estimated that between 30 and 60% of stroke patients have clinically significant depression, the highest prevalence and severity occurring in the first 2 years after stroke.[96] Diagnosis of mood disorders in patients with acute stroke is difficult because changes in appetite, sleep or interest (all indicative of depression) may be a normal adjustment response to physical disability and changed roles. The diagnosis of depression in stroke is further hampered by the presence of dysphasia and impairments in attention or concentration which make assessment difficult. A pooled estimate from population-based studies of individuals who have had a stroke indicated a prevalence of depression of about 33% at any time during follow-up.[97] There are no precise estimates on severity of depression after stroke, although most patients seem to have minor symptoms of depression. Women, younger patients and those with greater disabilities are at a higher risk of developing post-stroke depression.[98] Post-stroke depression also appears to be more common in patients with a family or personal premorbid history of depression.

Post-stroke depression may last for 7–8 months or more without treatment and is highly correlated with failure to resume premorbid social and physical activities. Depression also has a negative effect on functional and cognitive recovery, integration into the family environment, and caregiver stress in stroke patients.[99] There is growing evidence suggesting that early recognition of depression in stroke and early treatment with appropriate antidepressants can facilitate recovery.[100] Specific treatment strategies, including counselling, cognitive behavioural therapy and treatment with antidepressants, have been used for treating post-stroke depression with variable results. A systematic analysis involving 1655 patients with stroke who underwent treatment for depression after stroke showed some effect of pharmacotherapy (i.e. tricyclic antidepressants, selective serotonin re-uptake inhibitors, monoamine oxidase inhibitors, and others such as flupentixol/melitracen, reboxetine and trazadone) in improving mood but no effect on cognitive functions, activities of daily living or in reducing disability.[101] Psychotherapy was ineffective in improving mood or overall functioning in patients with stroke and depression and had no effect on activities of daily living or social functioning.

Pain

Pain assessment in stroke patients can be difficult but a population-based study has shown that nearly one third of stroke patients have moderate to severe pain in the first few months after stroke.[102] Although pain improves spontaneously in most cases, it can interfere with physical therapy, interrupt sleep and contribute to depression. Post-stroke pain can be caused by pre-existing arthritis, decreased mobility, changes in gait and abnormal body posture. Patients with spino-thalamic involvement may develop a central post-stroke pain syndrome, which is often associated with sensory loss.[103] Central post-stroke pain syndrome can be difficult to treat but may respond to amitriptyline or gabapentin.

Fatigue

Many patients suffer from fatigue after a stroke, which can be long lasting and cause functional limitations. Although post-stroke fatigue has been attributed to depression, physical deconditioning, associated medical ailments and effects of medications are likely to be contributory factors.[104] Treatment of post-stroke fatigue involves treatment of underlying causes; no specific treatment has been shown to be any benefit.[105]

Psychosocial aspects

Stroke is a major life event which presents major difficulties for patients, their spouses and their families. It may result not only in physical dependency but also requires a wide range of emotional and social adjustments within families, often leading to role reversals and establishment of new hierarchies.[106] The post-stroke phase is a period of considerable turmoil during which patients and their families need to be supported in order to achieve good outcomes. The reaction to stroke is akin to bereavement; a phase of shock and despondency is followed by a period of positive thinking and optimism as patients focus on the activities of the rehabilitation team. Many patients and caregivers harbour unrealistic hopes of recovery and it becomes important for the clinician to prevent unrealistic expectations and pave the way to more successful adaptation to the reality of residual disability. People who were very active and independent prior to stroke feel distressed when they need to rely on others for even the most basic personal tasks. This loss of esteem may lead to apathy and even depression and is more likely to happen in the paternalistic environment of hospitals. The attitude and approach of the medical team are crucial in enabling the patient to maintain dignity. Esteem plummets when patients are not given much attention on hospital rounds or are depersonalized by staff who refer to them as 'CVAs' or 'hemis' rather than considering them as unique individuals. Stroke patients may need counseling as well as practical support to cope with the fears of disfigurement, loss of physical function, falls, poverty and an uncertain future after returning home. Alterations in personality may occur after stroke and are a source of great distress to spouses and caregivers of stroke patients.

Conclusion

Stroke is a devastating illness and causes long-term disability which dramatically and irreversibly changes the lives of patients and their families. Although there is great optimism that improvements in preventive care and acute interventions will reduce the burden of stroke, their potential remains to be realized. Meanwhile, organized coordinated rehabilitation provided by specialists and in partnership with patients and their caregivers offers the only realistic hope of reducing disability and handicap after stroke. Despite its proven effectiveness, specialist stroke rehabilitation is not available to the majority of stroke patients who stand to gain from this input. A part of the problem is the lack of infrastucture, resources, staff and training to provide specialist care. This is compounded by the lack of awareness of the special needs of stroke patients and the benefits of dedicated rehabilitation amongst some professionals. Increased resources may be hard to achieve in the short term but improving the level of awareness amongst health professionals may prove a quicker, simpler and effective way of improving stroke outcome.

Key points

- Stroke is the leading cause of severe physical disability in adults.
- The brain is capable of significant recovery after stroke, provided that appropriate treatments are applied in adequate amounts and at the right time.
- Early and planned multidisciplinary rehabilitation remains the cornerstone of stroke management.
- Rehabilitation is a multidisciplinary problem-solving, educational process focusing on disability and intended to reduce handicap.
- Objectives of rehabilitation should include supporting and training caregivers in disability management.

References

1 Johnston SC, Mendis S and Mathers CD. Global variation in stroke burden and mortality: estimates from monitoring, surveillance, and modelling. *Lancet Neurol* 2009;**8**(4):345–54.

2 Truelsen T, Piechowski-Jozwiak B, Bonita R *et al.* Stroke incidence and prevalence in Europe: a review of available data. *Eur J Neurol* 2006;**13**(6):581–98.

3 Marini C, Baldassarre M, Russo T *et al.* Burden of first-ever ischemic stroke in the oldest old: evidence from a population-based study. *Neurology* 2004;**62**(1):77–81.

4 Evers SM, Struijs JN, Ament AJ *et al.* International comparison of stroke cost studies. *Stroke* 2004;**35**(5):1209–15.

5 Luengo-Fernandez R, Gray AM and Rothwell PM. Costs of stroke using patient-level data: a critical review of the literature. *Stroke* 2009;**40**(2):e18–e23.

6 Youman P, Wilson K, Harraf F and Kalra L. The economic burden of stroke in the United Kingdom. *Pharmacoeconomics* 2003;**21**(Suppl. 1):31–9.

7 Saka O, McGuire A and Wolfe C. Cost of stroke in the United Kingdom. *Age and Ageing* 2009;**38**(1):27–32.

8 Liebeskind DS. Imaging the future of stroke: I. *Ischemia. Ann Neurol* 2009;**66**:574–90.

9 Wardlaw JM, Murray V, Berge E and Del Zoppo GJ. (2009) Thrombolysis for acute ischaemic stroke. *Cochrane Database Syst Rev* **4** (Art. No.: CD000213).

10 Evans A, Perez I, Harraf F *et al.* Can differences in management processes explain different outcomes between stroke unit and stroke team care? *Lancet* 2001; **358**:1586–92.

11 Kalra L and Langhorne P. Facilitating recovery: evidence for organized stroke care. *J Rehabil Med* 2007;**39**(2):97–102.

12 del Zoppo GJ. Thrombolysis: from the experimental findings to the clinical practice. *Cerebrovasc Dis* 2004;**17**(Suppl. 1):144–52.

13 Teasell R, Foley N, Salter K *et al.* Evidence-based review of stroke rehabilitation: executive summary, 12th edition. *Top Stroke Rehabil* 2009;**16**(6):463–88.

14 Nudo RJ. Plasticity. *NeuroRx* 2006;**3**(4):420–7.

15 Cramer SC. Repairing the human brain after stroke: I. Mechanisms of spontaneous recovery. *Ann Neurol* 2008;**63**:272–87.

16 Steinberg BA and Augustine JR. Behavioural, anatomical and physiological aspects of recovery of motor function following stroke. *Brain Res Rev* 1997;**25**:125–32.

17 Wade D. Rehabilitation therapy after stroke. *Lancet* 1999;**354**:176–7.

18 Johnston MV. Plasticity in the developing brain: implications for rehabilitation. *Dev Disabil Res Rev* 2009;**15**(2):94–101.

19 Takahashi CD, Der Yeghiaian L and Cramer SC. Stroke recovery and its imaging. *Neuroimaging Clin N Am* 2005;**15**(3):681–95.

20 Pineiro R, Pendlebury S, Johansen-Berg H and Matthews PM. Functional MRI detects posterior shifts in primary sensorimotor cortex activation after stroke: evidence of local adaptive reorganization? *Stroke* 2001;**32**(5):1134–9.

21 Small SL, Hlustik P, Noll DC *et al.* Cerebellar hemispheric activation ipsilateral to the paretic hand correlates with functional recovery after stroke. *Brain* 2002;**125**: 1544–57.

22 Butefisch CM, Kleiser R and Seitz RJ. Post-lesional cerebral reorganisation: evidence from functional neuroimaging and transcranial magnetic stimulation. *J Physiol Paris* 2006;**99**(4–6):437–54.

23 Zhang ZG and Chopp M. Neurorestorative therapies for stroke: underlying mechanisms and translation to the clinic. *Lancet Neurol* 2009;**8**(5):491–500.

24 Minger SL, Ekonomou A, Carta EM *et al*. Endogenous neurogenesis in the human brain following cerebral infarction. *Regen Med* 2007;**2**(1):69–74.
25 Ratan RR, Siddiq A, Smirnova N *et al*. Harnessing hypoxic adaptation to prevent, treat, and repair stroke. *J Mol Med* 2007;**85**:1331–8.
26 Hodics T, Cohen LG and Cramer SC. Functional imaging of intervention effects in stroke motor rehabilitation. *Arch Phys Med Rehabil* 2006;**87**(12 Suppl. 2):S36–42.
27 Hamdy S, Rothwell JC, Aziz Q *et al*. Long-term reorganization of human motor cortex driven by short-term sensory stimulation. *Nat Neurosci* 1998;**1**(1):64–8.
28 Richards LG, Stewart KC, Woodbury ML *et al*. Movement-dependent stroke recovery: a systematic review and meta-analysis of TMS and fMRI evidence. *Neuropsychologia* 2008;**46**(1):3–11.
29 Tombari D, Ricciardi MC, Bonaffini N *et al*. Functional MRI, drugs, and poststroke recovery. *Clin Exp Hypertens* 2006;**28**(3–4):301–7.
30 Nudo RJ, Milliken GW, Jenkins WM and Merzenich MM. Use-dependent alterations of movement representations in primary motor cortex of squirrel monkeys. *J Neurosci* 1996;**16**:785–807.
31 Schallert T, Leasure JL and Kolb B. Experience-associated structural events, subependymal cellular proliferative activity, and functional recovery after injury to the central nervous system. *J Cereb Blood Flow Metab* 2000;**20**(11):1513–28.
32 Kozlowski DA, James DC and Schallert T. Use-dependent exaggeration of neuronal injury after unilateral sensorimotor cortex lesions. *J Neurosci* 1996;**16**:4776–86.
33 Biernaskie J, Chernenko G and Corbett D. Efficacy of rehabilitative experience declines with time after focal ischemic brain injury. *J Neurosci* 2004;**24**(5):1245–54.
34 Teasell RW and Kalra L. What's new in stroke rehabilitation: back to basics. *Stroke* 2005;**36**(2):215–7.
35 Feys H, De Weerdt W, Verbeke G *et al*. Early and repetitive stimulation of the arm can substantially improve the long-term outcome after stroke: a 5-year follow-up study of a randomized trial. *Stroke* 2004;**35**:924–9.
36 Kwakkel G, van Peppen R, Wagenaar RC *et al*. Effects of augmented exercise therapy time after stroke: a meta-analysis. *Stroke* 2004;**35**:2529–39.
37 Meinzer M, Elbert T, Wienbruch C *et al*. Intensive language training enhances brain plasticity in chronic aphasia. *BMC Biol* 2004;**2**:20.
38 Bode RK, Heinemann AW, Semik P and Mallinson T. Relative importance of rehabilitation therapy characteristics on functional outcomes for persons with stroke. *Stroke* 2004;**35**:2537–42.
39 Pariente J, Loubinoux I, Carel C *et al*. Fluoxetine modulates motor performance and cerebral activation of patients recovering from stroke. *Ann Neurol* 2001; **50**(6):718–29.
40 Wade DT and Hewer RL. Functional abilities after stroke: measurement, natural history and prognosis. *J Neurol Neurosurg Psychiatry* 1987;**50**:177–82.
41 Skilbeck CE, Wade DT, Hewer RL and Wood VA. Recovery after stroke. *J Neurol Neurosurg Psychiatry* 1983;**46**:5–8.
42 Kotila M, Waltimo O, Niemi ML *et al*. The profile of recovery from stroke and factors influencing outcome. *Stroke* 1984;**15**:1039–44.
43 Harvey RL. Tailoring therapy to a stroke patient's potential. *Postgrad Med* 1998; **104**:78–88.
44 Centers for Disease Control and Prevention. (2011) *Classification of Diseases, Functioning, and Disability*. Available at: www.cdc.gov/nchs/about/otheract/icd9/icfhome.htm (last accessed June 2012).

45 Duncan PW, Jorgensen HS and Wade DT. Outcome measures in acute stroke trials: a systematic review and some recommendations to improve practice. *Stroke* 2000; **31**:1429–38.

46 Wade DT and de Jong BA. Recent advances in rehabilitation. *BMJ* 2000;**320**: 1385–8.

47 Wade DT. (1992) *Measurement in Neurological Rehabilitation*, Oxford University Press, Oxford.

48 Stinear CM, Barber PA, Smale PR *et al.* Functional potential in chronic stroke patients depends on corticospinal tract integrity. *Brain* 2007;**130**:170–80.

49 Wade DT. Evidence relating to goal planning in rehabilitation. *Clin Rehab* 1998;**12**:273–5.

50 Dewey HM, Thrift AG, Mihalopoulos C *et al.* Informal care for stroke survivors: results from the North East Melbourne Stroke Incidence Study (NEMESIS). *Stroke* 2002;**33**:1028–33.

51 Kalra L, Evans A, Perez I *et al.* Training carers of stroke patients: randomised controlled trial. *BMJ* 2004;**328**:1099.

52 Kalra L and Walker MF. Stroke rehabilitation in the United Kingdom. *Top Stroke Rehabil* 2009;**16**(1):27–33.

53 Teasell RW, Foley NC, Salter KL and Jutai JW. A blueprint for transforming stroke rehabilitation care in Canada: the case for change. *Arch Phys Med Rehabil* 2008;**89**(3):575–8.

54 Kalra L. Stroke rehabilitation 2009: old chestnuts and new insights. *Stroke* 2010;**41**(2):e88–90.

55 Fjaertoft H, Indredavik B, Johnsen R and Lydersen S. Acute stroke unit care combined with early supported discharge. Long-term effects on quality of life. A randomized controlled trial. *Clin Rehabil* 2004;**18**(5):580–6.

56 Diserens K, Michel P and Bogousslavsky J. Early mobilisation after stroke: review of the literature. *Cerebrovasc Dis* 2006;**22**(2–3):183–90.

57 Kalra L and Ratan R. What's new and exciting in stroke regenerative medicine. *Stroke* 2008;**39**(2):273–5.

58 Stewart KC, Cauraugh JH and Summers JJ. Bilateral movement training and stroke rehabilitation: a systematic review and meta-analysis. *J Neurol Sci* 2006;**244**(1–2): 89–95.

59 Pohl M, Mehrholz J, Ritschel C and Ruckriem S. Speed-dependent treadmill training in ambulatory hemiparetic stroke patients: a randomized controlled trial. *Stroke* 2002;**33**(2):553–8 .

60 Wolf SL, Winstein CJ, Miller JP *et al.* Effect of constraint-induced movement therapy on upper extremity function 3 to 9 months after stroke: the EXCITE randomized clinical trial. *JAMA* 2006;**296**:2095–104.

61 Wolf SL. Revisiting constraint-induced movement therapy: are we too smitten with the mitten? Is all nonuse 'learned'? and other quandaries. *Phys Ther* 2007;**87**(9): 1212–23.

62 van der Lee JH. Constraint-induced therapy for stroke: more of the same of something completely different? *Curr Opin Neurol* 2001:**14**(6):741–4.

63 Brown JA, Lutsep HL, Weinand M and Cramer SC. Motor cortex stimulation for the enhancement of recovery from stroke: a prospective, multicenter safety study. *Neurosurgery* 2006;**58**(3):464–73.

64 Lefaucheur JP. Stroke recovery can be enhanced by using repetitive transcranial magnetic stimulation (rTMS). *Neurophysiol Clin* 2006;**36**(3):105–15.

65 Braun SM, Beurskens AJ, Borm PJ *et al.* The effects of mental practice in stroke rehabilitation: a systematic review. *Arch Phys Med Rehabil* 2006;**87**(6):842–52.

66 Sütbeyaz S, Yavuzer G, Sezer N and Koseoglu BF. Mirror therapy enhances lower-extremity motor recovery and motor functioning after stroke: a randomized controlled trial. *Arch Phys Med Rehabil* 2007;**88**(5):555–9.
67 He BJ, Snyder AZ, Vincent JL *et al.* Breakdown of functional connectivity in frontoparietal networks underlies behavioral deficits in spatial neglect. *Neuron* 2007;**53**:905–18.
68 Hillis AE. Rehabilitation of unilateral spatial neglect: new insights from magnetic resonance perfusion imaging. *Arch Phys Med Rehabil* 2006;**87**(12 Suppl. 2):S43–9.
69 Kalra L. The influence of stroke unit rehabilitation on functional recovery from stroke. *Stroke* 1994;**25**:821–5.
70 Langhorne P, Cadilhac D, Feigin V *et al.* How should stroke services be organised? *Lancet Neurol* 2002;**1**(1):62–8.
71 Stroke Unit Trialists' Collaboration. Collaborative systemic review of the randomised trials of organised inpatient (stroke unit) care after stroke. *BMJ* 1997;**314**: 1151–8.
72 Stroke Unit Trialists' Collaboration. (2002) Organised inpatient (stroke unit) care for stroke. *Cochrane Database Syst Rev* **1** (Art. No.: CD000197).
73 Irwin P, Hoffman A, Lowe D *et al.* Improving clinical practice in stroke through audit: results of three rounds of National Stroke Audit. *J Eval Clin Pract* 2005;**11**(4): 306–14.
74 Stegmayr B, Asplund K, Hulter-Asberg K *et al.* Stroke units in their natural habitat. Can results of randomised trials be reproduced in routine clinical practice? *Stroke* 1999;**30**:709–14.
75 Langhorne P for Stroke Unit Trialists' Collaboration. The effect of different types of organised inpatient (stroke unit) care. *Cerebrovasc Dis* 2005;**19**(Suppl. 2):17.
76 Bernhardt J, Dewey H, Thrift A and Donnan G. Inactive and alone: physical activity within the first 14 days of acute stroke unit care. *Stroke* 2004;**35**(4):1005–9.
77 De Wit L, Putman K, Schuback B *et al.* Motor and functional recovery after stroke: a comparison of 4 European rehabilitation centers. *Stroke* 2007;**38**:2101–7.
78 De Wit L, Putman K, Dejaeger E *et al.* Use of time by stroke patients: a comparison of four European rehabilitation centers. *Stroke* 2005;**36**:1977–83.
79 Kwakkel G, Wagenaar RC, Kollen BJ and Lankhorst GJ. Predicting disability in stroke: a critical review of the literature. *Age and Ageing* 1996;**25**:479–89.
80 Kumar S, Selim MH, Caplan LR. Medical complications after stroke. Lancet Neurol 2010; 9: 105–18.
81 Kalra L. (2007) Medical complications after stroke, in *Textbook of Stroke Recovery and Rehabilitation* (ed. J Stein, R Harvey, R Macko and R Zorowitz), Demos Medical Publishing, New York.
82 Martino R, Foley N, Bhogal S *et al.* Dysphagia after stroke: incidence, diagnosis, and pulmonary complications. *Stroke* 2005;**36**(12):2756–63.
83 Ramsey DJC, Smithard DG and Kalra L. Early assessments of dysphagia and aspiration risk in acute stroke patients. *Stroke* 2003;**34**(5):1252–7.
84 Smithard DG, O'Neill PA, Park C *et al.* Complications and outcome after acute stroke: does dysphagia matter. *Stroke* 1997;**27**:1200–4.
85 Sharma JC, Fletcher S, Vassallo M and Ross I. What influences outcome of stroke – pyrexia or dysphagia? *Int J Clin Pract* 2001;**55**(1):17–20.
86 Singh I, Vilches A and Narro M. Nutritional support and stroke. *Hosp Med* 2004; **65**(12):721–3.
87 Smithard DG, Smeeton NC and Wolfe CD. Long-term outcome after stroke: does dysphagia matter? *Age and Ageing* 2007;**36**(1):90–4.
88 Healthcare for London. (2007) *A Framework for Action*, 2nd, NHS London, UK.

89 Mann G, Hankey J and Cameron D. Swallowing function after stroke. *Stroke* 1999; **30**:744–8.

90 Martino R, Pron G and Diamant N. Screening for oropharyngeal dysphagia in stroke: insufficient evidence for guidelines. *Dysphagia* 2000;**15**:19–30.

91 Ramsey DJC, Smithard DG and Kalra L. Can pulse oximetry or a bedside swallowing assessment be used to detect aspiration following stroke? *Stroke* 2006;**37**(12): 2984–8.

92 Warnecke T, Teismann I, Oelenberg S *et al.* Towards a basic endoscopic evaluation of swallowing in acute stroke – identification of salient findings by the inexperienced examiner. *BMC Med Educ* 2009;**9**:13.

93 Pomeroy VM and Tallis RC. Physical therapy to improve movement performance and functional ability post-stroke. Part I. Existing evidence. *Rev Clin Gerontol* 2000;**10**:261–90.

94 Hesse S and Werner C. Poststroke motor dysfunction and spasticity: novel pharmacological and physical treatment strategies. *CNS Drugs* 2003;**17**(15):1093–107.

95 Elia AE, Filippini G, Calandrella D and Albanese A. Botulinum neurotoxins for post-stroke spasticity in adults: a systematic review. *Mov Disord* 2009;**24**(6):801–12.

96 Rao R. Cerebrovascular disease and late life depression: an age old association revisited. *Int J Geriatr Psychiatry* 2000;**15**:419–33.

97 Hackett, ML, Yapa C, Parag V and Anderson CS. Frequency of depression after stroke: a systematic review of observational studies. *Stroke* 2005;**36**:1330–40.

98 Carota A, Berney A, Aybek S *et al.* A prospective study of predictors of poststroke depression. *Neurology* 2005;**64**:428–33.

99 Robinson-Smith G, Johnston MV and Allen J. Self-care, self-efficacy, quality of life, and depression after stroke. *Arch Phys Med Rehabil* 2000;**81**:460–4.

100 Rigler SK. Management of poststroke depression in older people. *Clin Geriatr Med* 1999;**15**:765–83.

101 Hackett ML, Anderson CS, House A and Xia J. (2008) Interventions for treating depression after stroke. *Cochrane Database Syst Rev* **8** (Art. No.: CD003437).

102 Jönsson AC, Lindgren I, Hallström B *et al.* Prevalence and intensity of pain after stroke: a population-based study focusing on patients' perspectives. *J Neurol Neurosurg Psychiatry* 2006;**77**:590–5.

103 Andersen G, Vestergaard K, Ingeman-Nielsen M and Jensen TS. Incidence of central post-stroke pain. *Pain* 1995;**61**:187–93.

104 Choi-Kwon S, Han SW, Kwon SU and Kim JS. Poststroke fatigue: characteristics and related factors. *Cerebrovasc Dis* 2005;**19**:84–90.

105 McGeough E, Pollock A, Smith LN *et al.* (2009) Interventions for post-stroke fatigue. *Cochrane Database Syst Rev* **8** (Art. No.: CD007030).

106 Robinson RG, Murata Y and Shimoda K. Dimensions of social impairment and their effect on depression and recovery following stroke. *Int Psychogeriatr* 1999; **11**:375–84.

CHAPTER 13

Communication Disorders and Dysphagia

Pamela M. Enderby

University of Sheffield, Sheffield, UK

Communication

Effective communication allows an individual to convey successfully a message or meaning to another person and for that meaning to be correctly interpreted. Communication is one of the most fundamental characteristics of higher cognitive functioning and is dependent upon symbolic encoding, either in sounds, script or gesture. These complex acts are supported by virtually every aspect of brain function, with the afferent sensory stimuli being processed through associated regions, being integrated with stored memories and emotions along with immediate factors relating to attention, arousal and motivation which can stimulate a verbal or gestural response governed by different environmental and behavioural conditioning.

In its simplest form, communication requires one individual to be able to receive a message from another, either auditorily or visually, to interpret this message and to generate an appropriate response which is encoded into sounds, gestures or written letters in order to respond. Thus, the term 'language' refers to a code used to represent and communicate ideas and feelings. Language may be verbal or non-verbal, for example written words, sign language, gestures. However, all modes are governed by rules shared within cultures. Speech is the verbal expression of language which comprises both the meaning (semantics) and sounds (phonology). Language can also be expressed through writing using symbols (as in letters) or agreed body movements for signs (e.g. sign language or gestures).

Ageing and communication

There is evidence that language is an inherent capacity and that the neural basis for language is not only a dynamic process but prewired biologically.[1]

Cardiovascular Disease and Health in the Older Patient: Expanded from 'Pathy's Principles and Practice of Geriatric Medicine, Fifth edition', First Edition. Edited by David J. Stott and Gordon D.O. Lowe.

Researchers have investigated the capacity for language in different animal species and although some animals, particularly apes, can be taught to use symbols, humans appear to be specifically, physically and neurologically adapted for the integrated neurocognitive requirements for complex speech and language. Much work has been done on the development of language from birth during its rapid acquisition stage. Less work has been conducted examining the effects of ageing on communication processes later in life.[2] However, it is clear that changes in vision and hearing, laryngeal function and cognitive function impact upon the effectiveness of communication. For example, less cognitive agility may reduce the facility to make inferences when complex language structures are used; the use of stereotypical phrases to fill in language when original vocabulary is less easily accessed and a slight deepening and huskiness in the voice may all be associated with normal communication changes associated with age. Many of these will be subtle and will not be evident in casual conversation.[3]

The impact of age-associated changes on the sensory systems is likely to have a profound effect on communication, but it is difficult to define exactly when the normal deterioration in hearing and eyesight becomes pathological and affects communication more extremely.[4]

Hearing

The prevalence of hearing impairment depends upon the criteria used to define it. However, many studies have indicated that between 30 and 40% of older people (over the age of 70 years) have a hearing loss of 25 dB hearing level. This level would affect the ability to hear normal conversation. Although men are more likely to have more severe hearing level loss than women, increasing age is by far the major determinant in predicting who is likely to have a hearing difficulty. A decrease in overall hearing acuity is often accompanied by disproportionate difficulty in discriminating higher frequency sounds and a lowering of the threshold at which sounds cause discomfort. These age-related changes are called *presbycusis*. Distortions of the speech signal result in misinterpretation and misunderstanding, which have implications for easy and effective communication and also cognition and mood.

Hearing loss can be profoundly isolating and reduce enjoyment in many activities, and is frequently associated with depression.[5] For many elderly individuals, communication problems and related psychosocial difficulties resulting from hearing impairments could be reduced significantly by the use of hearing aids.[6] However, a high proportion of those provided with hearing aids do not use them. One study indicated that only 21% of hearing-impaired elderly individuals provided with a hearing aid used them. Improved usage is associated with the provision of a hearing aid accompanied by an education program. This should include information on how physically to manipulate the aid itself in addition to giving encouragement to develop the necessary tolerance in order to become accustomed to the different auditory input provided through a hearing aid. Thus, provision of a hearing aid is not an end in itself and is unlikely to lead to successful improvement in communication.[7]

Vision

This chapter would be incomplete without mentioning the contribution of vision to communication but, as this is less central, only an outline is given. Visual changes occur with age and affect depth perception, colour sensitivity, the ability to focus and the ability to adapt to changes in lighting. In addition, a number of visual impairments, such as cataract, glaucoma and macular degeneration, are associated with increasing age. Vision obviously affects reading and writing, but reduced ability to see gestures and facial expressions or to recognize people can impair the communication process in a more subtle manner.[8] One of the concerns to speech and language therapists is that visual and hearing impairments can profoundly affect an individual's response to rehabilitation of acquired dysphasia or dysarthria. Detailed speech and language assessments usually require reasonable vision and hearing; hence patients with defects in these may be more difficult not only to treat but also to evaluate and diagnose.

Cognition

There is a close relationship between thought and language and it has been suggested that various types of cognitive decline, including specific dementia types, lead to fundamentally different communicative symptoms. However, with cognitive decline, pragmatic dysfunction leading to incompetence in communicative processes is more frequently evident than linguistic difficulty. Thus, a person may have appropriate language structure, but may use the language in a way that does not communicate effectively, either by ignoring the context, lacking coherence or showing difficulty in sticking to a topic.

Studies have indicated that certain cognitive abilities, such as accessing vocabulary, may be insensitive to age-related changes until the age of 75–85 years.[9] The main difficulty in normal ageing is associated with slowing of processing time and less resistance to distraction.[10] However, the prevalence of dementia increases with age, rising from around 1% at age 65 years to 35% at 85 years. The rate of increase for both genders is marked throughout ageing.[11] It is estimated that 30% of those with dementia do not get a diagnosis, particularly in the young onset group (aged under 65 years) who are usually diagnosed late in the course of their dementia.[12]

Dementia can be seen as going through three stages, progressing from mild, through moderate to severe loss of function. Language can be affected at each stage, causing difficulties in understanding and expression and may, along with memory problems, be an early indicator of the condition. Individuals may demonstrate word-finding difficulties, particularly for objects and people's names, and use empty phrases (i.e. without meaning). Additionally, the individual has difficulty in focusing on a topic of conversation and may start in the middle of a topic, with no reference to the listener's knowledge or understanding of the subject. This difficulty in providing relevant information for the listener causes communication to break down and is frequently misunderstood by the communication partner.[13,14]

Persons with age-related cognitive disorders affecting communication can be assisted by speech and language therapists. The therapist will undertake a differential communication assessment and advise the patient and carers on strategies to improve effectiveness of interaction. These strategies include reducing the use of pronouns such as 'he' or 'she' and referring to people or things by name; avoiding open-ended questions, for example giving definite options; encouraging gesture and using communication prompts such as pictures and charts.[15]

A review of recent research indicates that multi-modality intervention that included physical exercise, volunteer work and exercises to help memory and language can have beneficial effects provided that participants are physically able to complete the intervention. The training of caregivers of patients with Alzheimer's disease about the disease, communication strategies and the use of memory books and wallets can help to improve their communication interactions with patients with this disease.

Motor speech

The power and range of movement may be affected by age; this can subtly change respiration, phonation and articulation, allowing the listener frequently to identify a speaker that they cannot see as being older or younger. The voice becomes less robust with the onset of tremulous, frail or a thinned quality. It is possible that these changes are associated with some adaptation of the laryngeal cartilages, thickening of the vocal folds and reduction in respiratory support.

Depression

There is a high prevalence of depression in older people and this has been found to be higher than that of dementia.[16] It has an impact on communication, leading to reduced communication, less interest in the communication of others and a general withdrawal from social groups. Depression has been associated with grieving over loss of functions (such as hearing and physical dependence), loss of autonomy and control over life, loneliness and anxiety about the future. Depression can be so profound that it can mimic a cognitive dysfunction or aphasia and in all cases will mean that rehabilitation of another specific communication disorder will be rendered more difficult. Identifying whether depression is a component of the communicative disorder is essential as its treatment can assist with general management of other physical deficits.

Diagnosis and assessment of communication disorders

The specific communication disorders associated with age-related pathologies, such as stroke, progressive neurological disease or dementia, are dysphasia, dysarthria and dyspraxia. Dysphasia is commonly a consequence of left-hemisphere stroke which can also give rise to dyspraxia. Dysarthria is more commonly a symptom with bilateral hemisphere damage or damage to the cerebellum or extra-pyramidal system as a consequence of head injury, brain tumour or progressive neurological diseases such as Parkinson's disease.

Dysphasia

Dysphasia is a disorder of language which affects the ability to understand or to express oneself in speech or writing. While the term 'aphasia' denotes a greater severity, the terms are now frequently used interchangeably. Dysphasia is usually of sudden onset and results from focal brain damage. One third of stroke survivors are affected by aphasia and between 30 and 43% of those affected will remain severely affected in the long term.[17]

Traditionally, aphasia has been classified according to localization theory. Wernicke aphasia is correlated with damage to the left posterior region of the perisylvan cortex or primary language area. A lesion in this area frequently produces disturbances of auditory comprehension, inability to repeat and name objects, but with the preservation of verbal fluency. Paraphasic errors and indefinite pronouns pervade expressive language of Wernicke aphasic patients, who often retain inappropriate, but rich, intonation. In contrast, Broca aphasia is classically associated with lesions localized to the left anterior region of the perisylvan cortex. Broca aphasia is associated with less disordered comprehension, severe word-finding problems and marked impairment of fluency. Thus, the patient will give the appearance of struggling for speech. Studies have indicated that the more profound, debilitating aphasia (Wernicke) is associated with increasing age. Thus, a high proportion of stroke patients over the age of 80 years will have Wernicke aphasia profoundly affecting their comprehension ability. One of the hypotheses for this age-related shift in aphasia type is that cerebral damage has a more posterior focus with advancing age, which could be associated with aetiological changes.

More recently, speech and language therapists have adopted a cognitive neuropsychological model for diagnosing and managing dysphasia as this approach is of more direct assistance in planning and targeting therapeutic intervention. This model is based on the assumption that the language system is organized in an integrated and modular manner and that this can be selectively impaired by brain damage. Thus, once the particular modules have been identified by assessment, then treatment can either stimulate the use of this linguistic deficit or teach strategies to overcome or bypass that aspect of the system. Much research, most of which is based on single case studies, has identified particular patterns of language associated with disruptions to the neurolinguistic structure and has reported varying degrees of success in focusing therapeutic intervention.[18–20]

There is no universally accepted treatment which can be applied to every aphasic person.[21] This is due to the great variation of persons with aphasia, in terms of symptoms and their severity, and in individual differences in lifestyle needs and preferences. A Cochrane review by Greener *et al.*[22] emphasized the importance of functional approaches to therapy, stating that 'The aim of rehabilitation in aphasia is primarily to maximise successful communication in day-to-day interactions' (p. 35).

In general, aphasia therapy strives to improve an individual's ability to communicate through multiple strategies by aiming to

- help the person to use remaining abilities;
- restore language abilities as much as possible by developing strategies;
- compensate for language problems;
- learn other methods of communicating;
- coach others (family, health and social care staff) to learn effective communication skills to maximize the aphasic patient's competence.

About half of recovery from stroke occurs within the first month, but it can continue up to 6 months post-stroke (according to Wade, 1997, cited by Greener *et al.*[22]) and beyond. However, single and group case studies have demonstrated improvements in language recovery after many years post-stroke.[18,23,24] There is evidence for the potential of neuroplasticity in the brain, that is, the ability of the brain to use other regions for functions where the original region has been damaged and that early, intense treatment can enhance this.[17]

It is important for all healthcare professionals to be able to have a good understanding of the communicative ability of a patient with aphasia – particularly confidence in the level of comprehension, in order that the patient is engaged in decisions and engaged in giving informed consent appropriately. There are several bedside screening tests that can assist with identifying the level and nature of dysphasia, for example the Frenchay Aphasia Screening Test.[25] The more formal speech and language therapy assessments provide a detailed description of the neurolinguistic and functional aspects of the aphasia which would inform speech therapy intervention, for example the Comprehensive Aphasia Test.[26]

A review of recent research indicates that when all other factors (e.g. health, education and social status) are held constant, chronological age alone is not a good predictor of either severity or prognosis in aphasia, with some very elderly patients improving and recovering remarkably well. However, the risk of concomitant problems is greater with increasing age and these may well contribute to a less good outcome. For example, patients who have aphasia alongside age-related memory problems or hearing loss provide more challenges to rehabilitation.

A recent Cochrane review of the impact of speech and language therapy for persons with dysphasia[27] along with two meta-analyses[28,29] indicate that speech language therapy is effective for people with aphasia. There are features of therapy that may make treatment more successful, for example timing, intensity and involvement of family and friends. More intense therapy of longer duration results in greater gains for aphasic individuals. There seems to be little difference between different types of aphasia therapy. Family and volunteer involvement is successful and results in better outcomes for individuals with aphasia. Laypersons can be effectively trained to deliver some aphasia therapies. Novel computer-based therapies can reduce therapist time, are acceptable to patients and are effective. Augmentative and alternative communication (AAC) devices can be successfully used with aphasic individuals, some of whom may be more suited to the use of such devices. It is important to remember that the effectiveness of therapy relies strongly on patient participation and motivation.

The use of computers to deliver therapy to people with aphasia is growing in popularity. Many studies indicate that language treatment can be made accessible for frequent practice and can be adapted to address different deficits and language styles and can implement structured approaches to neurolinguistic learning. Single case and group studies using both qualitative and quantitative methodologies indicate encouraging progress with computer-delivered treatment.[30] Additionally, there is growing recognition relating to the social consequences of aphasia to the patient and the family and increasing evidence that a holistic life-long approach to support a person with aphasia improves the quality of life, preventing isolation, depression and withdrawal from society.[31]

Assessment of mental competence and comprehension is important in some cases where the need for informed consent, power of attorney or testamentary capacity is being considered. While observation and subjective opinion may lead to a particular conclusion, it is essential to support and/or test this with objective tests and consider other influences, for example social pressures, perseveration, fatigue and poor attention span which may affect ability.[15]

Dyspraxia of speech

Dyspraxia of speech refers to the inability to carry out fine voluntary movements necessary for speech, while voluntary and automatic movements of the same muscles often remain intact. Thus, a patient may be unable to stick their tongue out on command but can lick their lips to remove a crumb (oral dyspraxia). Muscular weakness may be absent or insufficient to account for the speech difficulty and the patient may produce expletives or automatic speech (as in counting) clearly but is unable to imitate sounds and words (verbal dyspraxia). Speech is characterized by effortful groping and patients have difficulty in imitating and repeating sounds and words. Patients with dyspraxia frequently do not have difficulty with other oral motor tasks such as controlling saliva or swallowing, and this can help distinguish dyspraxia from dysarthria where those functions are frequently abnormal. Dyspraxia rarely exists without some degree of dysphasia and may lead to individuals being thought of as having more language impairment than is the case; it is primarily associated with cortical damage.

Dysarthria

Speech requires accurate motor programming, initiation and control of fine movements of the lips, tongue, palate and larynx, which act in harmony with timing of inspiration and expiration. This results in the precise articulation, pitch and tonal quality, resonance and phrasing which are associated with normal speech.[32] Impairment of the central peripheral nervous system can affect this choreography and produce a motor speech disorder termed *dysarthria*. Again, the term anarthria usually indicates a more severe form of the disorder.

The different types of abnormal speech can indicate the level of underlying neurobiological dysfunction (Table 13.1).

Traditionally, speech and language therapists have managed dysarthria by assisting in differential diagnosis, treating the speech problem and preventing secondary complications by facilitating participation in normal activities (Yorkston, 1996, cited in Sellars *et al.*[34]). Evaluation of speech and language therapy of this kind of group has been deeply problematic given the heterogeneous nature of the underlying impairments, making single

Table 13.1 Speech symptoms associated with underlying pathology.

Type	Features
Spastic	Strained and hoarse voice, hypernasality and slow, imprecise articulation (Aronson, 1993, cited in Palmer *et al.*[33]). Often accompanied by swallowing and drooling difficulties[33]
Flaccid	Isolated areas of involvement depending on which motor neurone is affected (Enderby, 1983, cited in Palmer *et al.*[33])
Ataxic	Excess loudness, tremor and irregular articulatory breakdowns (Aronson, 1993, cited in Palmer *et al.*[33]). Intonation, pitch and volume can also be affected (Enderby, 1983, cited in Palmer *et al.*[33]), in addition to difficulty with alternate tongue movements
Hypokinetic	Breathy monotone voice with reduced loudness (Enderby, 1983, cited in Palmer *et al.*[33]) and articulation tends to be accelerated and imprecise (Yorkston *et al.*, 1999, cited in Palmer *et al.*[33])
Hyperkinetic	Features strained hoarseness and voice arrests
Mixed	Similar symptoms to spastic dysarthria and tends to be accompanied by a wet-sounding voice with rapid tremor, poor laryngeal and tongue movements and poor control of lips (Enderby, 1983, and Aronson, 1993, cited in Palmer *et al.*[33])

case studies the most usual method for evaluation. Frequently people with dysarthria benefit from augmentative or alternative communication methods.

Augmented and alternative communication

Augmentative and alternative communication (AAC) refers to any system of communication that is used to supplement or replace speech, to help people with oral communication impairments to communicate. For individuals with aphasia or dysarthria, this could range from 'low-tech' aids such as drawing and writing or communication books, to 'high-tech' aids such as computerized voice output communication aids.

The objectives of introducing AAC to a patient with an acquired communication problem is to maximize their communicative function in the areas of life that are seen as a priority by the patient and to continually review the changing needs of the patient. It is necessary to[35]

- identify participation and communication needs;
- assess capabilities in order to determine appropriate options;
- assess external constraints;
- find strategies for evaluating the success of interventions.

To ensure appropriate access to the range of resources available, individuals who may benefit from communication aids should have access to an AAC specialist or team, who are skilled in assessment, planning, intervention and continuing support in this area.

Swallowing

The normal swallow

Swallowing involves a process of transporting saliva, food and drink from the mouth to the stomach and it involves the protection of the respiratory system from being entered by anything other than air. Normal swallowing is easy, quick and unconsciously performed, but it is a highly complex process carried out more than 1000 times per day in normal adults just to clear saliva from the mouth to the oesophagus. In the one second that it takes to swallow to clear the mouth of saliva, over 40 paired muscles are used.[36] The mouth, nose and pharynx are passages for food and air in addition to being involved in speech. The mechanisms for using these pathways appropriately can be affected by central and peripheral neural or structural damage. Swallowing necessitates cessation of respiration with closure of the airway, while the pharynx is being used to transport saliva, liquids or foodstuff. Alterations in tone, pressure or timing can cause aspiration, that is, the leakage of food or fluid into the airway. This will commonly cause coughing or choking as the system acts in a coordinated fashion to expel the foreign material and return it to the pharynx. However, silent aspiration can occur where food or liquid does not stimulate coughing or choking and penetration of the material is unimpeded.

Oral phase

Swallowing is frequently described as having three phases, the oral phase, the pharyngeal phase and the oesophageal phase. In the oral phase, sometimes termed the preparatory phase, food is taken into the mouth, chewed and moved back to the opening of the pharynx. The lips seal the oral cavity and the hyoid rises. At the start of the oral propulsion phase, the soft palate will seal off the nose prior to the tongue propelling the bolus into the pharynx. The oral phase is mainly under voluntary control and can be disturbed if the lips are affected and unable to make a good seal – this delays the initiation of the swallow. Facial palsy can lead to some of the bolus being deposited within the buccal sulcus and poor tongue movements will result in poor bolus control (Figure 13.1).

Pharyngeal/oesophageal phases

The pharyngeal phase is considered to start when the bolus touches the posterior pharyngeal wall. The nasal pharynx is sealed more tightly through the raising of the soft palate and the laryngeal inlet is sealed through raising the larynx, closure of the vocal folds and tilting of the epiglottis. Descending movements of the pharyngeal constrictor muscles squeeze the bolus down. The oesophageal phase is seen as the last phase

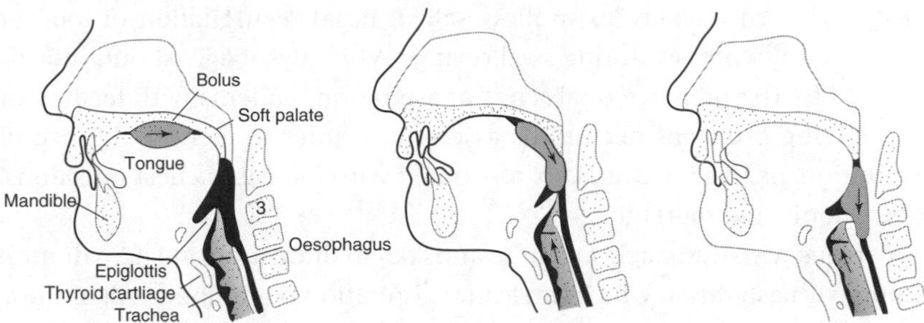

Figure 13.1 Normal swallowing process.

of swallowing; it is the involuntary transport of the bolus through the oesophagus to reach the stomach. Anatomically, the oesophagus starts at the upper oesophageal sphincter; this sphincter is frequently called the PE (pharyngoesophageal) segment or is otherwise known as the *cricopharyngeal sphincter*. This sphincter at rest is contracted and the bolus alone will not stimulate its release. It relaxes in concert with the pharyngeal bolus transport and opens in unison with the anterior movement of the larynx. This protects the pharynx from regurgitated food and prevents air from entering the oesophagus during breathing. The timing of the opening and closure of this sphincter can be problematic in many neurological diseases. If this sphincter is not released in a timely fashion, patients will complain that they have difficulty in pushing food down into their throat or they may have overspill aspiration with the bolus not clearing through the pharynx into the oesophagus before the airway becomes patent.

The ageing process alone affects deglutition with an increase in chewing movements in order to form a bolus and to initiate swallowing, a slowed swallowing propulsion time and a reduction in pharyngeal and oesophageal peristalsis. There is evidence that, with increasing age, the normal elderly person aspirates increasingly, but this may not give rise to any symptoms. The mechanisms for tolerating increasing aspiration are not fully understood. However, targeted assistance for those with dysphagia can reduce symptoms and improve weight gain and quality of life.[37]

Dysphagia

The broad term 'dysphagia' can encompass problems at the oral, pharyngeal or oesophageal stages of swallowing and should not be confused with difficulties with feeding or eating, which may be associated with anorexia, depression or other psychological problems or difficulties in transporting food from the plate to the mouth. Symptoms associated with dysphagia include choking during eating or drinking, difficulty in swallowing certain food types, an inability to swallow saliva, nasal regurgitation of food or drink and discomfort during swallowing. While dysphagia should not be defined by the presence or absence of aspiration, patients with feeding or swallowing problems need to be assessed in order to identify the risk of aspiration, as this is particularly associated with increased chest infections, pneumonia and mortality.

Persons with dysphagia are more at risk of malnutrition and dehydration along with aspiration which can lead to aspiration pneumonia. All of these complications can lead to poor outcome and can ultimately be the cause of death, but additionally there are profound social and psychological effects of swallowing disorders. Coughing and choking can be frightening for both the patient and carers. Dribbling/drooling can be socially offensive and embarrassing and have a severe effect on the quality of life of the patient.

Clinically, dysphagia is common with 78% of people having had a stroke initially presenting with this symptom and a high percentage of those with dementia and progressive neurological disease also having dysphagia. It presents a 'major diagnostic and therapeutic challenge'.[38] Interdisciplinary management of dysphagia is advocated[39]; the aim of this management is to protect the patient from complications of dysphagia, maintain adequate nutrition and ensure that patients and carers are fully aware of the nature of deficit and methods of managing the problems.

Assessment will in the first instance be done at the bedside (see Box 13.1) and will take account of the oral and laryngeal structures and movements, dental state, cognition, posture and other issues which can contribute to the safety of the patient to progress with oral feeding. It is important to note that the absence of the gag reflex does not automatically indicate a major swallowing problem, just as the presence of the gag does not indicate safe swallowing. Other factors, such as the bolus control, clarity of the voice (is it wet and gurgly after a test swallow?) and the effectiveness of the cough (is the cough firm and effective?) are all important. A therapist will frequently give different trial swallows of food substances (semisolid, firm, etc.) and liquid. Certain food substances may be more easily and safely transported and, therefore, there could be recommendations on the consistency of oral intake. If it is clear from the bedside assessment that there is a danger of aspiration, it may be necessary to request further assessment in a videofluoroscopy clinic which can determine more objectively the type and nature of the aspiration and whether positioning the patient or changing the consistency of the bolus can moderate such risk. However, there are certain guidelines that can assist with the management of any person with dysphagia. It is important to remember that it is very difficult to swallow safely if one is not fully conscious and aware. Furthermore, if a patient is unable to sit upright or cough purposefully, the likelihood

Box 13.1 Bedside swallow assessment

Risk indicators

- Weak, husky voice (dysphonia)
- Inability to cough voluntarily
- Weak cough – no effective expulsion
- Pooling of food or saliva in mouth/cheek
- Frequent coughing/choking even on saliva
- History of recent chest infection
- Complaints of difficulty with swallowing
- Reports having to gulp/or abnormal sensation
- Reports difficulty with some types of food

Observation

Try teaspoons of water, and if successful try teaspoons of soft purée, and then if successful try foods with more substance

Observe:

- Patient reports negative sensation
- Poor lip closure/degree of leakage
- Untimely or absent elevation of larynx
- Residue in mouth following swallow
- Lack of clarity of voice, following swallow
- Choking/coughing before, during or after swallow

of aspiration is increased. Any of the above would indicate a necessity for more in-depth dysphagia assessment.

Videofluoroscopy to assess swallowing is not infallible. The procedure can produce both false positives and false negatives. For example, the trial swallows may not produce, at the time of recording, evidence of dysphagia which in some patients occurs only with fatigue after several mouthfuls – a false negative. However, on other occasions, aspiration may be observed, which is asymptomatic or induced by the tension of the situation or unpleasantness of the radiopaque material – a false positive. The indications from videofluoroscopy must be placed in the context of the history of the patient.

Some patients are able to eat certain food textures more efficiently and safely. For example, persons with either reduced oral sensation, buccal control or inadequate laryngeal lift may aspirate more on fluids than on semisolids. Fluids do not stimulate the swallow reflex so rapidly, cannot be formed into a bolus, overflow into the pharynx and larynx without needing propulsion and leak into the larynx more readily. Therefore, some patients may be advised to avoid liquids, but may manage a soft puréed diet. Other patients may have difficulty in manoeuvring or forming a bolus due primarily to the involvement of tongue, lips and jaw and these patients may need to avoid foods that require chewing.

Problems with communication and/or swallowing are profoundly disabling to the patient and cause great anxiety to relatives. While some of these components may not resolve spontaneously or with treatment, they all deserve appropriate assessment and intervention aimed at improving the management of the symptoms, improving the quality of life by maximizing function and reducing secondary sequelae.

Key points

- Communication and swallowing impairments are profoundly disabling and impact upon the quality of life.
- Discriminating between dysphasia, dysarthria and dyspraxia is important for neurological diagnosis and therapeutic intervention.
- Patients need their level of comprehension to be assessed objectively by the speech and language therapist as it is frequently not what it seems.
- There is evidence that some patients continue to improve communication skills and swallowing function with therapy beyond the period of spontaneous recovery.
- Appropriate identification and management of dysphagia reduces mortality and morbidity.

References

1 Banich MT and Mack M (eds). (2003) *Mind, Brain and Language.* Multidisciplinary Perspectives, Lawrence Erlbaum Associates, Mahwah, NJ.

2 Heine C and Browning C. Communication and psychosocial consequences of sensory loss in older adults: overview and rehabilitation directions. *Disabil Rehabil* 2002;**24**:763–73.

3 Civil RH and Whitehouse PJ. (1991) Neurobiology of the aging communication system, in *Handbook of Geriatric Communication Disorders* (ed. DN Ripich), Pro-Ed Press, Austin, TX, pp. 5–19.

4 Gulya AJ. (2002) Disorders of hearing, in *Oxford Textbook of Geriatric Medicine* (eds JG Evans, TF Williams and BL Beattie), Oxford University Press, Oxford, pp. 893–8.

5 Dalton DS, Cruickshanks KJ, Klein B *et al.* The impact of hearing loss on the quality of life in older adults.. *Gerontologist* 2003;**43**:661–8.

6 Smeeth L, Fletcher A, Ng ES *et al.* Reduced hearing, ownership and use of hearing aids in elderly people in the UK – the MRC Trial of the Assessment and Management of Older People in the Community: a cross-sectional survey. *Lancet* 2002;**359**:1466–70.

7 Lesner SA and Kricos PB. Candidacy and management of assistive listening devices: special needs of the elderly. *Int J Audiol* 2003;**41**(Suppl. 2):2568–76.

8 Gravell R and Stevens S. (1998) *Communication disorders and dysphagia, in* Principles and Practice of Geriatric Medicine *(ed. M Pathy),* John Wiley & Sons Ltd, Chichester, p. 976.

9 Bouchard-Ryan E. (1991) Normal ageing and language, in *Dementia and Communication* (ed. R Lubinski), Singular Publishing, San Diego, p. 86.

10 Vliet E, Manly J, Tang MX *et al*. The neuropsychological profiles of mild Alzheimer's disease and questionable dementia as compared to age related cognitive decline. *J Int Neuropsychol Soc* 2003;**9**:720–32.

11 Knapp M, Prince M, Albanese E *et al*. (2007) *Dementia UK*, Alzheimer's Society, London.

12 Metcalfe S and Curtice M. (2008) *We Can No Longer Ignore Dementia – The National Dementia Strategy*. Available at: http://www.bgs.org.uk/index.php?option=com_content&view=article&id=730:curticedementiastrategy&catid=77:mentalhealth&Itemid=315 (last accessed June 2012).

13 Feyereisen P, Berrewaerts J and Hupet M. Pragmatic skills in the early stages of Alzheimer's disease: an analysis by means of a referential communication task. *Int J Lang Commun Disord* 2007;**42**:1–17.

14 Carlomagno S, Santoro A, Menditti A *et al*. Referential communication in Alzheimer's type dementia. *Cortex* 2005;**41**:520–34.

15 Enderby P. (1997) *Promoting communication in patients with dementia, in* Working with Dementia *(eds G Stoke and F Goudie)*, Winslow Press, Windsor.

16 Alexopoulos GS. Depression in the elderly. *Lancet* 2005;**365**:1961–70.

17 Bakheit AMO, Shaw S, Barrett L *et al*. A prospective, randomized, parallel group, controlled study of the effect of intensity of speech and language therapy on early recovery from post-stroke aphasia. *Clin Rehabil* 2007;**21**:885.

18 Hicklin J, Best W, Herbert R *et al*. Phonological therapy for word finding difficulties: a re-evaluation. *Aphasiology* 2002;**16**:981–99.

19 Nickels LA. Therapy for naming disorders: revisiting, reviving and reviewing. *Aphasiology* 2002;**16**:935–79.

20 Franklin SE, Buerk F and Howard D. Generalised improvement in speech production for a subject with reproduction conduction aphasia. *Aphasiology* 2002;**16**:1087–114.

21 Greener J, Enderby P, Whurr R and Grant A. Treatment for aphasia following stroke: evidence for effectiveness. *Int J Lang Commun Disord* 1998;**33**(Suppl.):158–62.

22 Greener J, Enderby P and Whurr R. (2000) Speech and language therapy for aphasia following stroke. *Cochrane Database Syst Rev* **2** (Art. No.: CD000425).

23 Fillingham JK, Sage K and Lambon Ralph MA. Further explorations and an overview of errorless and errorful therapy for aphasic word-finding difficulties : the number of naming attempts during therapy affects outcome. *Aphasiology* 2005;19:597–614.

24 Mortley J, Wade J and Enderby P. Superhighway to promoting a client–therapist partnership? Using the Internet to deliver word-retrieval computer therapy, monitored remotely with minimal speech and language therapy input. *Aphasiology* 2004;**18**:193–211.

25 Enderby P, Wood V, and Wade D. (2012) *Frenchay Aphasia Screening Test*, third edition. Stass Publications, St Mabyn, Cornwall, UK.

26 Swinburn K, Porter G and Howard D. (2004) *Comprehensive Aphasia Test*, Psychology Press, Hove.

27 Kelly H, Brady MC and Enderby P. (2010) Speech and language therapy for aphasia following stroke. *Cochrane Database Syst Rev* **5** (Art. No.: CD000425).

28 Robey RR. A meta-analysis of clinical outcomes in the treatment of aphasia. *J Speech Lang Hearing Res* 1998;**41**:172–87.

29 Whurr R, Lorch MP and Nye C. A meta-analysis of studies carried out between 1946 and 1988 concerned with the efficacy of speech and language therapy treatment for aphasic patients. *Eur J Disord Commun* 1992;**27**:1–17.

30 Petheram B (ed.). Computers and Aphasia: Special Issue of *Aphasiology*. *Aphasiology* 2004;**18**(3).

31 Parr S, Byng S, Gilpin S and Ireland C. (2007) *Talking About Aphasia*, Open University Press, Buckingham.

32 Palmer R and Enderby P. Methods of speech therapy treatment for stable dysarthria: a review. *Adv Speech Lang Pathol* 2007;**9**:140–53.

33 Palmer R, Enderby P and Cunningham S. The effect of three practice conditions on the consistency of chronic dysarthric speech. *J Med Speech Lang Pathol* 2005;**12**:183–8.

34 Sellars C, Hughes T and Langhorne P. (2005) Speech and language therapy for dysarthria due to non-progressive brain damage. *Cochrane Database Syst Rev* **3** (Art. No.: CD002088).

35 Beukelman DR and Mirenda P. (1998) *Augmentative and Alternative Communication: Management of Severe Communication Disorders in Children and Adults*, 2nd edn, Paul H. Brookes Publishing, Baltimore, MD.

36 Rubin JS and Bradshaw CR. (2000) The physiologic anatomy of swallowing, in *The Swallowing Manual* (eds JS Rubin, M Broniatowski and J Kelly), Singular Publications, San Diego, pp. 1–20.

37 Wright L, Cotter D and Hickson M. The effectiveness of targeted feeding assistance to improve the nutritional intake of elderly dysphagic patients in hospital. *J Hum Nutr Diet* 2008;**21**:555–62.

38 Nilsson HO, Eckberg R, Olsson R and Hindfelt B. Dysphagia in stroke: a prospective study of quantitative aspects of swallowing in dysphagia patients. *Dysphagia* 1998;**13**:32–8.

39 Carrau RL and Murry T. (1999) *Comprehensive Management of Swallowing Disorders*, Singular Publishing, San Diego.

CHAPTER 14
Peripheral Arterial Disease

Leocadio Rodríguez-Mañas, Marta Castro Rodríguez and Cristina Alonso Bouzón
Hospital Universitario de Getafe, Madrid, Spain

Introduction

Peripheral arterial disease (PAD) occurs when blood flow reaching limbs is insufficient to fulfill the metabolic necessities of the tissue. This often comes from the presence of occlusive arterial disease, the underlying disease process being atherosclerosis.

Epidemiology

Risk factors for PAD

The factors leading to PAD are mainly the same as those leading to atherosclerosis, a process that directly or indirectly accounts for 70% of all deaths in people older than 70 years. These factors are multiple: genetic factors, age, type 2 diabetes mellitus, hypertension, dyslipidaemia, smoking, physical inactivity and abdominal obesity.

The prevalence of PAD varies depending upon the characteristics of the population and the criteria used to define its presence.[1] There are two main methods to define PAD: the clinical one and the ankle-brachial index (ABI). The clinical method is based on the presence of the most classic symptoms of PAD, namely intermittent claudication (IC), characterized by the presence of exertional calf pain that causes the patient to stop walking, resolves within 10 minutes of rest, does not resolve while the patient is walking, and does not begin at rest. The ankle-brachial index (ABI), a ratio of the systolic blood pressures in the lower and upper extremities obtained by Doppler, is the most widely used diagnostic test for detecting PAD. Among the participants in the Cardiovascular Health

Cardiovascular Disease and Health in the Older Patient: Expanded from 'Pathy's Principles and Practice of Geriatric Medicine, Fifth edition', First Edition. Edited by David J. Stott and Gordon D.O. Lowe.

Table 14.1 Stages and symptoms of PAD.

Fontaine's stages Stage	Clinical
I	Asymptomatic
IIa	Mild claudication (more than 150 metres)
IIb	Moderate–severe claudication (less than 150 metres)
III	Ischaemic rest pain
IV	Ulceration or gangrene

Study, an epidemiological evaluation of 5084 community-dwelling men and women ≥65 years, the prevalence of PAD as defined by ABI was 12%, whereas only 2% of participants had IC.[2] The PARTNERS (PAD Awareness, Risk, and Treatment: New Resources for Survival) study, with 6979 men and women from primary care (aged 50–69 years with a history of diabetes mellitus or cigarette smoking and ≥70 years), which also used the ABI as the diagnostic criteria, found a prevalence of 29%. Only 11% of these patients with PAD had IC.[3] The majority of the men and women diagnosed with PAD based on the ABI do not have classic symptoms of IC. The prevalence of classic symptoms (Table 14.1) varies from ~10–30% in patients with PAD based on the ABI value.

The prevalence of PAD increases dramatically with age. The Cardiovascular Health Study found a prevalence of PAD around 30% in men >85 years while it was lower than 10% in men ranging from 65–69 years old. The prevalence of PAD in women aged from 65–69 years old was lower than 5%, but exceeded 35% in those aged 85 or older. This association between older age and higher prevalence of PAD was also observed in both women and men with a history of heart disease and stroke.[2] Data from 2174 subjects aged 40 years and older from The National Health and Nutrition Examination Survey 1999–2000 show a PAD prevalence of 4.3% (95% CI, 3.1–5.5%) in the whole sample, but among those 70 years or over the prevalence was 14.5% (95% CI, 10.8–18.2%).[4]

The pattern of the disease changes according to age: aorto-iliac disease occurs usually in younger subjects and is more rapidly progressive than distal disease.

Other risk factors besides age are smoking, diabetes, hypertension, dyslipidaemia and black race. In the National Health and Nutrition Examination Survey 1999–2000,[4] more than 60% of individuals with PAD had hypercholesterolaemia, 74% were hypertensive, 26% had diabetes and 33% were current smokers. Approximately 95% had, at least, one of these cardiovascular risk factors and 72% had two or more. When adjusted by age and gender, current smoking (OR 4.46; 95% CI, 2.25–8.84), diabetes (OR 2.71; 95% CI, 1.03–7.12), black race/ethnicity (OR 2.83; 95% CI,

1.48–5.42), low kidney function (OR 2.00; 95% CI, 1.08–3.70), hypertension (OR 1.75; 95% CI, 0.97–3.13) and hypercholesterolaemia (OR 1.68; 95% CI, 1.09–2.57) remained positively associated with prevalent PAD. After adjustment for smoking status, BMI, hypertension, hypercholesterolemia, diabetes and glomerular filtration rate, the smoking status (OR 4.23; 95% CI, 1.95–9.17), black ethnicity (OR 2.39; 95% CI, 1.11–5.12), diabetes (OR 2.08; 95% CI, 1.08–4.28) and low kidney function (OR 2.17; 95% CI, 1.10–4.30) remained significantly associated with the presence of PAD.

Smoking is a major and modifiable risk factor for PAD. Smoking not only predisposes to develop PAD but also increases its severity and affects the prognosis of revascularization interventions. In patients who smoke, PAD affects predominantly proximal arteries, especially the aorta and iliac arteries.[5]

The prevalence of PAD is approximately twice as high for individuals with diagnosed diabetes. Diabetes mellitus is not only a qualitative risk factor but also a quantitative one. In fact, glycaemic control is one of the strongest risk factors of illness: a positive, graded and independent association between HbA1c and PAD risk has been described in adult people with diabetes.[6] This association is stronger for clinical (symptomatic) PAD, where manifestations may be related to the existence of microvascular disease, than for asymptomatic PAD. The glycaemic control is also associated with the worst consequence of this disease: amputation. In this regard, amputation is 10 times more frequent in diabetic than in non-diabetic patients. This suggests that efforts to improve glycaemic control in persons with diabetes may substantially reduce the risk of PAD. However, the efficacy of an intensive glycaemic control (reaching HbA1c values lower than 7%) to prevent PAD as compared with other less stringent therapeutic goals (~8%) is not established and, in fact, may have adverse consequences. Another important risk factor to develop PAD in diabetic patients is the presence of albuminuria, whatever its magnitude. Diabetes causes predominantly distal occlusive disease, including the arteries of the calves and feet.[5]

Although arterial hypertension contributes to the development of PAD to a lesser extent than either of the two previously mentioned factors, it is also a risk factor that must be controlled. There are limited data regarding the association between hypertension and PAD according to lesion localization.[5]

Black ethnicity is a strong and independent risk factor for PAD. At first, some epidemiological studies suggested a differential relationship between risk factors and prevalence of lower peripheral disease in people from different ethnicities. However, data from recent studies cannot explain the excess risk of PAD in black people by a higher prevalence of diabetes or hypertension, increased BMI or higher levels of some of the new cardiovascular risk factors (interleukin-6, fibrinogen, D-dimer, homocysteine). This suggests that unknown factors may account for the residual differences. In clinical series, PAD in blacks is associated with poorer prognosis after revascularization because of the greater presence of distal lesions involved.[5]

The Cardiovascular Health Study assessed the incidence rate of abnormal ABI over time in a community population (5888 participants, men and women ≥65 years, without PAD) and tried to identify what cardiovascular risk factors were predictors of ABI decline. ABI decline occurred in 9.5% of this elderly cohort over 6 years and was associated with modifiable vascular disease risk factors: current cigarette use (OR 1.74; 95% CI, 1.02–2.96), hypertension (OR 1.64; 95% CI, 1.18–2.28), diabetes (OR 1.77; 95% CI, 1.14– 2.76), higher low-density lipoprotein cholesterol (LDL-C) level (OR 1.60; 95% CI, 1.03–2.51), and lipid-lowering drug use (OR 1.74; 95% CI, 1.05–2.89).[7]

Consequences of PAD

Peripheral arterial disease increases the risk of total mortality. Among these patients, more severe disease, as measured by the ABI, is associated with increased mortality. For example, mortality is higher in patients with an ABI less than 0.50 than in those with an ABI between 0.50 and 0.90. Traditionally, an ABI greater than 1.40 has been considered of little diagnostic value because it was believed that it indicates the presence of non-compressible lower extremity arteries. However, non-compressible arteries may be the manifestation of the presence of calcification of the media layer of the artery, a common condition in patients with diabetes and chronic kidney disease that is associated with increased mortality. Individuals with ABI values greater than 1.40 have a higher prevalence of intermittent claudication and atypical leg symptoms, suggesting an increased prevalence of PAD among these individuals. In fact, an ABI index higher than 1.40 is associated with an increased mortality. In this regard, the Cardiovascular Health Study found an increase in total mortality in patients with basal ABI greater than 1.40 compared with a normal ABI. The magnitude of this increased mortality risk in people with an ABI greater than 1.40 was similar to that observed in people with an ABI less than 0.90. This suggests that across the spectrum of ABI values, the association between the ABI and mortality appears to be 'U' shaped.[1]

Peripheral arterial disease is a strong predictor of subsequent cardiovascular morbidity and mortality. Associations between PAD and cardiovascular mortality are independent of age, BMI, cigarette smoking, LDL-C, HDL-C, blood pressure, fasting glucose levels and history of angina, myocardial infarction, stroke or other heart problems. This association has been observed in multiple populations (clinical and community settings, general population and special groups like elderly or diabetic patients, subjects with and without classic intermittent claudication, etc.). It has been reported over relatively short-term (3–4 years) and long-term (10 years) follow-up. Like the association between PAD and total mortality, the Strong Heart Study found a higher cardiovascular mortality risk if ABI was <0.90 or >1.40, describing a 'U' shaped line too. PAD is associated with prevalent cardiovascular disease and adverse cardiovascular disease risk factor profiles. Prospective studies using the ABI show in people with a low ABI, a higher incidence of stroke (mainly in older people), fatal and non-fatal coronary disease, heart failure and a poor prognosis in all forms of cardiovascular disease. Because of that, identifying persons at both ends of the ABI distribution may be a useful method for cardiovascular risk stratification and may also be an indication for a comprehensive management of cardiovascular risk factors.[8] However, in the cardiovascular risk stratification, it is not just the grade of PAD that is important. The progression of PAD, measured as the changes in ABI over time, can add information in this evaluation of the cardiovascular risk. Criqui *et al.* demonstrated that progressive PAD (ABI decline >0.15) was significantly and independently associated with an increased cardiovascular risk.[9]

In addition to the classical implications of PAD on cardiovascular disease, in elderly people PAD also plays a crucial role in determining an impaired functional status. Specifically, elders with PAD have lower physical activity levels, slower walking speed, poorer balance and poorer walking endurance. Data obtained from 1798 participants 60 years and older who participated in the population-based National Health and Nutrition Examination Survey,[10] showed several relevant findings about the relationship between PAD and physical function. Participants were asked about their dependence in performing several tasks (basic activities of daily living, instrumental activities, social activities, general physical activities and capacity to walk one-quarter mile and to walk up 10 steps). Trained health technicians measured ABI, maximal right leg force and gait speed. There were differences in both self-reported functional dependence and performance-based physical measures. Gardner and Montgomery[11] compared two groups of subjects 65 years and older, the first group with symptomatic PAD and the second one without illness. PAD patients had 28% shorter unipedal stance time, 86% higher prevalence of ambulatory stumbling and unsteadiness, and 73% higher prevalence of falling than non-PAD patients. Instability in patients with PAD was exacerbated in those with a worse ambulatory function and lower levels of physical activity. These findings remind us of the old scheme about the theoretical model of the pathway to late-life dependence proposed by Verbrugge.[12] He defined four related but different categories that represent the causal connection between pathology and actual dependence. These are: 'active pathology' (such as PAD), 'impairment' (such as low leg force or low ABI), 'functional limitation' (such as slow gait speed) and 'disability' (such as dependence in activity daily living). As a consequence, for a complete evaluation of an elderly patient with suspected PAD, performance-based physical measures (gait speed, strength, unipodal time, full tandem stance time, etc.) must be included.

Gardner *et al.*[13] followed 43 men limited by intermittent claudication (mean age, 69 years ±7) during 18 months to understand the natural evolution of physical performance in patients with PAD. They experienced a decline in 6-minute walk performance, monitored and self-reported physical activity, physical performance, measured and self-reported stability and calf blood flow despite no change in ABI. While it may be assumed that all these changes could cause an impaired balance and a higher prevalence of falling, putting PAD patients at higher risk for serious injury, restricted physical activity, higher cost and more frequent hospitalizations, higher nursing home admissions and greater mortality, the actual clinical consequences and prognostic significance of functional impairment in persons with PAD was unknown until the study by McDermott *et al.*[14] They carried out a prospective observational study with 638 participants followed for a median of 50 months. Among PAD participants, the risk of mobility loss, measured as the hazard ratio (HR), in the lowest versus the two highest quartiles of baseline performance for the 6-minute walk test was 9.65 (95% CI, 3.35–27.77, $p < 0.001$). For the Short Physical Performance Battery the adjusted HR was 12.84 (95% CI, 4.64–35.55, $p < 0.001$). They concluded that differences in the rate of mobility loss between PAD persons and healthy subjects appear to be primarily related to poorer lower extremity performance at baseline. The measures of lower extremity performance predict risk of mobility lost and risk of mortality;[15] they are simple and easy to perform in the office. So, they can be used to identify PAD persons at highest risk of mobility loss.

The 'vulnerability' of these patients could suggest a possible relationship between PAD and frailty. In The Cardiovascular Health Study the ABI was inversely related to frailty status, in elderly people with or without clinical cardiovascular disease.[16] The prevalence of progressively lower levels of ABI increased in each level of frailty (non-frail, pre-frail, frail). These data, along with the other results in the CHS, suggest that cardiovascular disease appears to be an important, but not sole, contributor to frailty.

Finally, the association between PAD and other apparently unlinked diseases must be emphasized. This is the case for depression and dementia. An increased prevalence of depression in patients with PAD has been detected. One explanation could be that the functional impairment accompanying PAD affects quality of life and may lead to depressive symptoms.

ABI is associated with the incidence of total dementia, vascular dementia and Alzheimer's disease,[17] as is shown in the data from the Honolulu-Asia Aging Study, a prospective community-based study of Japanese-American men, older than 70 years at baseline. The analysis included 2588 men who were free of dementia at the first assessment, had an ABI measurement, and were examined up to twice more for dementia. After adjustment for education, year of birth, high blood pressure, BMI, diabetes mellitus, cholesterol concentration, smoking status, alcohol consumption and apolipoprotein E4 allele, a low ABI was associated with an increased risk of dementia (HR, 1.66; 95% CI, 1.16–2.37) and vascular dementia (HR, 2.25; 95% CI, 1.07–4.73). ABI was weakly associated with Alzheimer's disease (HR, 1.57; 95% CI, 0.98–2.53), particularly in the apolipoprotein E4 carriers (HR, 1.43; 95% CI, 1.02–1.96).

The public is poorly informed about PAD. Current data suggest that PAD detection and treatment are lower than other forms of atherosclerotic disease, although there is evidence to support a prognostic significance and an impact on quality of life comparable to other forms of cardiovascular disease.[18] As a consequence it is essential to detect PAD as well as ischaemic heart disease and cerebrovascular disease.

Pathophysiology

Atherosclerosis is a long-lasting process of thickening and stiffness of the arteries, whose basic lesion is the atherosclerotic plaque. The evolution of atheroma involves several stages, which once breached, cause the 'harm'. Unfortunately this complex process does not follow an ordered fashion, because even if the lesions develop gradually, the first symptom of many injuries occurs suddenly. Therefore, early diagnosis of atherosclerosis is important. To that end, it is essential to detect disorders associated with endothelial dysfunction and its progression toward atherothrombosis long before they are visible obstructive lesions, which highlights the importance of early detection and treatment of vascular risk factors. It must be remembered that vascular disease is not simply a local process in a concrete plaque, but this is a widespread process that affects the entire vascular tree. This concept has therapeutic implications because it calls for an integrated treatment. Another important aspect of the pathophysiology of atherosclerosis in elderly people, and more specifically of the endothelial dysfunction, is which processes that occur at the endothelium are due to physiological ageing and which ones to the presence of other cardiovascular risk factors. In fact, some of the mechanisms involved in the development of endothelial dysfunction are shared by both ageing and cardiovascular risk factors (diabetes, hypertension, hypercholesterolemia),[19] as shown in

Figure 14.1. Moreover, the mechanisms by which vascular risk factors lead to vascular disease may be different in the elderly population.

Atherosclerosis is a universal process, although it shows some pathophysiological differences depending on the anatomical location of the occurrence. The atherosclerotic plaques located in the lower limbs are very fibrous and may result in strictures. When associated with a hypercoagulable state this gives rise to the acute event. By contrast, when present at the coronary arteries, the atherosclerotic plaque usually consists of a large extracellular lipid core and a large number of foam cells, coated with a thin cover susceptible to breakage, which is the ultimate cause triggering the acute event. Whatever the underlying process, the final consequence is the same: an imbalance between the needs of the tissues and the support of oxygen and nutrients. If this mismatch happens suddenly, as in the thrombotic event, it leads to acute ischaemia. If the establishment of the stenosis is gradual, allowing the development of collateral circulation, metabolic adaptation of the muscle mass involved and the use of non-ischaemic muscle groups, ischaemia may persist as a chronic state. From the pathophysiological point of view, one can talk about functional ischaemia when blood flow is insufficient to cope with the demand that involves the exercise but it is enough at rest. This functional ischaemia translates clinically into intermittent claudication. The critical ischaemia occurs when the flow is insufficient even at rest, appearing as pain and trophic lesions in the extremities. In this situation there is a need to intervene to restore an adequate blood flow, to avoid the risk of amputation. However, the symptoms will largely depend on the number of affected territories and the level of physical activity performed by each person.

The importance of inflammation in the genesis, progression and outcome of the atherosclerotic disease has emerged over the last two decades, adding to the classic concept according to which atherosclerosis is a mechanical accumulation of lipids and a fibrodegenerative response of the arterial wall by changes in its structure, leading to a progressive failure of tissue perfusion. Currently, atherosclerosis is regarded as a multifactorial disease where metabolic, inflammatory, haemodynamic and haemostatic factors are involved, with both local and systemic roles.

Glyco-oxidation contributes to the development of atherosclerosis in the below-the-knee peripheral artery tree in type 2 diabetes, and very probably also in elderly patients without diabetes. Advanced glycosylation end-products (AGEs) levels increase with ageing and in patients with diabetes. AGEs are elevated in type 2 diabetic patients with PAD as compared with diabetic patients without PAD and control subjects. More precisely, among AGEs components, pentosidine appears to be strongly associated with the peripheral artery status of diabetic patients. In addition,

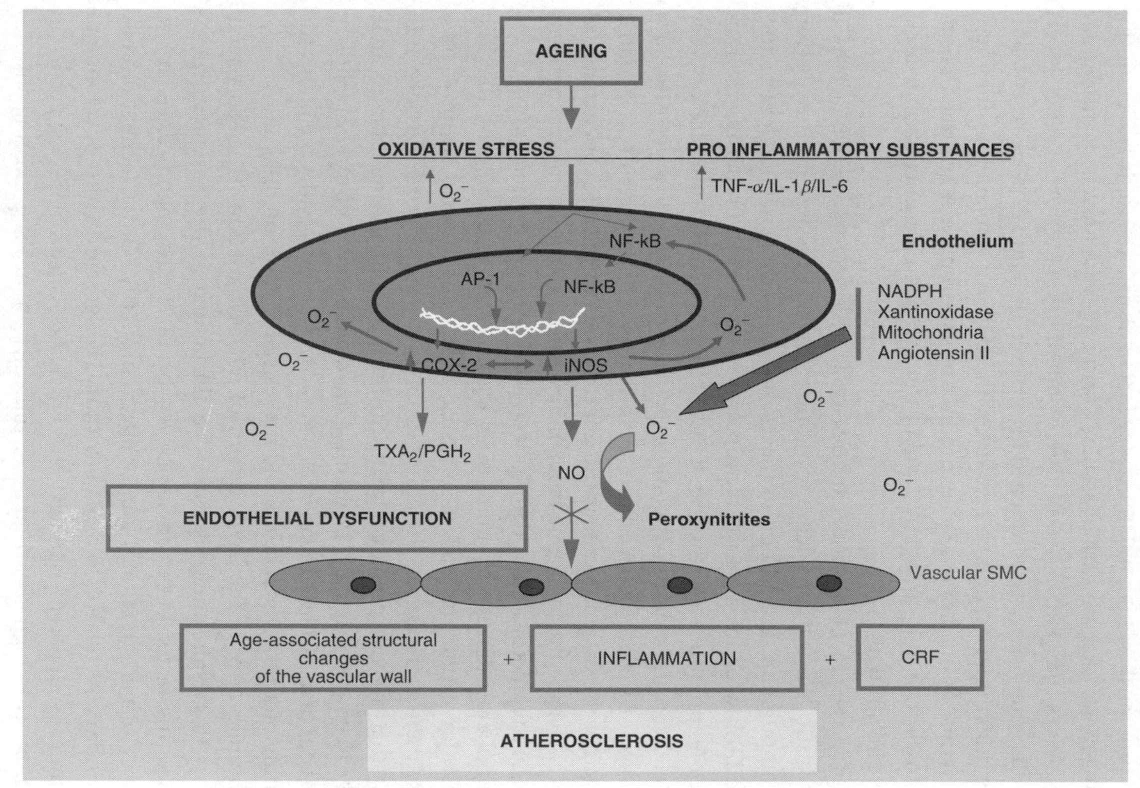

Figure 14.1 Mechanisms of endothelial dysfunction and atherosclerosis in ageing. COX-2, cyclooxygenase-2; CRF, cardiovascular risk factors; IL, interleukin; iNOs, inducible nitric oxide synthase; NO, nitric oxide; O_{2-}, superoxide anions.

lipid oxidation, estimated by the serum levels of malondialdehyde (MDA), is associated with diabetic peripheral angiopathy. On the other hand, both TRAP and vitamin E levels, which estimate antioxidant capacity, are lower in type 2 diabetic patients with PAD than in those who are diabetic without PAD, and in healthy subjects.

As previously stated, inflammatory mechanisms are also involved in the pathogenesis of acute cardiovascular events. Elevated levels of inflammatory factors may encourage plaque instability and rupture. Higher levels of inflammation are associated with greater functional impairment and faster functional decline in persons with PAD. An explanation for these associations is not still available, but inflammation plays a key role in both atherosclerosis and sarcopenia, and in the age-related reduction in muscle mass and strength.

The presence of several cardiovascular risk factors, which act in a synergistic way, is the main condition for progression of the disease and amputation. In addition to these, there are other independent factors contributing to increased risk of amputation: sensory neuropathy, previous minor amputations and the use of insulin. Furthermore, other factors very prevalent in the elderly population (physical disability, loss of vision or a shortage of social resources), act as facilitators. As is the rule in geriatric medicine, the final outcome is the effect of the pathogenic concurrence of several factors, the main one being involvement of the peripheral nervous system, the microvascular damage and a superimposed infection.

Peripheral neuropathy diminishes algesic perception, putting the skin at risk for conditions such as pressure ulcers and muscle atrophy. As a consequence, changes in the points of support occur, placing pressure onto areas that are not prepared for it. So the heads of the metatarsals may suffer ischaemic necrosis, facilitating the development of osteomyelitis in the event of an underlying ulcer. The autonomic neuropathy facilitates the opening of artery-vein shunts and makes skin hydration difficult.

The relevance of the involvement of microcirculation has been widely discussed. Despite the existence of a thickening of the basement membrane, this factor does not appear to be of clinical significance in the absence of peripheral and autonomic neuropathy. Other factors, directly and indirectly related to vascular injury, cooperate in the development of clinically apparent damage: the ischaemia causes pain, especially in patients with high blood-glucose, difficulty in healing existing injuries and delay in the sterilization of infected lesions. Other mechanisms that can hinder healing include training AGEs or zinc shortfall related to its increased renal elimination in patients with poor glycaemic control. It is quite possible that this mechanism should be enhanced in elderly people. Ischaemia also hinders antibiotic response to infected ulcers.

Diagnosis

Assessment

Diagnosis of PAD is based mainly on clinical evaluation and the patient's medical history. Patients frequently minimize symptoms, attributing them to normal ageing. Because of this an active search for intermittent claudication or atypical presentation of PAD must be carried out, distinguishing them from non-vascular causes (pseudoclaudication).[20] The 2011 ACC/AHA guidelines on PAD[20] and the 2007 TASC II consensus document on the management of PAD[21] recommend that the standard review of symptoms should include questions related to a history of walking impairment, symptoms of claudication, ischaemic rest pain, or non-healing wounds in patients ≥65–70 years of age, those ≥50 years of age with a history of smoking and/or diabetes, or, in TASC II, those with a Framingham risk score of 10–20% at 10 years. A careful history including a comprehensive geriatric assessment should reveal functional impairment when this is the clinical presentation.

Clinical presentation

Adult patients with PAD often present with the classic symptoms of leg ischaemia. However, elderly patients are often asymptomatic, and among symptomatic patients, atypical symptoms are more common than claudication.[3]

Many patients with PAD have unrecognized disease as illustrated by the following observations. In the PARTNERS programme cited above, around 45% of the patients with a new diagnosis of PAD had no history of leg symptoms and only 5.5% had classic claudication. In another study that included 239 men and women aged 55 and over with no history of PAD who were recruited from a general internal medicine practice, the ABI was abnormal (<0.90) in 14%. Most of these patients did not report exertional leg symptoms. However, they were not able to walk as far in 6 minutes as a group of patients without PAD (1362 vs 1539 feet).

Older patients with PAD have atypical symptoms, usually focused on functional issues, mainly as a result of comorbidities, physical inactivity and alterations in pain perception. Functional capacity is diminished in some patients with PAD even in the absence of claudication, being the principal manifestation of the disease. In addition, a gradual decline in activity level or a progressive loss of independence in the activities of daily life may mask the symptoms of PAD in elderly people.

This issue was addressed in a study of 417 patients with PAD and 259 without disease who underwent measurement of ABI and assessment of functional capacity at baseline and 1 and 2 years later.[22] Patients with an ABI <0.50 had a significantly greater annual decline in 6-minute walk distance than those with an ABI of 0.50 to <0.90 or those with an ABI of 0.90–1.50 (73 vs 59 and 13 feet, respectively). In addition, patients with PAD who reported no exertional pain had a greater annual decline in 6-minute walk distance than those with typical intermittent claudication (77 vs 36 feet).

These findings suggest that activity level is an important factor in the evaluation of patients with PAD. Patients with evidence of PAD who report no or few symptoms should be asked about functional capacity and decline in activity over time.

Finally, some patients have atypical symptoms that may mimic other disorders[20] including nerve root compression, spinal stenosis and hip arthritis.

Physical examination

The physical assessment should include an examination with shoes and socks off, paying special attention to pulses (femoral, poplital, posterior tibial and pedal), bruits, hair loss, skin colour, temperature, ulcers and trophic skin changes.

We can measure the functional impairment using several validated tests and scores. Walking velocity, time to arise from a seated position or the standing balance score have been related to the presence of subclinical disease and its prognosis.[14,15] The most frequently suggested instruments are the Short Physical Performance Battery (SPPB) and the 6-metre walking speed.

The Clinical Guidelines for Type 2 Diabetes Mellitus (European Diabetes Working Party for Older People 2011)[23] suggest that a Comprehensive Geriatric Assessment should be a routine measure in older people with type 2 diabetes at diagnosis and at regular intervals, and recommend as a minimum an annual inspection of the feet by a healthcare professional, including a vascular and neurological examination, even if no symptoms are present. When available, an ABI determination should be done (see below).

Detection of asymptomatic PAD has value because it identifies patients at increased risk of atherosclerosis at other sites. As many as 50% of patients with PAD have at least a 50% stenosis in one renal artery. Thus, patients with asymptomatic PAD, most often detected by ABI, should be assessed to detect clinically significant atherosclerosis in other vascular territories apart from the legs.

Non-invasive tests

These tests help to establish an accurate diagnosis of PAD, to quantify the severity of the disease, to localize the stenosis, to organize a treatment plan and to determine the progression of the disease or its response to treatment.

A variety of non-invasive examinations are available to assess the presence and degree of PAD. They include ABI, exercise treadmill test, segmental limb pressures, segmental volume plethysmography and ultrasonography. Magnetic resonance imaging may become an important non-invasive method for assessment; however, at the present time costs and time considerations limit its use as a routine screening modality. The two most used methods in the clinical setting are the ABI and ultrasonography.

A relatively simple and inexpensive method to confirm the clinical suspicion of arterial occlusive disease is to measure the resting systolic blood pressures in the ankle and arm, and calculate the ABI, which provides a measure of the severity of PAD.

Calculation of the ABI is performed by measuring the systolic blood pressure (by Doppler probe) in the brachial arteries and in posterior tibial or dorsalis pedis arteries (Figure 14.2). The highest of the four measurements in the ankles and feet is divided by the higher of the two brachial measurements. Depending on the value of this index, several categories are defined[20]:

- Normal ABI: 1.0–1.4. Values above 1.4 suggest a non-compressible calcified vessel.
- ABI ≤0.9 has 95% sensitivity (and 100% specificity) for detecting angiogram-positive PAD and is associated with ≥50% stenosis in one or more major vessels.
- ABI of 0.91–0.99 represents borderline values.
- ABI >1.4 represents noncompressible arteries.

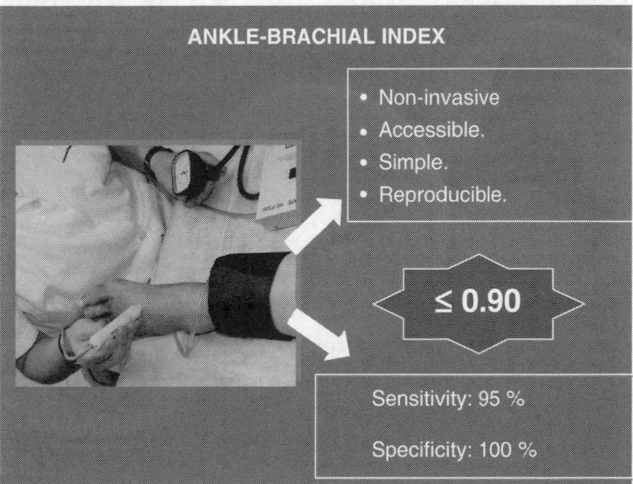

Figure 14.2 Measurement and diagnostic characteristics of the ankle-brachial index (ABI).

If ABI is normal at rest but symptoms strongly suggest claudication, ABI and segmental pressures should be obtained before and after exercise on a treadmill.

As previously stated, the ABI correlates with clinical measures of lower extremity function such as walking distance, velocity, balance and overall physical activity. In addition, a low ABI has been associated with a higher risk of coronary heart disease, stroke, TIA, progressive renal insufficiency and all-cause mortality.[8]

A potential source of error with ABI is that calcified vessels may not compress normally, possibly resulting in falsely elevated Doppler signals. Thus, an ABI above 1.3 is suspicious for a calcified vessel. An abnormally high ABI (>1.4) is also associated with higher rates of leg pain, cardiovascular risk and heart failure.

The examination of the lower extremity using the duplex ultrasonography (Doppler) begins at the common femoral artery and proceeds distally to the popliteal artery. An area of stenosis is localized with colour Doppler and assessed by measuring Doppler velocities at several arterial sites. It has been suggested that the main purpose of duplex ultrasonography is to avoid the diagnostic angiography before intervention in patients with arterial disease proximal to the calf. A meta-analysis of 14 studies found that sensitivity and specificity of this technique for $\geq 50\%$ stenosis or occlusion were 86% and 97% for aortoiliac disease and 80% and 98% for femoropopliteal disease.

Invasive tests

At the present time, contrast angiography is the 'gold standard' for the diagnosis of PAD. It is the definitive method before revascularization procedures. Although it is relatively secure, it is associated with a higher risk of medical complications (bleeding, infection, contrast allergy, etc.) than non-invasive techniques and should be performed only in selected patients (surgical patients).[20]

Treatment

The main aim when treating elderly people with PAD is to avoid the consequences of atherosclerotic disease in lower limbs and other vascular territories, and to prevent the functional decline associated with vascular disease.

Once the diagnosis is established, the patient can be treated medically by means of risk factor modification, exercise, foot care and drugs. If the disease progresses and/or the patient meets a number of established criteria, percutaneous intervention or surgery should be performed.

Risk factors modification

The principal risk factors for the development of PAD are ageing, cigarette smoking, diabetes mellitus, hypertension and hyperlipidaemia. With regard to the reduction of cardiovascular risk in elderly patients with PAD it must be stated that there is no conclusive evidence about the relation between the control of risk factors and PAD prognosis. Nevertheless, the role of control of cardiovascular risk factors in the manifestations of atherosclerosis is well established. For this reason, treatment of cardiovascular risk factors is a priority in all patients with PAD, whatever their clinical manifestations.

Cigarette smoking

Cessation of cigarette smoking reduces the progression of disease as shown by lower amputation rates and lower incidences of rest ischaemia among those who quit. It is not clear whether smoking cessation reduces the severity of symptoms of claudication.

According to the recommendations of the 2007 TASC II consensus document, all patients should be strongly advised to stop smoking by their physicians and all patients should be offered nicotine replacement and group counselling sessions. Many patients may benefit from the addition of antidepressant drug therapy, but in older patients special attention should be paid to the adverse effects of this kind of drug on functional status.

Diabetes mellitus

There is no evidence on what is the best control level of cardiovascular risk factors in elderly diabetic patients with PAD. Because of this, treatment goals are similar to those in diabetic elderly patients.[20] No controlled trials have directly evaluated the effects of hypoglycaemic therapy upon the natural history of PAD. Aggressive control of blood glucose in both type 1 and type 2 diabetes reduces the risk of microvascular complications (e.g. nephropathy, retinopathy and neuropathy). However, in the Diabetes Control and Complications Trial of patients with type 1 diabetes, intensive insulin therapy had no effect upon the risk of PAD. The results were similar in the United Kingdom Prospective Diabetes Study in patients with type 2 diabetes.[24]

The 2007 TASC II consensus document on the management of PAD, recommends aggressive control of blood glucose levels with an HbA1c goal of <7% and as close to 6% as possible in adult patients. However, as previously stated at the beginning of this chapter, less stringent goals may be appropriate for elderly patients (around 7.5–8%, depending on the frailty status) and in those with comorbid conditions.[23]

Hypertension

Hypertension is a major risk factor for PAD. However, there are no data evaluating whether antihypertensive therapy modifies the progression of claudication. Nevertheless, hypertension should be controlled in these patients to reduce morbidity from cardiovascular and cerebrovascular disease.

There has been some concern in the past about the use of beta-blockers in the treatment of hypertension among patients with intermittent claudication, but there appears to be no adverse effect of beta-1 selective blockers on claudication symptoms. As a result, these drugs are not contraindicated in patients with PAD.[20]

There are no therapeutic groups that provide a differential benefit in these patients. Although the HOPE trial suggested that the angiotensin-converting enzyme (ACE) inhibitor ramipril provided added protection against cardiovascular events in patients with cardiovascular disease, including PAD, these benefits are likely to be a consequence of blood pressure reduction in this placebo-controlled trial, rather than a specific benefit of ACE inhibition although there is some evidence that ACE inhibitor therapy may increase walking distance in selected patients with PAD.

The blood pressure goal in these patients should be the same as that in patients with hypertension and established cardiovascular disease: below 130/80, as recommended by the American Heart Association and the European Society of Hypertension-European Society of Cardiology (ESH-ESC), or a higher goal of <140/90 mmHg if we adhere to the recommendations set by the 2007 TASC II consensus document. It must be highlighted than in the very old person (≥80 yrs) with systolic hypertension there is no evidence about the benefits of decreasing blood pressure below 140 mmHg. By contrast, some studies have raised worries about the possibility of harm when blood pressure is reduced below that threshold.

Hyperlipidaemia

A number of cholesterol-lowering trials in patients with hyperlipidaemia and coronary and/or PAD have evaluated the effects of lipid-lowering therapy on PAD. A 2000 Cochrane meta-analysis of old trials mostly carried out before statins use, which specifically evaluated patients with lower limb atherosclerosis, concluded that lipid-lowering therapy reduced disease progression (as measured by angiography) and alleviated symptoms. Subsequent studies confirmed these benefits in patients treated with statin therapy. Regression of femoral atherosclerosis, a lower rate of new or worsening intermittent claudication, and improvements in walking distance and pain-free walking time have all been described.

The Scandinavian Simvastatin Survival Study (4S), found that treatment with 20–40 mg day^{-1} of simvastatin reduced the incidence of new or worsening intermittent claudication by 38% (2.3 vs 3.6% with placebo).[25] Another randomized, double-blind trial included 354 patients with claudication attributable to PAD who were assigned to atorvastatin (10 or 80 mg day^{-1}) or placebo. At 12 months, there was a significant improvement in pain-free walking time with high-dose atorvastatin and in community-based physical activity with both doses of atorvastatin but there was no change in ABI.

With regard to the goals for lipid levels in elderly patients with PAD, there are no specific recommendations and the recommendations for adult patients[21] can be applied, with some caution. For instance, the recommendation for all patients with PAD to have their LDL-cholesterol lowered to $<100\,mg\,dl^{-1}$ (2.6 mmol l^{-1}), should be qualified in frail patients, where the risk of malnutrition is very high.

Exercise rehabilitation

Several studies have demonstrated the benefit of exercise rehabilitation programmes in reducing symptoms of claudication. A meta-analysis that included only randomized, controlled trials found that lower limb exercise produced a significant increase in maximum walking time (mean difference 6.5 minutes); the benefit was greater than that seen with angioplasty at 6 months (mean difference 3.3 minutes).[26]

The effect of upper limb exercise was assessed in a subsequent trial in which 104 patients with stable PAD were randomly assigned to twice weekly aerobic exercise training with upper limb or lower limb exercise or a non-exercise training control group. At 6 months, upper and lower limb exercise was associated with similar increases in claudication distance (51% and 57%), maximal walking distance (29% and 31%), and peak oxygen consumption.

There are several mechanisms by which exercise training may improve claudication, although the available data are insufficient to reach firm conclusions regarding their relative importance: improved endothelial dysfunction via increases in nitric oxide synthase and prostacyclin, reduced local inflammation, increased exercise pain tolerance, induction of vascular angiogenesis, improved muscle metabolism by favourable effects on muscle carnitine metabolism and other metabolic pathways, and reductions in blood viscosity and red cell aggregation.

A separate issue is whether patients with asymptomatic PAD benefit from exercise rehabilitation. This issue was addressed in a study of 156 patients with an ABI $\leq$0.95, most of whom were asymptomatic (81%), who were randomly assigned to one of three intervention groups: supervised treadmill exercise, lower extremity resistance training, or usual management (control group). At 6 months participants in the treadmill exercise group significantly increased in their distance walked (36 metres) during a 6-minute walk test compared to those in the placebo group.[27]

Although less well studied, exercise may also improve survival. This issue was addressed in a prospective observational study of 225 men and women with PAD evaluated in whom physical activity was measured with a vertical accelerometer.[28] Patients were followed for a mean duration of 57 months at which time 75 patients (33%) had died. Individuals in the highest quartile of accelerometer-measured activity had a significantly lower mortality than those in the lowest quartile (HR 0.29; 95% CI, 0.10–0.83).

Exercise prescription must be done following some guidelines. Patients should be referred to a claudication exercise rehabilitation programme. These programmes consist of a series of sessions lasting 45–60 minutes per session, involving the use of either a motorized treadmill or a track to permit each patient to achieve symptom-limited claudication. The initial session usually includes 35 minutes of intermittent walking; after that, walking is increased by 5 minutes in each session until 50 minutes of intermittent walking can be accomplished, surrounded by warm-up and cool-down sessions of 5 to 10 minutes each. Ideally, the patient must attend at least 3 sessions per week, with a programme length greater than 3 months.

Foot care

The use of appropriate footwear to avoid pressure injuries, the use of moisturizing cream to prevent dryness and fissuring, daily inspection and cleansing by the patient and chiropody, are necessary measures to reduce the risk of skin ulceration, necrosis and amputation. Although these measures are recommended based on the results of some work analysing their effects in diabetic patients, there are no studies evaluating their impact on elderly diabetic patients with PAD.

Pharmacological therapy

Drug therapy of claudication is aimed at symptomatic relief or slowing progression of the natural disease. A number of drugs[20] have been evaluated but, as will be seen, the evidence of benefit is convincing only for antiplatelet agents, mainly aspirin and cilostazol.

Antiplatelet therapy

Patients with symptomatic atherosclerosis in the lower limbs or in other vascular beds should usually be prescribed an antiplatelet drug (assuming no contra-indications). Aspirin (75–325 mg/day) is the agent of choice; clopidogrel (75 mg/day) may be used if aspirin cannot be tolerated or in the subgroup of patients with symptomatic PAD. Aspirin has not been shown to reduce cardiovascular risk in asymptomatic patients with a low ABI.[29] Anticoagulant therapy has not been shown to improve cardiovascular outcomes in patients with PAD.

Cilostazol

This is a phosphodiesterase inhibitor approved by the Food and Drug Administration (FDA) for the treatment of intermittent claudication. It suppresses platelet aggregation and is a direct arterial vasodilator. The efficacy of cilostazol has been demonstrated in several studies and in a meta-analysis of eight randomized, placebo-controlled trials that included 2702 patients with stable, moderate to severe claudication.[30] In this meta-analysis, treatment with 100 mg twice daily for 12–24 weeks increased maximal and pain-free walking distances by 50% and 67%, respectively. Benefit may be noted as early as 4 weeks. Side effects noted in clinical studies included headache, loose and soft stools, diarrhoea, dizziness (increasing risk of falls) and palpitations, and it is contraindicated in heart failure. It should be taken half an hour before or 2 hours after eating, because high-fat meals markedly increase absorption. Several drugs such as diltiazem and omeprazol, as well as grapefruit juice, can increase serum concentrations of cilostazol if taken concurrently. All these features hamper its use in elderly patients.

Pentoxifylline

This is a rheologic modifier approved by the FDA for the symptomatic relief of claudication. It is less effective than cilostazol.

Naftidrofuryl

Naftidrofuryl is a 5-hydroxytryptamine-2-receptor antagonist that is currently available only in Europe. The mechanisms of action of this drug are unclear but it is thought to promote glucose uptake and increase adenosine triphosphate levels. A meta-analysis of four trials showed an increase in the time to initial pain development on treadmill-walking over a 3- to 6-month period. This conclusion was also found in a 2008 Cochrane systematic review.[31] The 2007 TASC II consensus document on the management of PAD concluded that naftidrofuryl (600 mg day^{-1} orally) can be considered for the treatment of intermittent claudication.[21]

Revascularization

There are two important criteria for revascularization: severe disability that limits the patient's ability to work or to perform other activities that are important to the patient, and failure (or predicted failure) to respond to exercise rehabilitation and pharmacological therapy. Endovascular or surgical revascularization therapy is reserved for patients whose functional capacity is compromised only by claudication (not for other comorbidities), patients who do not have a response to exercise and pharmacotherapy and patients for whom the risk-benefit ratio with revascularization is favourable.[20] These patients (and the patients with critical and acute limb ischaemia) should be referred to a vascular surgeon.

Acknowledgments

Supported by grants from Instituto de Salud Carlos III (Ministerio de Ciencia e Innovación) RD06/0013; PI07/90306; PI08/1649 and from FIMMM2008.

References

1 McDermott M. The magnitude of the problem of peripheral arterial disease: epidemiology and clinical significance. *Cleve Clin J Med* 2006;**73**(Suppl. 4):S2–S7.

2 Newman AB, Siscovick DS, Manolio TA *et al.* Ankle-arm index as a marker of atherosclerosis in the Cardiovascular Health Study. *Circulation* 1993;**88**:837–45.

3 Hirsch AT, Criqui MH, Treat-Jacobson D *et al.* Peripheral arterial disease detection, awareness, and treatment in primary care. *JAMA* 2001;**286**:1317–24.

4 Selvin E and Erlinger TP. Prevalence of and risk factors for peripheral arterial disease in the United States: Results from the National Health and Nutrition Examination Survey, 1999–2000. *Circulation* 2004;**110**:738–43.

5 Aboyans V, Lacroix P and Criqui MH. Large and small vessels atherosclerosis: similarities and differences. *Prog Cardiovasc Dis* 2007;**50**:112–25.

6 Selvin E, Wattanakit K, Steffes MW *et al.* HbA_{1c} and peripheral arterial disease in diabetes. *Diabetes Care* 2006;**29**:877–82.

7 Kennedy M, Solomon C, Manolio TA *et al.* Risk factors for declining Ankle-Brachial Index in men and women 65 years or older. The Cardiovascular Health Study. *Arch Intern Med* 2005;**165**:1896–1902.

8 Resnick HE, Lindsay RS, McDermott MM *et al.* Relationship of high and low ankle brachial index to all-cause and cardiovascular disease mortality: The Strong Heart Study. *Circulation* 2004;**109**:733–9.

9 Criqui MH, Ninomiya JK, Wingard DL *et al.* Progression of peripheral arterial disease predicts cardiovascular disease morbidity and mortality. *JACC* 2008;**52**:1736–42.

10 Kuo HK and Yu YH. The relation of peripheral arterial disease to leg force, gait speed and functional dependence among older adults. *J Gerontol* 2008;**63A**:384–90.

11 Gardner AW and Montgomery PS. Impaired balance and higher prevalence of falls in subjects with intermittent claudication. *J Gerontol* 2001;**56A**:M454–M458.

12 Verbrugge LM and Jette AM. The disablement process. *Soc Sci Med* 1994;**38**:1–14.

13 Gardner AW, Montgomery PS and Killewich LA. Natural history of physical function in older men with intermittent claudication. *J Vasc Surg* 2004;**40**:73–8.

14 McDermott MM, Guralnik JM, Tian L *et al.* Baseline functional performance predicts the rate of mobility loss in persons with peripheral arterial disease. *JACC* 2007;**50**:974–82.

15 McDermott MM, Tian L, Liu K *et al.* Prognostic value of functional performance for mortality in patients with peripheral arterial disease. *JACC* 2008;**15**:1482–9.

16 Newman AB, Gottdiener JS, McBurnie MA *et al.* for The Cardiovascular Health Study Research Group. Associations of subclinical cardiovascular disease with frailty. *J Gerontol* 2001;**56A**:M158–M166.
17 Laurin D, Masaki KH, White LR and Launer LJ. Ankle-to-brachial index and dementia: the Honolulu-Asia Aging Study. *Circulation* 2007;**116**:2269–74.
18 Regensteiner JG, Hiatt WR, Coll JR *et al.* The impact of peripheral arterial disease on health-related quality of life in the Peripheral Arterial Disease Awareness, Risk and Treatment: New Resources for Survival (PARTNERS) Program. *Vasc Med* 2008;**13**:15–24.
19 Rodríguez-Mañas L, El-Assar M, Vallejo S *et al.* Endothelial dysfunction in aged humans is related with oxidative stress and vascular inflammation. *Aging Cell* 2009;**8**:226–38.
20 2011 Writing Group Members; 2005 Writing Committee Members; ACCF/AHA Task Force Members. HYPERLINK "http://www.ncbi.nlm.nih.gov/pubmed/21959305" 2011 ACCF/AHA Focused Update of the Guideline for the Management of patients with peripheral artery disease (Updating the 2005 Guideline): a report of the American College of Cardiology Foundation/American Heart Association Task Force on practice guidelines. Circulation. 2011 Nov 1;124(18):2020–45. Epub 2011 Sep 29.
21 Norgren L, Hiatt WR, Dormandy JA *et al.* Inter-Society Consensus for the Management of Peripheral Arterial Disease (TASC II). *J Vasc Surg* 2007;**45**(Suppl. S):S5–S67.
22 McDermott MM, Liu K, Greenland P *et al.* Functional decline in peripheral arterial disease: associations with the ankle-brachial index and leg symptoms. *JAMA* 2004;**292**:453–61.
23 Sinclair AJ, Paolisso G, Castro M *et al.* European Diabetes Working Party for Older People 2011 Clinical Guidelines for Type 2 Diabetes Mellitus. Executive Summary. *Diabetes & Metabolism* 2011;**37**:S27–S38.
24 UK Prospective Diabetes Study Group. Intensive blood-glucose control with sulphonylureas or insulin compared with conventional treatment and risk of complications in patients with type 2 diabetes (UKPDS 33). *Lancet* 1998;**352**:837–53.
25 Pedersen TR, Kjekshus J, Pyorala K *et al.* Effect of simvastatin on ischemic signs and symptoms in the Scandinavian Simvastatin Survival Study (4S). *Am J Cardiol* 1998;**81**:333–5.
26 Leng GC, Fowler B and Ernst E. (2000) Exercise for intermittent claudication. *Cochrane Database Syst Rev* **2** (Art. No.: CD000990).
27 McDermott MM, Ades P, Guralnik JM *et al.* Treadmill exercise and resistance training in patients with peripheral arterial disease with and without intermittent claudication: a randomized controlled trial. *JAMA* 2009;**301**:165–74.
28 Garg PK, Tian L, Criqui MH *et al.* Physical activity during daily life and mortality in patients with peripheral arterial disease. *Circulation* 2006;**114**:242–8.
29 Fowkes FG, Price JF, Stewart MC *et al.* Aspirin for Asymptomatic Atherosclerosis Trialists. Aspirin for prevention of cardiovascular events in a general population screened for a low ankle-brachial index: a randomized controlled trial. *JAMA* 2010;**303**: 841–8.
30 Thompson PD, Zimet R, Forbes WP and Zhang P. Meta-analysis of results from eight randomized, placebo-controlled trials on the effect of cilostazol on patients with intermittent claudication. *Am J Cardiol* 2002;**90**:1314–19.
31 De Backer TL, Vander Stichele R, Lehert P and Van Bortel L. (2008) Naftidrofuryl for intermittent claudication. *Cochrane Database Syst Rev* **2** (Art. No.: CD001368).

CHAPTER 15
Venous Thromboembolism

Gordon D.O. Lowe

Institute of Cardiovascular and Medical Sciences, University of Glasgow, Glasgow Royal Infirmary, Glasgow, Scotland, UK

Epidemiology and pathogenesis

Thromboembolism (venous, cardiac, or arterial) is the commonest cause of death, and a major cause of morbidity, in later life. Like cardiac and arterial thromboembolism, the incidence of venous thromboembolism increases exponentially with age approaching 1% per year by 90 years (Figure 15.1).[1] Almost half of cases occur between 60 and 79 years; and almost a quarter after 80 years (Figure 15.2).[1] This may reflect age-related increases in risk factors and comorbidities (Table 15.1), and in activation of inflammation, endothelium, platelets and coagulation[2,3] combined with age-related decreases in coagulation inhibition,[2,4] fibrinolytic activity and in general mobility.

Venous thromboembolism (VTE) may present as deep vein thrombosis of the leg (DVT) or pulmonary embolism (PE). Case-fatality is largely due to PE; and increases to over 10% in elderly people.[1] Treatment of VTE is also more hazardous in elderly patients: the risk of major haemorrhage during anticoagulation increases by nearly 50% for each decade of age.[5,6] Hence prophylaxis of VTE is especially important in older people. Because about half of cases occur within 3 months of hospitalization, routine prophylaxis against hospital-acquired thrombosis is important.

Risk factors for VTE in older patients are similar to those in younger patients, with the obvious exception of pregnancy and the puerperium (Table 15.1). There is increasing evidence that the pathogenesis of DVT involves a 'multiple hit model', which starts at conception with multiple, interacting, genetic predispositions (thrombophilias) which thereafter interact throughout life with acquired risk factors which may precipitate thrombosis (Figure 15.3).[7] Once venous thrombosis has occurred, it acts as a strong predictor of the risk of recurrence, especially if idiopathic.

Cardiovascular Disease and Health in the Older Patient: Expanded from 'Pathy's Principles and Practice of Geriatric Medicine, Fifth edition', First Edition. Edited by David J. Stott and Gordon D.O. Lowe.

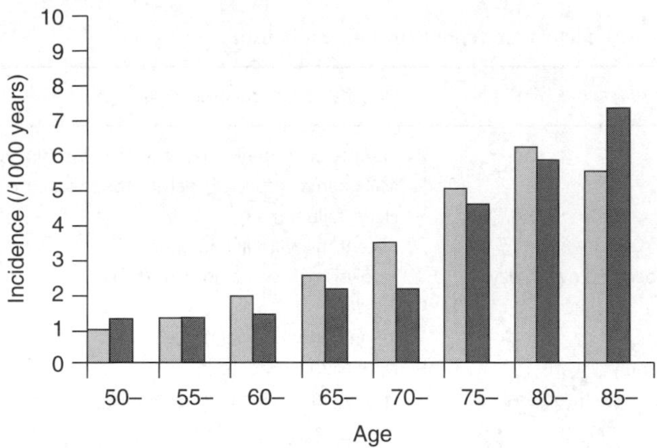

Figure 15.1 Incidence of first venous thromboembolism by age and sex. Rates are shown per 1000 per year, for men (striped bars), for women (solid bars). Reproduced from Rosendaal *et al.*[1], with permission from Wiley-Blackwell.

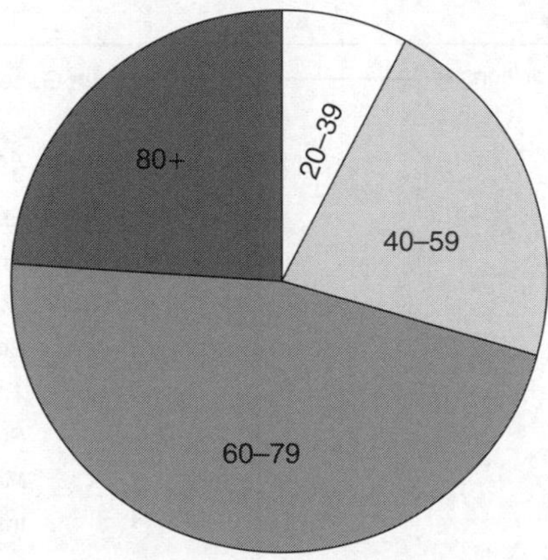

Figure 15.2 Age distribution of patients with venous thromboembolism. Percentage of patients by age group: 20-39 years, 7.5%; 40-59 years, 21.5%; 60-79 years, 45.9%; 80+ years, 23.6%. Reproduced from Rosendaal *et al.*[1], with permission from Wiley-Blackwell.

Genetic thrombophilias

Genetic thrombophilias should be suspected clinically if there is a past history, or a family history in blood relatives, of 'premature' (e.g. onset before 40–45years) DVT, PE or recurrent fetal loss (spontaneous abortion or stillbirth); if there is recurrent VTE or thrombophlebitis; or if thromboembolism occurs at an unusual site (upper limb veins, retina, cerebral venous sinuses, mesenteric, portal or hepatic veins).[8] Protein C or protein S deficiency may also present with coumarin-induced skin necrosis.[8] Congenital deficiencies of the three coagulation inhibitors (antithrombin, protein C,

Table 15.1 Risk factors for venous thromboembolism.

Patient factors	Disease or surgical procedure
Age	Trauma or surgery, especially of pelvis, hip, lower limb
Smoking	Malignancy, especially pelvic, abdominal, metastatic
Obesity	Heart failure
Blood lipids	Recent myocardial infarction
Immobility (bed rest over 4 days)	Paralysis of lower limb (e.g. stroke)
(Pregnancy)	Infection
(Puerperium)	Inflammatory bowel disease
Estrogen therapy	Nephrotic syndrome
Previous deep vein thrombosis or pulmonary embolism	Polycythemia Homocysteinaemia
Genetic thrombophilias	Paraproteinemia
Varicose veins	Paroxysmal nocturnal haemoglobinuria
	Bechet's disease

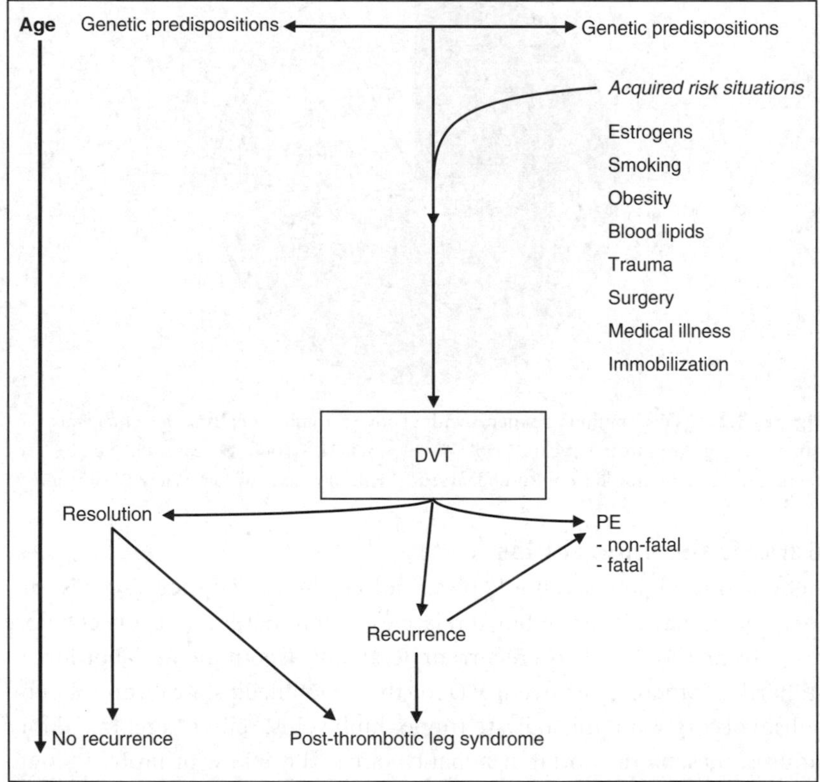

Figure 15.3 Multiple hit model for DVT.

or protein S) are usually due to heterozygosity for autosomal dominant gene defects; they increase the risk of VTE about two- to threefold.[9] The low prevalence of these mutations in non-Western countries may explain their low incidence of DVT and PE.

DVT in the population is also associated with increased plasma levels of the von Willebrand factor – coagulation factor VIII complex;[9] and probably explains why non-O blood group increases the risk of VTE by about 80% (non-O blood group elevates plasma levels of this complex by about 30%).[10] Homozygous homocystinuria has long been recognized as a risk factor for premature arterial and venous thrombosis. More recently, hyperhomocysteinaemia has also been associated with increased risk of both venous and arterial thrombosis: this is partly due to heterozygosity for cystein synthase or methylene-tetrahydrofolate reductase (MTHRF) deficiency (whose cumulative prevalence in the general population is 0.4–1.5%) and partly due to deficiencies of vitamins (folate, cobalamine and pyridoxine) especially in elderly people.[11] There is much current interest in the possibility that dietary supplementation of these vitamins could have a major impact on venous as well as arterial thrombosis, particularly in the elderly population; however, randomized trials have to date been inconclusive.[12]

Acquired risk factors

In recent years it has been increasingly appreciated that risk factors for arterial thrombosis (tobacco-smoking, obesity, diabetes and increased levels of blood lipids) are also risk factors for VTE.[9] As with genetic thrombophilias, increased activation of blood coagulation is the most likely explanation.[9] Reduction in blood lipids by statin therapy appears to reduce the risk of VTE, as well as of arterial thrombosis.[13] Aspirin prophylaxis in high-risk persons reduces the risk of VTE, as well as of arterial thrombosis, by about 24%.[14]

Varicose veins increase the risk of post-operative DVT,[15] possibly because they may be a marker of previous (often asymptomatic) DVT in older persons. The increased risks of DVT and PE with increased estrogens, for example hormone replacement therapy,[16,17] suggest common mechanisms, including activated protein-C resistance, low levels of antithrombin and protein S, and high levels of factor IX.[17] These risks are increased in women with thrombophilias.[16,17]

Immobilization (at home or in hospital) in older persons is often due to medical illness (e.g. infection, malignancy, heart failure, myocardial infarction and stroke), trauma or surgery. The cumulative risk of VTE increases with the duration of immobility, suggesting a role for venous stasis in the inactive leg in the pathogenesis of VTE. Venous stasis also increases in patients with paralysed legs, heart failure or polycythemia, which are also risk factors for VTE. Activation of blood coagulation also occurs following trauma, surgery and immobilizing illnesses including infection, malignancy, infarction and haemorrhage. The hypothesis that the combination of immobility and coagulation activation predisposes to DVT formation is supported by the prophylactic efficacy of both mechanical measures which increase leg vein blood flow, and antithrombotic drugs especially anticoagulants, and by the increased efficacy of combinations of mechanical with anticoagulant prophylaxis.

The elderly population has a high prevalence of malignant disease, which activates blood coagulation and increases the frequency of both 'spontaneous' and recurrent VTE. While the *relative* risk may be lower in patients aged >70 years, about 5% of VTE events in elderly people can be attributed to cancer.[1] Whether or not a routine detailed work-up for cancer (beyond routine history, physical examination, routine blood tests and chest X-ray) improves prognosis is not yet established.

Less common acquired conditions which are associated with increased risk of VTE include lupus anticoagulants, which are antiphospholipid antibodies and which usually occur in persons without systemic lupus erythematosis (SLE); inflammatory bowel disease, nephrotic syndrome, Bechet's disease, hyperviscosity (polycythemias, paraproteinemias), and paroxysmal nocturnal haemoglobinuria (Table 15.1).

Primary prophylaxis of VTE

In the great majority of patients dying from PE, previous VTE was not diagnosed or treated. DVT is often non-occlusive and hence clinically silent prior to embolization; while non-fatal PE occurring prior to fatal PE may not be recognized clinically, especially in older patients who frequently have pre-existing cardiorespiratory symptoms, for example from heart failure or chronic obstructive airways disease.[18]

The clinical non-recognition of VTE prior to fatal PE implies that its detection and treatment cannot have a major impact on its mortality: hence, identification of, and primary prophylaxis in, hospitalized patients (medical and surgical) at high absolute risk of DVT is required for its prevention. Increasingly, healthcare systems in developed countries (including the United Kingdom and North America) mandate routine assessment of all patients admitted to hospital for risk of hospital-acquired thrombosis.[19–22] A risk assessment tool is currently mandated in the United Kingdom.[21,22] Subcutaneous unfractionated or low molecular weight (LMW) heparin prevents about two in three cases of DVT; and also reduces the risk of PE (including fatal PE) in both medical and surgical hospitalized patients.[20–22] All hospital units and services should establish, (and regularly update), local protocols for prophylaxis, based on their national evidence-based guidelines and standards; and audit their performance.

Management of suspected DVT or PE

As with prophylaxis of VTE, evidence-based guidelines for diagnosis and management have been published in the United Kingdom and North America[22–24] from which local protocols, standards and audit should be developed. There is good evidence from randomized trials that full-dose anticoagulation (initially with heparins, followed by oral anticoagulants such as warfarin) is effective in secondary prophylaxis of recurrent thromboembolism, reducing morbidity and mortality. In patients for whom full-dose anticoagulants are contraindicated (usually due to high risk of bleeding), insertion of an inferior vena caval (IVC) filter should be considered to reduce PE risk. However, the costs and morbidity risks of both long-term anticoagulants and IVC filters require that they should be prescribed only to the minority of patients with clinically suspected DVT or PE in whom venous thromboembolism is confirmed by objective tests.

Venous thromboembolism should be suspected in patients with:

1 congenital or acquired risk factors (Table 15.1) and
2 clinical symptoms or signs suggestive of either DVT – leg (usually calf, usually unilateral) pain, tenderness, swelling, oedema, warmth, distended superficial veins and/or PE – breathlessness, chest pain, cough, haemoptysis, wheeze, tachycardia, tachypnea, syncope, shock, or cardiac arrest.

In outpatients, the need for routine imaging studies can be reduced in the Accident and Emergency Department by clinical scoring, and a rapid test for fibrin D-dimer. In patients with a low clinical score and normal D-dimer, DVT and PE can be excluded. Other patients should receive heparin therapy (unless strongly contraindicated, e.g. by high risk of bleeding) until diagnostic imaging is performed.

For suspected DVT[22,23] *compression ultrasound* or *Duplex ultrasound scanning* are non-invasive, specific and sensitive to proximal DVT, but less sensitive to calf DVT. A negative ultrasound test does not exclude the presence of calf DVT, which in about 20% of patients may extend proximally over the subsequent few days and increase the risk of PE. Hence, a negative ultrasound test in patients with clinically suspected DVT should be repeated (usually after 5–7 days), or followed immediately by venography to exclude calf DVT.

Diagnosis of clinically suspected PE [22–24] includes:

1 *chest X-ray and ECG* to exclude alternative diagnoses such as myocardial infarction, pneumothorax or pneumonia;
2 *ventilation perfusion isotope lung scanning* which may be exclusive (normal) or diagnostic (high probability – 'mismatched' major lung segments that are ventilated but not perfused); but which in about 50% of cases is non-diagnostic (intermediate probability);

3 *computerized tomographic pulmonary angiography* (CTPA), contrast pulmonary *angiography* (invasive and not widely available), or *echocardiography* (suspected massive PE).

In contrast to unfractioned heparin, *LMW heparins* do not require routine coagulation monitoring and have been shown in meta-analyses of randomized trials to have greater efficacy (lower rates of DVT extension, recurrence and mortality) and lesser risk of major bleeding than unfractionated heparin in the initial treatment of DVT.[22–25] Their efficacy as daily, unmonitored subcutaneous injections allows the possibility of outpatient treatment of acute DVT in many cases, provided this is acceptable to patients and their hospital and general practitioners. Many centres now have guideline-based local protocols for this.

Oral anticoagulants (usually warfarin) are required as maintenance treatment following initial heparin treatment of DVT or PE, to reduce the risk of recurrence. They can be started as soon as objective diagnosis is obtained; concomitant heparin treatment should be continued until the target therapeutic range of the international normalized ratio (INR) (2.0–3.0) has been achieved for 2 consecutive days. The routine recommended duration of oral anticoagulant therapy following a first episode of VTE is at least 3 months.

Newer oral anticoagulants (e.g. dabigatran, rivaroxaban) have advantages, compared to warfarin, of efficacy in fixed dosage hence no need for coagulation monitoring; and lack of interaction with diet or other drugs. They are currently in evaluation.[25]

A significant percentage of patients develop recurrent VTE after discontinuation of oral anticoagulant drugs. Risk factors for recurrence include idiopathic presentation (no recent precipitating risk factors); male sex; continuing risk factors (e.g. estrogen therapy, cancer) and persistently elevated fibrin D-dimer levels.[26–28] Genetic thrombophilias do not appear useful in prediction of recurrence.[26,27] While clinical decision rules are under development and evaluation,[26,27] the decision on prolonged oral anticoagulant therapy, especially in older patients, often requires individualized assessment of risk factors, patient preferences and the risks and burdens of anticoagulants.[27] There are ongoing studies of antiplatelet agents in secondary prevention.[29]

Compression stockings should be prescribed routinely to be worn on the affected leg(s) during the day, long term, to reduce the risk of the post-thrombotic leg syndrome.[22,23]

Considerations in elderly patients

Practical considerations when prescribing oral anticoagulants to elderly patients include:[6]

1 Sensitivity to the anticoagulant effect of a given dose increases with age: for example, an average warfarin dose of 4 mg day^{-1} was required

in patients 74–90 years old to achieve the same target INR as an average dose of 8 mg day^{-1} in patients aged 19–35.[30]

2 Polypharmacy (including self-medications) increases the risk of drug interactions which alter oral anticoagulant effect, or which increase the risk of bleeding (e.g. aspirin and other non-steroidal anti-inflammatory drugs).
3 Increased prevalence of concurrent or intercurrent illness also increases risk of bleeding (e.g. severe anaemia, renal failure, gastrointestinal bleeding, haemorrhagic stroke, bleeding disorder).
4 Decreased compliance or decreased access to monitoring – whether performed by the general practitioner or hospital anticoagulant clinic - also increases risk of bleeding.

Key points

- Venous thromboembolism is common in elderly patients, especially with obesity, malignancy, heart failure, immobility, trauma, surgery and acute medical illness.
- Consider primary prophylaxis (low-dose heparin, aspirin or stockings) in acutely immobilized patients, especially those with other risk factors, previous DVT or PE, or known thrombophilia.
- Diagnosis of suspected non-massive DVT or PE involves a formal clinical score and rapid D-dimer in outpatients; proceeding to initial heparin therapy and diagnostic imaging.
- If diagnosis is confirmed, oral anticoagulation with warfarin (target INR 2.0–3.0) is usually given for at least 3 months.
- Older patients are at increased risk of bleeding on oral anticoagulants.

References

1 Rosendaal FR, van Hylckama Vlieg A and Doggen CJM. Venous thrombosis in the elderly. *J Thromb Haemost* 2007;**5**(Suppl.1):310–17.

2 Lowe GDO, Rumley A, Woodward M *et al.* Epidemiology of coagulation factors, inhibitors and activation markers: the Third Glasgow MONICA Survey. I. Illustrative reference ranges by age, sex and hormone use. *Br J Haematol* 1997; **97**:775–84.

3 Woodward M, Rumley A, Tunstall-Pedoe H and Lowe GDO. Associations of blood rheology and interleukin-6 with cardiovascular risk factors and prevalent cardiovascular disease. *Br J Haematol* 1999;**104**:246–57.

4 Lowe GDO, Rumley A, Woodward M *et al.* Activated protein C resistance and the FV: R506Q mutation in a random population sample: associations with cardiovascular risk factors and coagulation variables. *Thromb Haemost* 1999;**81**:918–24.

5 Van der Meer FJM, Rosendaal FR, Vandenbroucke JP and Briet E. Bleeding complications in oral anticoagulant therapy: an analysis of risk factors. *Arch Intern Med* 1993;**153**:1557–62.

6 Lowe GDO and Stott DJ. (1996) Oral anticoagulation in the elderly, in *Oral Anticoagulants* (eds L Poller and J Hirsh), Arnold, London, pp. 239–45.

7 Rosendaal FR. Venous thrombosis: a multicausal disease. *Lancet* 1999; **353**:1167–73.

8 Walker ID, Greaves M and Preston FE, on behalf of the Haemostasis and Thrombosis Task Force, British Committee for Standards in Haematology. Guideline: investigation and management of heritable thrombophilia. *Br J Haematol* 2001;**114**:512–28.

9 Lowe GDO. Can haematological tests predict cardiovascular risk? The 2005 Kettle Lecture. *Br J Haematol* 2006;**133**:232–50.

10 Wu O, Bayoumi N, Vickers MA and Clark P. ABO (H) blood groups and vascular disease: a systematic review and meta-analysis. *J Thromb Haemost* 2008;**6**:62–9.

11 Boushey CJ, Beresford SAA, Omenn GS and Motulsky AG. A quantitative assessment of plasma homocysteine as a risk factor for vascular disease: probable benefits of increasing folic acid intakes. *JAMA* 1995;**274**:1049–57.

12 den Heijer M, Willems HPO, Blom HJ *et al.* Homocysteine lowering by B vitamins and the secondary prevention of deep vein thrombosis and pulmonary embolism: a randomized, placebo-controlled, double-blind trial. *Blood* 2007;**109**:139–44.

13 Glynn RJ, Danielson E, Fonseca FA *et al.* A randomized trial of rosuvastatin in the prevention of venous thromboembolism. *New Engl J Med* 2009;**360**:1851–61.

14 Antithrombotic Trialists' Collaboration. Collaborative meta-analysis of randomised trials of antiplatelet therapy for prevention of death, myocardial infarction and stroke in high risk patients. *BMJ* 2002;**324**:71–86.

15 Lowe GDO, Haverkate F, Thompson SG *et al.*, on behalf of the ECAT DVT Study Group. Prediction of deep vein thrombosis after elective hip replacement surgery by preoperative clinical and haemostatic variables: The ECAT DVT Study. *Thromb Haemost* 1999;**81**:879–86.

16 Rosendaal FR, van Hylckama VA, Tanis BC and Helmerhorst FM. Estrogens, progestogens and thrombosis. *J Thromb Haemost* 2003;**1**:1371–80.

17 Lowe GDO. Hormone replacement therapy and cardiovascular disease: increased risks of venous thromboembolism and stroke, and no protection from coronary heart disease. *J Intern Med* 2004;**256**:361–74.

18 Goldhaber SZ, Hennekens CH, Evans DH *et al.* Factors associated with correct antemortem diagnosis of major pulmonary embolism. *Am J Med* 1982;**73**:822.

19 Lowe GDO, Greer IA, Cooke TG *et al.* (Thrombo-embolic Risk Factors [THRIFT] Consensus Group). Risk of and prophylaxis for venous thromboembolism in hospital patients. *Br Med J* 1992;**305**:567–74.

20 Geerts WH, Bergqvist D, Pineo GF *et al.* Prevention of venous thromboembolism. *Chest* 2008;**133**(6 Suppl.):381S–453S.

21 National Institute for Health and Clinical Excellence (NICE). (2010) Reducing the risk of venous thromboembolism (deep vein thrombosis and pulmonary embolism) in patients admitted to hospital. Available at www.nice.org.uk (last accessed 21 November 2011).

22 Scottish Intercollegiate Guidelines Network (SIGN). (2010) *Prevention and management of venous thromboembolism and antithrombotics: Indications and management*, December 2010 (No. 122). Available at www.sign.ac.uk (last accessed 19 April 2011).

23 Segal JB, Strieff MB, Hoffman LV *et al.* Management of venous thromboembolism. *Ann Intern Med* 2007;**146**:396.

24 The Task Force for the Diagnosis and Management of Acute Pulmonary Embolism of the European Society of Cardiology (ESC). Guidelines on the diagnosis and management of acute pulmonary embolism. *Eur Heart J* 2008;**29**:2276–315.

25 Schulman S, Kearon C, Kakkar AK *et al*. Dabigatran versus warfarin in the treatment of acute venous thromboembolism. *New Engl J Med* 2009;**361**:2342–52.

26 Eichinger S and Kyrle PA. Duration of anticoagulation after initial idiopathic venous thrombosis – the swinging pendulum: Risk assessment to predict recurrence. *J Thromb Haemost* 2009;**7**:291–5.

27 Kearon C. Balancing risks and benefits of extended anticoagulant therapy for idiopathic venous thrombosis. *J Thromb Haemost* 2009;**7**:296–300.

28 Verhovsek M, Douketis JD, Yi Q *et al*. Systematic review: D-dimer to predict recurrent disease after stopping anticoagulant therapy for unprovoked venous thromboembolism. *Ann Intern Med* 2008;**149**:481–90.

29 Hovens MM, Snoep JD, Tamsma JT and Huisman MV. Aspirin in the prevention and treatment of venous thromboembolism. *J Thromb Haemost* 2006;**4**:1470–5.

30 Routledge PA, Chapman PH, Davies DM and Rawlins MD. Factors affecting warfarin requirements. *Eur J Clin Pharmacol* 1979;**15**:319–22.

CHAPTER 16

Planning Cardiovascular Investigations and Management of Older People

Jennifer K. Harrison[1], *Terence J. Quinn*[2] *and David J. Stott*[2]

[1]Glasgow Royal Infirmary, Glasgow, Scotland, UK

[2]Institute of Cardiovascular and Medical Sciences, University of Glasgow, Glasgow Royal Infirmary, Glasgow, Scotland, UK

Introduction

Determining an appropriate plan for the investigation and management of cardiovascular disease in an older person can be a challenging task. Although comprehensive clinical guidelines are available for most common cardiovascular conditions, their focus is often single-organ pathology. The relevance of such guidelines to the frail, older patient is often limited. This chapter aims to discuss the challenges of assessment and management of cardiovascular disease, with a particular focus on planning investigations in frail older people. Considerations that will often influence decision-making include overlapping areas of functional and cognitive decline; frailty; comorbidity and the non-specific presentation of disease. For each, general guidance is given as to how these can be assessed. Recommendations are evidence based where an evidence base exists, but the lack of original research in older adults is widely recognized and attention is drawn to important 'evidence gaps'. Finally a practical approach to planning investigations in older people is suggested, illustrated with a case study.

Demographics and economics

The increasing life expectancy of the global population is one of the major successes of modern society. Those over the age of 65 make up a greater proportion of the population than ever before: 8% in 1950, projected to rise to 21% of global population by 2050.[1] Within this cohort the

Cardiovascular Disease and Health in the Older Patient: Expanded from 'Pathy's Principles and Practice of Geriatric Medicine, Fifth edition', First Edition. Edited by David J. Stott and Gordon D.O. Lowe.

proportion of adults aged over 80 is increasing faster still, current estimates suggest a 3.8% annual proportional increase.[1] The potential challenges of this demographic shift are well described and have generated considerable research.[2] The United Nations World Population Ageing Report describes global ageing as 'unprecedented, pervasive, enduring (and with) profound implications for many facets of human life'.[1]

These substantial demographic changes occur in the context of global financial uncertainty. The financial implications of societal ageing go beyond direct medical care and encompass societal costs, retirement provision, care provision and research.[3] However, with a worldwide trend towards the reduction of healthcare costs as a proportion of government spending,[4,5] consideration of the economic implications of ageing is warranted. A common misconception is that healthcare spending is increasing due solely to the ageing of the population. Certainly those aged over 65 years account for a greater proportion of healthcare expenditure compared with young and middle-aged populations.[6] However, closer analysis reveals that 'elderly' people are not a homogeneous group, their health states are highly varied and age itself is not the key driver of healthcare costs.[7] Greatest healthcare expenditure for an individual is seen in the final year of life regardless of age[8] with substantial variation in costs depending on cause of death and level of care required.[9] Retrospective recognition that a series of expensive investigations and interventions did not prolong or improve a subject's life is relatively straightforward; however, prospective rationalizing of management, recognizing when an individual is unlikely to benefit is more challenging and further research in this area is urgently required. Rational use of investigations is an economic, ethical and scientific imperative that does not solely apply to older adults. Recent guidance from a collective of nine specialist medical societies has described lists of tests or procedures that are commonly used but are of no benefit to patients; these include cardiac stress testing in asymptomatic subjects and routine follow-up echocardiography for subjects with native valve disease.[10]

Impairment, activity and participation

The most recent update of the World Health Organization's International Classification of Functioning, Disability and Health (WHO-ICF)[11] gives us a framework to evaluate the older adult that encapsulates the wider consequences of ill-health (Figure 16.1). As well as the pathology and consequential impairment associated with disease, the WHO-ICF also considers activity limitation (previously termed disability) and restriction in societal participation (previously handicap). For example, an older

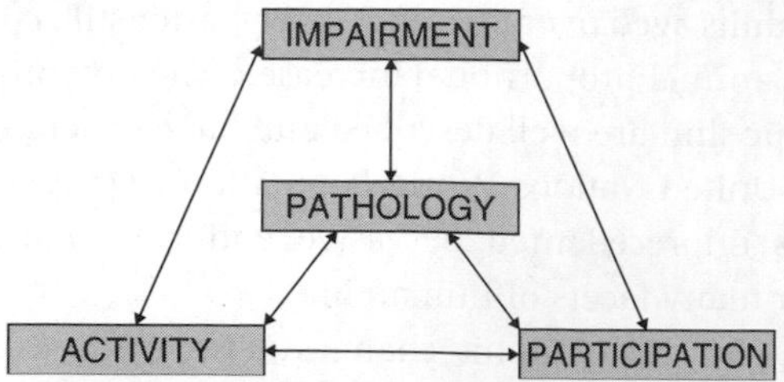

Figure 16.1 World Health Organization International Classification of Function.

person with angina may suffer from reduced exercise capacity due to chest pain (impairment), which may stop them from doing their own shopping (activity limitation) which leads to dependence on others, additional financial costs and limits their social engagement with friends and family (participation restriction).

The traditional medical model of investigation and management often has a focus on pathology and impairment, while for many older adults it is prolonging or restoring activity and participation that are of most importance. The relationship between the levels of WHO-ICF is non-linear and it should not be assumed that attending to the pathology and impairment will necessarily ameliorate problems of activity and participation. For example, an older adult with disease of the cardiac conducting system (pathology) may experience frequent injurious falls related to syncope and fear of falling may limit their activity, for example not going outdoors. A cardiac pacemaker may prevent the syncope but on its own may not improve the mobility problems caused by fear of falling (activity limitation) and the related social isolation as the subject is afraid to leave their house (participation restriction).

Specific challenges

Older adults are a heterogeneous group; however, a number of fundamental issues are common in old age, these include: functional and cognitive impairment; frailty; comorbidity; and the non-specific presentation of disease. These processes often coexist and interact (Figure 16.2). Consideration of each of these aspects can help shape the clinician's approach to investigation and management.

Functional status

To appreciate how to incorporate functional status into a management plan we must first define the concept in terms relevant to the clinician. Spector's definition of functional assessment as inclusive of three domains: activities of daily living (ADLs), instrumental activities of daily living (IADLs)

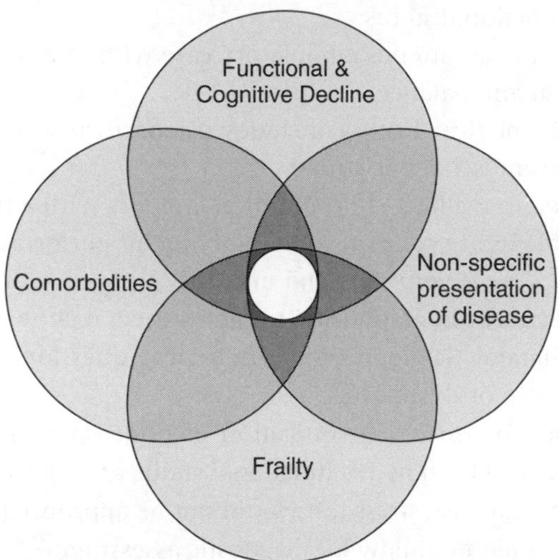

Figure 16.2 Diagrammatic representation of the inter-linked factors to be considered when investigating the older adult.

and mobility, is a useful paradigm.[12] ADLs are those tasks an individual performs for self-care, for example feeding, toileting and dressing. Various scales exist to formally describe ADL with the Barthel Index one of the better validated instruments.[13] IADLs are a wider group of tasks, incorporating the functioning of the individual within society and including shopping, cooking and medication management. An example IADL instrument is the Lawton and Brody tool.[14] Mobility includes components of walking speed, strength, balance, stair climbing and transfer skills.[15] Again a range of tools are available to describe mobility, however for clinical assessment a basic screen such as the timed 'up and go' test (Box 16.1) can be as useful as more comprehensive and sophisticated gait analysis.[16]

Box 16.1 The timed 'up and go' test

With the patient in normal footwear and using their customary walking aid, ask the patient to:

Rise independently from an armless chair or with arms folded
Stand still
Then walk 10 feet/3 metres
Turn 180°
Return to chair
Sit down

The whole process should be completed in 10 s. Unsteadiness, need for external support or time to complete greater than 20 s will signal need for more detailed gait and balance assessment.

Case study functional status:

- An 80-year-old man attends ambulatory care with falls in the context of disordered gait and balance.
- Relevant past medical history includes osteoarthritis and residual left hemiparesis from ischaemic stroke.
- He is restricted to walking short distances indoors with a tripod stick.
- Mobility problems are confirmed in observing his performance in the 'up and go' test[17] – he is very slow and unsteady.
- A 12-lead electrocardiograph (ECG) is performed; it shows sinus rhythm with antero-lateral ST depression. On repeat questioning the patient denies chest pain or dyspnoea.

Here the plan for further investigation of underlying ischaemic heart disease is influenced both by his functional status and lack of symptoms.

- Referral for an exercise stress test would not be appropriate as it is likely his mobility would not allow for diagnostic assessment.
- A pharmacological stress test would be feasible, but carries some risks and is unlikely to provide useful prognostic information or alter his management plan.
- In discussion with the patient, the decision may be made to forego definitive diagnostic investigation for underlying ischaemic heart disease but to offer secondary prevention with antiplatelet, statin and blood pressure control.
- However these decisions may need to be revised, for example if the patient develops exertional chest pain, when a more invasive investigation and management strategy should be reconsidered.

Cognitive status

Cognition can be considered as the over-arching term integrating the domains of attention, memory, language, visuo-spatial skills and frontal or executive functioning and can be assessed by mental state examination targeted to these domains.[18] If we include mild cognitive impairment as well as dementia, the population prevalence of chronic cognitive impairment in the over-65s is up to 24%, rising substantially in those aged >80 years.[19,20]

Delirium (sometimes called 'acute confusional state') is an important cause of cognitive impairment in older people.[21] Delirium is a clinical syndrome characterized by disturbed consciousness, cognitive function or perception, which has an acute onset and fluctuating course. It is a common but serious and complex clinical syndrome associated with poor outcomes including prolonged length of hospital stay, increased healthcare costs, raised mortality and risk of subsequent cognitive decline. Delirium may be present when a person presents for healthcare or may develop during a healthcare episode. It has an incidence of up to 20% in over-65s in acute hospital care. In addition to age, risk factors include prior dementia, current hip fracture or any severe illness (a clinical condition that is deteriorating or is at risk of deterioration). Common precipitants include cardio-respiratory failure and drugs with anticholinergic activity.[22]

Young *et al.* advocate the need for three components in assessing cognition: observation of the patient, collateral information from a carer, and use of standardized assessment tools.[23]

Subjective assessment by clinicians (including doctors and nurses) misses many patients with clinically significant cognitive impairment. Performance is greatly improved by use of brief patient questionnaires, such as the four-question Abbreviated Mental Test (AMT4; age, date of birth, current year and current location)[24] – any error should make the clinician consider whether the patient has a cognitive problem; where there is a high index of suspicion more detailed assessment is required such as with the Mini Mental State Examination (MMSE),[25] and may necessitate specialist psychiatric review and use of neuropsychological batteries such as Addenbrooke's Cognitive Examination--Revised (ACE-R).[26]

If indicators of delirium are identified, it is recommended that a clinical assessment is performed based on the Diagnostic and Statistical Manual of Mental Disorders (DSM-IV) criteria or short Confusion Assessment Method (CAM) to confirm the diagnosis.[22] The short CAM[27] requires observation of the following features:

1 Acute onset and fluctuating course
2 Inattention
3 Disorganized thinking
4 Altered level of consciousness.

For diagnosis of delirium, features 1 and 2 AND either feature 3 or 4 must be displayed.

There are also standardized tools that can be used to obtain collateral information. The Informant Questionnaire on Cognitive Decline in the Elderly (IQCODE) is a reliable, validated proxy questionnaire which aims to identify cognitive decline over a 5-year period.[28]

There are several reasons that recognition of cognitive impairment is so important in planning cardiovascular management. In people diagnosed with delirium, it is vital to identify and manage the underlying cause or combination of causes. Attention is also required to ensure effective communication and reorientation (e.g. explaining where the person is, who they are, and what your role is), attempting to provide a suitable care environment and reassurance for people diagnosed with delirium. Involving family, friends and carers can be helpful. Subjects with cognitive impairment are likely to have reduced capacity to make informed decisions about treatment. However, it is important to recognize that the presence of cognitive impairment (including dementia) does not necessarily render an individual incapable of making decisions nor, significantly, of expressing preferences regarding their investigation and management (see below). Lastly their dementia and delirium are important comorbidities in terms of longer term prognosis. Dementia in particular is associated with impaired quality of life and reduced life expectancy.

Frailty

A general concept of frailty will be familiar to most clinicians and those working with older adults will intuitively recognize frail patients. Rockwood describes a theoretical construct of frailty as: 'a failure to integrate responses in the face of stress'.[29] However, attempts to operationalize frailty have led to development of measurement tools that are complex and difficult to use;[30,31] there is no consensus on a standardized definition to use in clinical practice,[32] despite extensive international discussion.[33–35]

The most commonly used frailty measure was developed by Fried in the Cardiovascular Health Study; frailty was defined as three or more of: unintentional weight loss, self-reported exhaustion, weakness, slow walking speed and low physical activity.[36] However, this measure is predominantly used in research rather than in clinical practice.

Comorbidity

Increasing number and complexity of chronic disease states is common in older adults and accounts for differential mortality and health experience more than age alone. In industrialized countries around 80% of the elderly population have three or more comorbidities.[37] In an American community study, there was substantial and predictable overlap in comorbidities among those with hypertension, coronary artery disease, cerebrovascular disease and diabetes.[38]

With increasing age, large numbers of past medical disease labels can accumulate in a patient's medical file. Not all of these disease states will be active, symptomatic or relevant to the subject. Describing comorbidity as an absolute number of previous medical diagnoses is a crude measure of disease burden. More sophisticated tools that assign differential weighting to various diagnoses are described. The Charlson Index is one such instrument that has been validated in various healthcare settings.[39,40] Higher Charlson Index comorbidity scores have been shown to be associated with increased risk of mortality, hospitalization and institutionalization. The tool has also been validated as a predictor of mortality and hospitalization in the nursing home population, a particularly important subgroup where extensive comorbidity is common.[41]

In clinical practice, in a patient with multimorbidity, it is important to consider which of the underlying diseases is likely to be the biggest problem, in terms of symptom load, quality of life and prognosis. This requires fine clinical judgement, but is generally more useful than use of a formal score for assessing comorbidity in routine care.

Case study comorbidity

- An 82-year-old man with atrial fibrillation, vascular dementia and right above-knee amputation for peripheral vascular disease experiences a transient ischaemic attack (TIA), with sudden onset left arm and leg weakness lasting approximately 10 minutes.
- The recommended diagnostic 'work-up' for TIA would include vascular imaging to exclude symptomatic carotid artery stenosis.
- However, this man is unlikely to benefit from vascular surgery should he be found to have carotid stenosis, as his life-span is likely to be limited (particularly due to his vascular dementia), and with multiple competing morbidities he is unlikely to gain from carotid endarterectomy.
- Therefore it could be argued that carotid imaging is not needed, and that medication review is all that is required in this case.

Polypharmacy

With comorbidity often comes polypharmacy; indeed the number of prescribed medications has been used as a proxy measure for comorbidity and has some utility.[42] In older adults a 'less is more' approach to medication can be advocated, as prescribing new drugs increases both the chance of inappropriate or harmful effects (both predictable and idiosyncratic) and interaction with other prescribed therapies. In an Australian study of antidepressant medication prescribing in older adults, the authors found 87% had at least one comorbidity which could be worsened by the antidepressant medication and 35% had three or more relevant comorbidities, for example arrhythmia, ischaemic heart disease and heart failure.[43] Similarly in a study of diabetic patients, median number of comorbidities was 5 and 16% were prescribed medication with recognized adverse effects in diabetics.[44] Drugs are also an important cause of delirium; in a systematic review, benzodiazepines or opioids were found to be associated with highest risk, but there is also some evidence that dihydropyridines and antihistamine H1 antagonists cause delirium and it is recommended that these groups of drugs are used with caution in older people who are at risk.[45]

Prescribing guidelines do not adequately support clinicians in decision-making for patients with extensive comorbidity as the evidence base is usually derived from studies of subjects with single organ pathology.[46,47] Where payment for healthcare is based on conformity with such published guidance there is scope for harm amongst those with multiple comorbidities.[48,49] Clinicians must take care that the goal of prescribing according to guidelines and tariffs does not over-ride clinical judgement for the individual patient.

Non-specific presentation of disease

A challenge of caring for older adults is that pathology rarely presents in a 'textbook' fashion. Life-threatening problems such as myocardial infarction can present with vague symptoms of confusion and immobility. Atypical presentation of serious disease processes is further compounded by existing comorbidities and under-reporting of symptoms.[50] Regardless of the underlying problem, certain stereotyped responses are seen in older adults. Isaacs' 'geriatric giants'[51] of immobility, instability (falls), incontinence and intellectual impairment encompass the multifactorial syndromes[52] that affect many older adults.

Thus when an older adult presents to medical services it can be difficult to initially ascertain the important underlying disease processes. It is necessary to strike a balance between over-investigation in pursuit of possible but unlikely diagnoses and under-investigation where problems are inappropriately attributed to 'old age'. There is evidence that the latter approach is prevalent, with lack of engagement particularly seen among medical staff with no training in geriatric medicine. Labels such as 'acopia' or 'social admission' are unhelpful, intellectually lazy and may cause patient harm through missing the opportunity for investigation and intervention.[53,54]

A standard screen of investigations when a subject presents with one of the 'geriatric giants' may suggest the underlying problem or point to the need for further investigation.

Case study non-specific presentation of disease

- An 85-year-old woman is admitted from a care home after a fall, after which she has become agitated and more confused; she has a past history of dementia, but usually is mobile and physically independent.
- On examination she has a regular heart rate of 104/minute, respiratory rate is 20/minute, and on auscultation of her chest there are fine crackles at her lung bases.
- In this situation investigations should be kept simple, and care must be taken not to distress the patient with procedures she does not understand. However, it usually would be possible to obtain routine bloods, a 12-lead ECG and a chest X-ray. These investigations confirm pulmonary oedema and a non-ST elevation acute myocardial infarction.
- Confirmation of the cardiac cause of the delirium allows a rational management plan including active management of the pulmonary oedema with intravenous diuretics and oxygen administration.

Evidence for best practice

In light of the lack of certainty associated with investigation and management of older adults, the clinician may turn to the scientific evidence to help guide decision-making. Limited inclusion of older adults is prevalent in multicentre trials including for cardiovascular disease.[55] Taking acute ST-segment elevation myocardial infarction (STEMI) as an example, the American Heart Association acknowledge that older patients continue to be excluded from trials into myocardial infarction investigation and management and that this may have direct effects on clinical management.[56] Even accounting for the higher occurrence of contraindications, older STEMI patients are less likely to receive reperfusion therapy (either percutaneous intervention or fibrinolytic therapy).

Furthermore, those studies that are done often exclude frail, disabled, older adults with disability, comorbidity and cognitive decline.[57] Extrapolating evidence from 'healthy' trial participants to frail older adults may not be valid.

This unmet need has been recognized, with the United Kingdom,[58] United States[59] and Australia[60] all targeting research development towards the ageing population with a renewed focus on trials involving 'real world' older people. Increasing participation of older adults in clinical trials is not without challenges. Engagement of certain groups, such as care-home residents[61] and those with physical or cognitive impairments,[62] is potentially problematic. However, efforts to improve the evidence base in these frailer older groups are needed as they are frequent healthcare consumers.

General approach to investigations

When determining the appropriate investigation of a patient, it is vital to assess the attendant risks and benefits of the proposed action. This may involve assessment of the risks of the test itself, that is complication rate, tolerability, mortality, etc., but should also include an appraisal of the risks of false positive or negative results and consequences these pose. In recent guidance the American College of Physicians advocate consideration of the value, not simply monetary but also diagnostic, of a test to ensure the clinician is investigating their patient appropriately.[63]

An older patient may evaluate benefits of management in terms of quality of life and functional decline, rather than simple life expectancy. Mallery and Moorhouse[64] suggest a series of pertinent questions for evaluating 'success' of a proposed intervention in the frail elderly: proposed length of stay in hospital, potential impact on physical function and memory, and alternative options to promote comfort and dignity.

However, even if the likely benefits of an investigation *per se* outweigh the risks, there are other considerations particularly pertinent to older adults. Situations where investigation may not be appropriate can be described under two broad headings: when there is likely to be no beneficial effect on outcome in its broadest sense, and where investigation is against the wishes of the patient.

If the pursuit of a diagnosis will not result in a beneficial outcome for the patient, for example change in treatment, improved prediction of prognosis, for example development of disabling disease or reduced life expectancy, or the potential harms of investigating are greater than reaching a diagnosis, then there is limited value in pursuing investigation. This includes when there are one or more other comorbidities that are clearly the dominant problem for the individual.

While advocating the principle that an investigation should only be performed if it will alter patient management, it can be argued that, in older adults, the term 'management' should be considered in its broadest sense, including needs for health and social care. For example confirming a progressive, end-stage condition may help the individual and their family plan for the future. Exploring these concepts requires time and detailed enquiry in partnership with the patient, and often their family/carers. It also necessitates an attempt to understand their individual circumstances and wishes, rather than an approach restricted to the medical value of diagnosis.

Patient autonomy

Respecting patient autonomy and their wishes regarding management is paramount. However, in the older population respecting autonomy can be challenging if it is felt that the patient lacks capacity to fully evaluate the consequences of their decision. Assessment of capacity should be determined in relation to the proposed intervention and there are no absolutes. For example consent to history-taking and basic examination can be assumed if the subject voluntarily presents to medical services; whereas formal assessment of capacity would be required in a patient with mild cognitive impairment who refuses life-saving treatment. Assessment of capacity is more than simply assessment of cognition, although cognitive ability is an integral part of the assessment (Box 16.2). In addition capacity

Box 16.2 The key components of an assessment of capacity

Does the subject understand the nature of the proposed investigation?
Does the subject understand the potential consequences of accepting/refusing a proposed investigation?
Is the subject able to understand information relevant to this decision with no external pressure or duress?
Is the subject able to communicate their decision (this may need involvement of other professionals to facilitate communication)?

can change over the course of an illness, and therefore patients often will need to be reassessed.

We outline an algorithm to aid clinicians in assessing patient views regarding investigations. Clearly there will be international variance in the legal framework determining both assessment of capacity, mechanisms for establishing wishes/views and the role of relatives or proxies (Figure 16.3).

Advanced Care Planning

Advanced care planning (ACP) describes the formalized process by which a patient makes a plan about their future healthcare and treatment in conjunction with medical staff and their relevant support network.[65] Although the focus of ACP is on end-of-life care and decisions, it is of particular relevance in the older adult population with chronic disease, even in the absence of a defined terminal illness. The aim is to allow patients to express their views about their care as a whole, including but not limited to: the level of intervention they wish, escalation of care, resuscitation and decisions about place of care, including a preference for avoiding or declining hospital admission.

The legal framework regarding ACPs will vary between countries but all must be flexible and updated in accordance with change in a subject's circumstances. There is trial evidence to support the value of ACPs. In a nursing home setting, ACP can be delivered by non-medical staff with the overall effect of improving the experience of both patients and relatives in end-of-life care situations.[66] Once decisions have been taken regarding patient investigation and management, particularly if a decision has been made not to investigate a problem further, this too can be integrated into a care plan. It is necessary to share the decision between primary

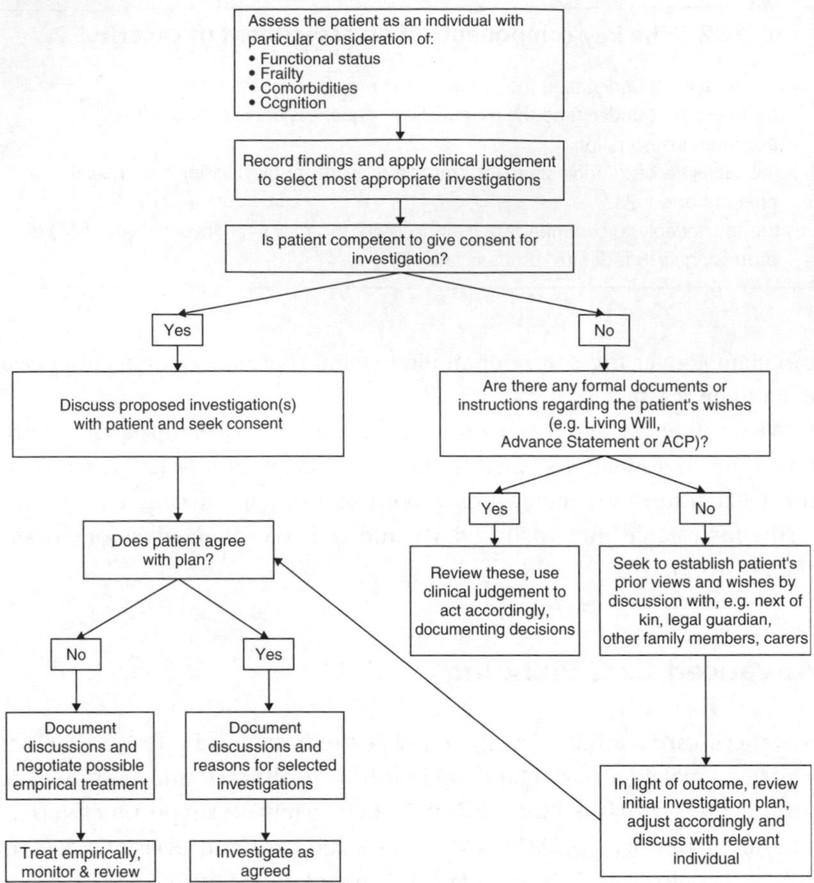

Figure 16.3 Algorithm to approach shared decision-making for investigations in the older adult.

and secondary care providers involved in that patient's care to prevent unnecessary repetition and burden to the patient.

Pragmatic management

Decisions about investigation in an older adult should be neither fixed nor absolute. Deciding how far to investigate does not have to be determined from the moment of presentation. Another approach which can be adopted for complex, non-specific presentations is that of a period of observation after initial assessment, often termed 'watchful waiting'. This approach with outpatient follow-up to observe the natural history of the symptom can help to minimize inappropriate, undirected investigation.[67] Another option is to modify the choice of investigation. Although this may mean a less sensitive test is chosen, it may be that the patient and clinician are prepared to accept the less burdensome investigation even if diagnostic yield is lower.

Case Study

To further illustrate a structured approach to the complexity of investigating the older adult, a common case scenario is presented and discussed.

- Murmurs

  An 82-year-old gentleman attends his primary care physician for routine review of Parkinson's disease. He had a TIA 10 years previously but no recent cardiovascular symptoms. His current drug treatment is of aspirin, simvastatin and madopar. On cardiac auscultation an ejection systolic murmur (grade III/VI) is heard, loudest at the aortic area radiating to the neck. How should the physician proceed?

- Evidence-based guidance

  The European Society of Cardiology guidance on the management of valvular heart disease recommend ECG and chest X-ray as initial assessment, with echocardiography the modality of choice for assessing cardiac structure and function.[68] However, systolic murmurs are prevalent in older adults and echocardiography of isolated systolic murmur is frequently normal.[69]

  It is important to consider when and why to investigate a systolic murmur. An initial starting point is clinical examination.[70] It is widely accepted that good clinical assessment should allow the delineation of benign from potentially pathological murmurs and that echocardiography with its attendant costs is not a replacement for clinical assessment in evaluating systolic murmurs.[71] Instead, it is advisable that clinicians apply clinical judgement.[72] The particular concern in older patients is potential aortic stenosis which can be rapidly progressive and fatal. However, directed questions on exertional symptoms can help rationalize the need for echocardiography.[73]

- Actions
  - The clinician performs a functional screening test using the timed 'up and go' test. The patient is able to rise unaided and mobilize across the consulting room, but is slow in movement and unsteady when changing direction.
  - A brief cognitive screen, using the 10-point Abbreviated Mental Test scores 10/10 and informal assessment suggests that the patient has capacity to make informed decisions about care.
  - Comorbidity is further assessed through review of the medical case file; Parkinson's disease is the main problem.

- The clinician discusses options for investigation, determining the patient's health priorities. Following discussion, the patient decides he does not want further investigation for his murmur.
- The history and examination, a record of the discussion and management plan is recorded in the case record.
- The patient is advised that this decision should be reconsidered should he develop troublesome symptoms, such as breathlessness on exertion.

Conclusions

Throughout this chapter we argue for a patient-centred, pragmatic approach which reflects outcomes of genuine importance to the older person. Tinetti and Fried highlight that if clinicians focus purely on disease and not on the individual patient, this leads to under-, over- and mis-treatment.[74]

We have highlighted various factors common to older people that should be considered when planning investigation or treatment of the older adult; we provide general guidance on options for evaluation of functional status, cognition and comorbidities; this approach should be combined with ascertainment of the views and opinions of the older person about their own health and healthcare.

References

1 World Health Organization (2002) World Population Ageing: 1950–2050. Available from: http://www.un.org/esa/population/publications/worldageing19502050/ (accessed 25 March 2012).

2 Ebrahim S. Ageing, health and society. *Int J Epidemiol* 2002;**31**:715–8.

3 Tinker A. The social implications of an ageing population. *Mech Ageing Dev* 2002;**123**:729–35.

4 Hussey PS, Eibner C, Ridgely S and McGlynn EA. Controlling U.S. health care spending – separating promising from unpromising approaches. *New Engl J Med* 2009;**361**(**22**):2109–11.

5 Appleby R, Crawford R and Emmerson, C. (2009) *How cold will it be? Prospects for NHS funding: 2011–2017*, The King's Fund, London, UK.

6 Seshamani M and Gray A. The impact of ageing in expenditures in the National Health Service. *Age and Ageing* 2002;**31**:287–94.

7 Zweifel P, Felder S and Meiers M. Ageing of population and health care expenditure: a red herring? *Health Econ* 1999;**8**:485–96.

8 Hoover DR, Crystal S, Kumar R, Sambamoorthi U and Cantor JC. Medical expenditures during the last year of life: findings from the 1992–1996 Medicare Current Beneficiary Study. *Health Serv Res* 2002;**37**(6):1625–42.

9 Polder JJ, Barendregt JJ and van Oers H. Health care costs in the last year of life – the Dutch experience. *Soc Sci Med* 2006;**63**:1720–31.

10 Choosing Wisely® – An initiative of the ABIM Foundation. Available from: http://choosingwisely.org/ (accessed June 2012).

11 World Health Organization (2002) Towards a Common Language for Functioning, Disability and Health: ICF, WHO, Geneva. Available from: http://www.who.int/classifications/icf/training/icfbeginnersguide.pdf (accessed 8 April 2012).

12 Spector WD. (1990) Functional disability scales, in *Quality of Life Assessments in Clinical Trials* (ed. R Spilker), Raven Press, New York.

13 Collin C, Wade DT, Davies S and Horne V. The Barthel ADL Index: a reliability study. *Int Disabil Stud* 1988;**10**(2):61–3.

14 Lawton MP and Brody EM. Assessment of older people: Self-maintaining and instrumental activities of daily living. *The Gerontologist* 1969;**9**(3):179–86.

15 Pearson VI. (2000) Assessment of function in older adults, in *Assessing Older Persons*, 1st (eds RL Kane and RA Kane), Oxford University Press.

16 Bischoff HA, Stahelin HB, Monsch AU *et al.* Identifying a cut-off point for normal mobility: a comparison of the timed 'up and go' test in community-dwelling and institutionalised elderly women. *Age and Ageing* 2003;**32**:315–20.

17 Mathias S, Nayak USL and Isaacs B. Balance in elderly patients: the "get-up and go" test. *Arch Phys Med Rehab* 1986;**67**:387–9.

18 Woodford HJ and George J. Cognitive assessment in the elderly: a review of clinical methods. *Q J Med* 2007;**100**:469–84.

19 Graham JE, Rockwood K, Beattie BL *et al.* Prevalence and severity of cognitive impairment with and without dementia in an elderly population. *Lancet* 1997; **349**:1793–6.

20 Ferri CP, Prince M, Brayne C *et al.*; Alzheimer's Disease International. Global prevalence of dementia: a Delphi consensus study. *Lancet* 2005; **366**(9503):2112–17.

21 Siddiqi N, Stockdale R, Britton AM, Holmes J. (2007) Interventions for preventing delirium in hospitalised patients. *Cochrane Database Syst Rev 2* (Art. No.: CD005563).

22 National Institute for Health and Clinical Excellence (NICE) (2010) Clinical Guideline 103: *Delirium: diagnosis, prevention and management*. Available from: http://www.nice.org.uk/nicemedia/live/13060/49909/49909.pdf (accessed June 2012).

23 Young J, Meagher D and MacLullich A. Cognitive assessment of older people. *BMJ* 2011;**343**:d5042.

24 Schofield I, Stott DJ, Tolson D *et al.*. Screening for cognitive impairment in older people attending accident and emergency using the 4-item Abbreviated Mental Test. *Eur J Emerg Med* 2010;**17**:340–2.

25 Folstein MF, Folstein SE and McHugh PR. "Mini-Mental State." A practical method for grading the cognitive state of patients for the clinician. *J Pyschiat Res* 1975;**12**:189–98.

26 Mioshi E, Dawson K, Mitchell J, Arnold R and Hodges JR. The Addenbrooke's Cognitive Examination Revised (ACE-R): a brief cognitive test battery for dementia screening. *Int J Geriatr Psychiatry* 2006;**21**(**11**):1078–85.

27 Inouye SK, van Dyck CH, Alessi CA *et al.* Clarifying confusion: the confusion assessment method. A new method for detection of delirium. *Ann Intern Med* 1990;**113**(12):941–8.

28 Jorm AF. The Informant Questionnaire on Cognitive Decline in the Elderly (IQCODE): a review. *Int Psychogeriatr* 2004;**16**(3):1–19.

29 Rockwood K and Hubbard R. Frailty and the geriatrician. *Age and Ageing* 2004;**33**:429–30.

30 Inouye SK, Studenski S, Tinetti ME and Kuchel GA. Geriatric syndromes: Clinical, research, and policy implications of a core geriatric concept. *J Am Geriatr Soc* 2007;**55**:780–91.

31 Conroy S. Defining frailty – The Holy Grail of geriatric medicine. *J Nutr Health Aging* 2009;**13**(4):389.

32 Rockwood K. What would make a definition of frailty successful? *Age and Ageing* 2005;**34**:432–34.

33 Bergman H, Ferrucci L, Guralnik J *et al.* Frailty: An emerging research and clinical paradigm – issues and controversies. *J Gerontol A Biol Sci Med Sci* 2007;**62A**(7):731–7.

34 Van Kan GA, Rolland Y, Bergman H *et al.* on behalf of the Geriatric Advisory Panel. The I.A.N.A. Task Force on Frailty Assessment of Older People in Clinical Practice. *J Nutr Health Aging* 2008;**12**(1):29–37.

35 Walston J, Hadley EC, Ferruci L *et al.* Research agenda for frailty in older adults: toward a better understanding of physiology and etiology: summary from the American Geriatrics Society/National Institute in Aging Research Conference on Frailty in Older Adults. *J Am Geriatr Soc* 2006;**54**:991–1001.

36 Fried LP, Tangen CM, Walston J *et al.* Frailty in older adults: evidence for a phenotype. *J Gerontol A Biol Sci Med Sci* 2001;**56A**(3):M146–56.

37 Caughey GE, Vitry AI, Gilbert AL and Roughead EE. Prevalence of comorbidity of chronic diseases in Australia. *BMC Public Health* 2008;**8**:221.

38 Fillenbaum GG, Pieper CF, Cohen HJ, Cornoni-Huntley JC and Guralnik JM. Comorbidity of five chronic health conditions in elderly community residents: determinants and impact on mortality. *J Gerontol A Biol Sci Med Sci* 2000;**55**(2):M84–9.

39 De Groot V, Beckerman H, Lankhorst GJ and Bouter LM. How to measure comorbidity: a critical review of available methods. *J Clin Epidemiol* 2003;**56**:221–9.

40 Charlson M, Szatrowski TP, Peterson J and Gold J. Validation of a combined comorbidity index. *J Clin Epidemiol* 1994;**47**(11):1245–51.

41 Buntinx F, Niclaes L, Suetens C *et al.* Evaluation of Charlson's comorbidity index in elderly living in nursing homes. *J Clin Epidemiol* 2002;**55**:1144–7.

42 Perkins AJ, Kroenke K, Unutzer J *et al.* Common comorbidity scales were similar in their ability to predict health care costs and mortality. *J Clin Epidemiol* 2004;**57**:1040–8.

43 Caughey GE, Roughead EE, Shakip S *et al.* Comorbidity of chronic disease and potential treatment conflicts in older people dispensed antidepressants. *Age and Ageing* 2010;**39**:488–94.

44 Caughey GE, Roughead EE, Vitry AI *et al.* Comorbidity in the elderly with diabetes: identification of areas of potential treatment conflicts. *Diabetes Res Clin Pr* 2010;**87**:385–93.

45 Clegg A and Young JB. Which medications to avoid in people at risk of delirium: a systematic review. *Age and Ageing* 2011;**40**(1):23–29.

46 Lugtenberg M, Burgers JS, Clancy C, Westert GP and Schneider EC. Current guidelines have limited applicability to patients with comorbid conditions: a systematic analysis of evidence-based guidelines. *PLoS ONE* 2011;**6**(10):e255987.

47 Mutasingwa DR, Ge H and Upshur REG. How applicable are clinical practice guidelines to elderly patients with comorbidities? *Can Fam Physician* 2011;**57**:e253–62.

48 Boyd CM, Darer J, Boult C *et al.* Clinical Practice Guidelines and quality of care for older patients with multiple comorbid diseases. Implications for pay for performance. *JAMA* 2005;**294**:716–24.

49 Heath I. Never had it so good? *BMJ* 2008;**336**:950–1.

50 Emmett KR. Nonspecific and atypical presentation of disease in the older patient. *Geriatrics* 1998;**53**:50–60.

51 Isaacs B. (1992) *The Challenge of Geriatric Medicine*, Oxford University Press, Oxford.

52 Inouye SK, Studenski S, Tinetti ME and Kuchel GA. Geriatric syndromes: clinical, research, and policy implications of a core geriatric concept. *J Am Geriatr Soc* 2007;**55**:780–91.
53 Oliver D. 'Acopia' and 'social admission' are not diagnoses: why older people deserve better. *J R Soc Med* 2008;**101**:168–74.
54 Kee Y-YK and Rippingale C. The prevalence and characteristic of patients with 'acopia'. *Age and Ageing* 2008;**38**(1):103–5.
55 Lee PY, Alexander KP, Hammill BG, Pasquali SK and Peterson ED. Representation of elderly persons and women in published randomized trials of acute coronary syndromes. *JAMA* 2001;**286**:708–13.
56 Alexander KP, Newby K, Armstrong PW *et al*. Acute coronary care in the elderly, Part II. *Circulation* 2007;**115**:2570–89.
57 Mody L, Miller DK, McGloin JM *et al*. Recruitment and retention of older adults in aging research. *J Am Geriatr Soc* 2008;**56**:2340–48.
58 The Academy of Medical Sciences. *Rejuvenating ageing research*, September 2009.
59 Norris SL, High K, Gill TM *et al*. Health care for older Americans with multiple chronic conditions: a research agenda. *J Am Geriatr Soc* 2008;**56**:149–59.
60 Anstey KJ, Bielak AAM, Birrell CL *et al*. and the DYNOPTA team. Understanding ageing in older Australians: The contribution of the Dynamic Analyses to Optimise Ageing (DYNOPTA) project to the evidence base and policy. *Aust J Ageing* 2011;**30**(2):24–31.
61 Hall S, Longhurst S and Higginson IJ. Challenges to conducting research with older people living in nursing homes. *BMC Geriatrics* 2009;**9**:38.
62 Warner J, McCarney R, Griffin M, Hill K and Fisher P. Participation in dementia research: rates and correlates of capacity to give informed consent. *J Med Ethics* 2008;**34**:167–70.
63 Qaseem A, Alguire P, Dallas P *et al*. Appropriate use of screening and diagnostic tests to foster high-value, cost conscious care. *Ann Intern Med* 2012;**156**:147–9.
64 Mallery LH and Moorhouse P. Respecting frailty. *J Med Ethics* 2011;**37**:126–8.
65 Singer PA, Robertson G and Roy DJ. Bioethics for clinicians: 6. *Advance care planning. Can Med Assoc J* 1996;**155**(12):1689–92.
66 Detering KM, Hancock AD, Reade MC and Silvester W. The impact of advance care planning on end of life care in elderly patients: randomised controlled trial. *BMJ* 2010;**340**:c1345.
67 McMinn J, Steel C and Bowman A. Investigation and management of unintentional weight loss in older adults. *BMJ* 2011;**342**:d1732.
68 Vahanian A, Baumgartner H, Bax J *et al*. Guidelines on the management of valvular heart disease. *Eur Heart J* 2007;**28**:230–68.
69 Etchells E, Bell C and Robb K. Does this patient have an abnormal systolic murmur? *JAMA* 1997;**277**(7):564–71.
70 Goroll AH and Mulley AG. (2009) Evaluation of the asymptomatic systolic murmur, in *Primary Care Medicine: Office Evaluation and Management of the Adult Patient*, Lippincott Williams & Wilkins.
71 Shub C. Echocardiography or auscultation? How to evaluate systolic murmures. *Can Fam Physician* 2003;**49**:163–7.
72 Jost CHA, Turina J, Mayer K *et al*. Echocardiography in the evaluation of systolic murmurs of unknown cause. *Am J Med* 2000;**108**:614–20.
73 Das P, Pocock C and Chambers J. The patient with a systolic murmur: severe aortic stenosis may be missed during cardiovascular examination. *QJM* 2000;**93**:685–88.
74 Tinetti ME and Fried T. The end of the disease era. *Am J Med* 2004;**116**:179–85.

Index

Cardiovascular Disease and Health in the Older Patient: Expanded from 'Pathy's Principles and Practice of Geriatric Medicine, Fifth edition', First Edition. Edited by David J. Stott and Gordon D.O. Lowe.